Feature Paper in Antibiotics for 2019

Feature Paper in Antibiotics for 2019

Editor

Jeffrey Lipman

MDPI • Basel • Beijing • Wuhan • Barcelona • Belgrade • Manchester • Tokyo • Cluj • Tianjin

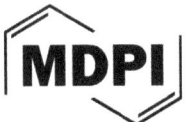

Editor
Jeffrey Lipman
The University of Queensland School of Medicine
Australia

Editorial Office
MDPI
St. Alban-Anlage 66
4052 Basel, Switzerland

This is a reprint of articles from the Special Issue published online in the open access journal *Antibiotics* (ISSN 2079-6382) (available at: https://www.mdpi.com/journal/antibiotics/special_issues/feature_paper_antibiotics).

For citation purposes, cite each article independently as indicated on the article page online and as indicated below:

LastName, A.A.; LastName, B.B.; LastName, C.C. Article Title. *Journal Name* **Year**, *Article Number*, Page Range.

ISBN 978-3-03943-122-9 (Hbk)
ISBN 978-3-03943-123-6 (PDF)

© 2020 by the authors. Articles in this book are Open Access and distributed under the Creative Commons Attribution (CC BY) license, which allows users to download, copy and build upon published articles, as long as the author and publisher are properly credited, which ensures maximum dissemination and a wider impact of our publications.

The book as a whole is distributed by MDPI under the terms and conditions of the Creative Commons license CC BY-NC-ND.

Contents

About the Editor . . . . **vii**

Dagan O Lonsdale and Jeffrey Lipman
Antimicrobial Resistance: We Must Pursue a Collaborative, Global Approach and Use a "One Health" Approach
Reprinted from: *Antibiotics* **2019**, *8*, 237, doi:10.3390/antibiotics8040237 . . . . **1**

Aleksandra J. Borek, Marta Wanat, Anna Sallis, Diane Ashiru-Oredope, Lou Atkins, Elizabeth Beech, Susan Hopkins, Leah Jones, Cliodna McNulty, Karen Shaw, Esther Taborn, Christopher Butler, Tim Chadborn and Sarah Tonkin-Crine
How Can National Antimicrobial Stewardship Interventions in Primary Care Be Improved? A Stakeholder Consultation
Reprinted from: *Antibiotics* **2019**, *8*, 207, doi:10.3390/antibiotics8040207 . . . . **5**

Shweta Rajkumar Singh, Alvin Qijia Chua, Sok Teng Tan, Clarence C. Tam, Li Yang Hsu and Helena Legido-Quigley
Combating Antimicrobial Resistance in Singapore: A Qualitative Study Exploring the Policy Context, Challenges, Facilitators, and Proposed Strategies
Reprinted from: *Antibiotics* **2019**, *8*, 201, doi:10.3390/antibiotics8040201 . . . . **21**

Júlia S. Vianna, Diana Machado, Ivy B. Ramis, Fábia P. Silva, Dienefer V. Bierhals, Michael Andrés Abril, Andrea von Groll, Daniela F. Ramos, Maria Cristina S. Lourenço, Miguel Viveiros and Pedro E. Almeida da Silva
The Contribution of Efflux Pumps in *Mycobacterium abscessus* Complex Resistance to Clarithromycin
Reprinted from: *Antibiotics* **2019**, *8*, 153, doi:10.3390/antibiotics8030153 . . . . **39**

Joana P. Costa, M. Joana F. Pinheiro, Sílvia A. Sousa, Ana M. Botelho do Rego, Fernanda Marques, M. Conceição Oliveira, Jorge H. Leitão, Nuno P. Mira and M. Fernanda N. N. Carvalho
Antimicrobial Activity of Silver Camphorimine Complexes against *Candida* Strains
Reprinted from: *Antibiotics* **2019**, *8*, 144, doi:10.3390/antibiotics8030144 . . . . **55**

Graeme Hood, Lina Toleikyte and Diane Ashiru-Oredope
Assessing National Antimicrobial Resistance Campaigns Using a Health Equity Assessment Tool (HEAT)
Reprinted from: *Antibiotics* **2019**, *8*, 121, doi:10.3390/antibiotics8030121 . . . . **69**

Marthe Sunde, Marthe Marie Nygaard and Sigurd Høye
General Practitioners' Attitudes toward Municipal Initiatives to Improve Antibiotic Prescribing—A Mixed-Methods Study
Reprinted from: *Antibiotics* **2019**, *8*, 120, doi:10.3390/antibiotics8030120 . . . . **77**

Larissa Grigoryan, Susan Nash, Roger Zoorob, George J. Germanos, Matthew S. Horsfield, Fareed M. Khan, Lindsey Martin and Barbara W. Trautner
Qualitative Analysis of Primary Care Provider Prescribing Decisions for Urinary Tract Infections
Reprinted from: *Antibiotics* **2019**, *8*, 84, doi:10.3390/antibiotics8020084 . . . . **85**

Annelies Colliers, Niels Adriaenssens, Sibyl Anthierens, Stephaan Bartholomeeusen,
Hilde Philips, Roy Remmen and Samuel Coenen
Antibiotic Prescribing Quality in Out-of-Hours Primary Care and Critical Appraisal of
Disease-Specific Quality Indicators
Reprinted from: *Antibiotics* **2019**, *8*, 79, doi:10.3390/antibiotics8020079 97

Rosa Elvira Gavilán, Carolina Nebot, Ewelina Patyra, Beatriz Vazquez, Jose Manuel Miranda
and Alberto Cepeda
Determination of Florfenicol, Thiamfenicol and Chloramfenicol at Trace Levels in Animal Feed
by HPLC–MS/MS
Reprinted from: *Antibiotics* **2019**, *8*, 59, doi:10.3390/antibiotics8020059 107

Eunice Ego Mgbeahuruike, Milla Stålnacke, Heikki Vuorela and Yvonne Holm
Antimicrobial and Synergistic Effects of Commercial Piperine and Piperlongumine in
Combination with Conventional Antimicrobials
Reprinted from: *Antibiotics* **2019**, *8*, 55, doi:10.3390/antibiotics8020055 117

Graeme Hood, Kieran S. Hand, Emma Cramp, Philip Howard, Susan Hopkins
and Diane Ashiru-Oredope
Measuring Appropriate Antibiotic Prescribing in Acute Hospitals: Development of a National
Audit Tool Through a Delphi Consensus
Reprinted from: *Antibiotics* **2019**, *8*, 49, doi:10.3390/antibiotics8020049 129

Helene L. Robertsen and Ewa M. Musiol-Kroll
Actinomycete-Derived Polyketides as a Source of Antibiotics and Lead Structures for the
Development of New Antimicrobial Drugs
Reprinted from: *Antibiotics* **2019**, *8*, 157, doi:10.3390/antibiotics8040157 141

Danitza Romero-Calle, Raquel Guimarães Benevides, Aristóteles Góes-Neto
and Craig Billington
Bacteriophages as Alternatives to Antibiotics in Clinical Care
Reprinted from: *Antibiotics* **2019**, *8*, 138, doi:10.3390/antibiotics8030138 193

Majdi N. Al-Hasan, Hana Rac Winders, P. Brandon Bookstaver and Julie Ann Justo
Direct Measurement of Performance: A New Era in Antimicrobial Stewardship
Reprinted from: *Antibiotics* **2019**, *8*, 127, doi:10.3390/antibiotics8030127 213

Lucía Fernández, Diana Gutiérrez, Pilar García and Ana Rodríguez
The Perfect Bacteriophage for Therapeutic Applications—A Quick Guide
Reprinted from: *Antibiotics* **2019**, *8*, 126, doi:10.3390/antibiotics8030126 233

Beatriz Suay-García and María Teresa Pérez-Gracia
Present and Future of Carbapenem-Resistant *Enterobacteriaceae* (CRE) Infections
Reprinted from: *Antibiotics* **2019**, *8*, 122, doi:10.3390/antibiotics8030122 249

Emily A. F. Holmes and Dyfrig A. Hughes
Challenges for Economic Evaluation of Health Care Strategies to Contain
Antimicrobial Resistance
Reprinted from: *Antibiotics* **2019**, *8*, 166, doi:10.3390/antibiotics8040166 265

About the Editor

Jeffrey Lipman is Executive Director of the Burns Trauma & Critical Care Research Centre, a professor of Anesthesiology & Critical Care at The University of Queensland, and until recently (for 23 years), he was Director of the Department of Intensive Care Medicine at Royal Brisbane and Women's Hospital. He currently holds honorary professorial positions at the Chinese University of Hong Kong, University of Witwatersrand (South Africa) and Queensland University of Technology. He has qualifications in anesthesia and intensive care, and set up and was in charge of a number of intensive care and trauma units in South Africa, before coming to Australia in 1997. he currently manages a large multidisciplinary research team with an output of over 120 peer-reviewed articles per annum. He has supervised dozens of Ph.D. students to completion and is currently supervising 6 Ph.D., 1 MPhil and 1 MBBS/Hons students. Prof Lipman has been instrumental in developing the anesthesiology and critical care component of a graduate medical program for Queensland, and continues to lecture to medical and postgraduate students. Prof Lipman is the author of over 550 peer reviewed publications, 30 book chapters and has been invited to deliver over 120 lectures at national and international conferences in many countries across the world. His research interests include all aspects of infection management in intensive care, and he has a special interest in the pharmacokinetics of antibiotic dosage, an area in which he received his MD in 2006. His research into antibiotic usage in acute situations has received international recognition and he is regarded as an expert in the field. As such, he and his research team have conducted and presently conduct a number of clinical trials in Australia, New Zealand, Hong Kong, Europe and the UK. Prof Lipman is an Editorial Board Member of 10 international journals, is Section Editor of four antibiotic-related journals, reviews for 23 journals, and is an external reviewer for NHMRC project grants (local), as well as the equivalent for a number of overseas countries. He is Chief Investigator on a 7000-patient international randomized controlled trial comparing bolus dosing versus continuous infusions of meropenem and piperacillin-tazobactam.

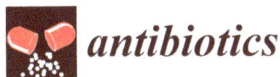

Editorial

Antimicrobial Resistance: We Must Pursue a Collaborative, Global Approach and Use a "One Health" Approach

Dagan O Lonsdale [1,2] and Jeffrey Lipman [3,4,*]

1. Department of Intensive Care Medicine, St George's University Hospitals NHS Foundation Trust, London SW17 0QT, UK; daganlonsdale@googlemail.com
2. Department of Clinical Pharmacology and Therapeutics, St George's, University of London, London SW17 0RE, UK
3. Royal Brisbane and Womens' Hospital, University of Queensland, Brisbane 4029, Australia
4. Nimes University Hospital, University of Montpellier, 30029 Nimes, France
* Correspondence: j.lipman@uq.edu.au; Tel.: +61-7-3636-8897; Fax: +61-7-3636-3542

Received: 14 November 2019; Accepted: 25 November 2019; Published: 27 November 2019

Treating infection is a key part of the work of most clinicians. Whilst new drug technologies like biologics have begun a revolution in the treatment of cancer and autoimmune disease, there has been a conspicuous absence of new classes of antibiotic over the last 30 years. This, coupled with the mass use of antibiotics in farming and the continued emergence of resistant pathogens has created a perfect storm, and antimicrobial resistance is now viewed as a global public health emergency [1,2]. Combating the threat posed by the failure of current antibiotics presents a unique need to co-ordinate research and intervention policy across the spectrum of primary and secondary care, the private and public sector, and public health alongside working with colleagues in agriculture and farming aiming towards a "one health" approach. In this issue of *Antibiotics*, a variety of articles are presented that cover the breadth of human research in this field from in vitro work on novel therapies to commentary on public health strategies.

The emerging crisis of antibiotic resistance and paucity of novel therapies, has led to a resurrection of historic drug development pipelines. Robertson and Musiol-Kroll [3] provide a comprehensive account of the part actinomycetes have played in the history of antimicrobial therapy. The origins of ß-lactams, macrolides, and tetracyclines (among others) lie in the exploration of these organisms in the mid twentieth century and the article details their discovery and utility, as well as outlining the potential discovery pipeline for future development of naturally occurring antimicrobials. Previously discarded treatment options are also undergoing a resurgence. In their articles, Romero-Calle and colleagues [4] and Fernandez et al. [5] discuss the potential of bacteriophages (bactericidal viruses) in comprehensive summaries that discuss the history, mechanism of action, and current state of early phase research of these therapies. Mgbeahurulike et al. [6] utilize another strategy for developing new antimicrobial treatments by combining a novel synergistic compound with an established antibiotic. They provide evidence in their in vitro work of the synergistic effect of the alkaloids piperine and piplartin with rifampicin against *Staphylococcus aureus*. Infection caused by carbapenem-resistant Enterobacteriaceae (CRE) provide a particular challenge to clinicians worldwide. Suay-Garcia and Pérez-Gracia [7] provide a concise summary of the history, epidemiology and resistance mechanisms of these pathogens, and outline the treatment strategies that may be employed to treat them. Old (fosfomycin), newer ('double carbapenem'), and novel (ceftazidime/avibactam) treatment strategies are described, with a clear message that global cooperation is paramount to combating CRE.

Antimicrobial stewardship, including the prevention of inappropriate antibiotic prescribing is key to preventing the continued rise and spread of resistant pathogens. However, there is currently no international consensus on the definition or accurate quantification of the global burden of inappropriate prescribing. Hood and colleagues [8] provide commentary on some of the audit tools available in Australia [9] and the USA [10] and present a novel approach, developed through an expert Delphi process, that they aim to use in UK secondary care. Al-Hasan et al. [11] in their review, argue for a more straightforward metric for antimicrobial stewardship performance–institutional antimicrobial use. In primary care, Colliers et al. [12] present an analysis of the burden of infection and antibiotic prescribing in out of hours contact between practitioners and patients in Belgium. They found that more than one in five out of hours appointments resulted in an antibiotic prescription. They also found that out of hours prescribing was often not in keeping with local guidelines. Sunde, Nygaard, and Høye [13] present some of the challenges faced by General Practitioners when deciding whether to give antimicrobial prescriptions, highlighting in their qualitative and quantitative study that patient expectations remain a significant driver of prescribing for practitioners. Grigoryan and colleagues [14] present a qualitative analysis of antimicrobial prescribing for perhaps one of the more common indications in primary care, urinary tract infections. They include a report on a wide variety of resources used by practitioners when making prescribing decisions, pointing out that stewardship interventions must consider where and how practitioners seek information. Borek et al. [15] further describe some of the barriers to success of antimicrobial stewardship interventions. They suggest some strategies, sourced from a stakeholder engagement exercise, to improve the success rates.

For many clinicians, the threat or challenge of managing infection due to antimicrobial resistant organisms is often focused on a single patient, ward or practice. In this issue, Holmes and Hughes discuss the wider health economic implications of failing to act to combat resistant pathogens [16]. The headline healthcare cost of no action, $100 trillion by 2050 [2], should prompt action from even the most skeptical of policymakers. However, the authors provide insightful commentary on the challenges in economic evaluation of interventions that may provide benefit to only individual patients or to populations over a long time period. They argue succinctly that economic assessment must be paired alongside evaluation of clinical efficacy of healthcare interventions to combat antimicrobial resistance, if funds are to be targeted efficiently and effectively. More broadly, it is clear that antimicrobial resistance is not an issue that is related to, or originates solely from humans. Although common sense dictates that policy and interventions to combat antimicrobial resistance must be multi-faceted and include stakeholders from public health, hospitals, and the community alongside colleagues from agriculture, farming and veterinary medicine. Singh et al. [17] provide a commentary of the situation in Singapore, pointing out that even in an economy with significant resource, combating antimicrobial resistance is complex and challenging to coordinate. Their work, based on a qualitative analysis from stakeholder interviews, highlights the need to understand and address cultural, social, and behavioral expectations of antibiotic use, alongside implementing public health policy.

Articles on in vitro work by Vianna et al. [18] on antimicrobial efflux pumps and Costa et al. [19] outlining the antimicrobial activity of silver camphro-imine complexes alongside work from Gavilán et al. [20] on a novel and sensitive assay for detecting low levels of antibiotic in animal feed, complete this innovative and exciting multi-disciplinary issue of *Antibiotics*.

Conflicts of Interest: The authors declare no conflict of interest.

References

1. WHO. Antibiotic resistance. 2018. Available online: https://www.who.int/news-room/fact-sheets/detail/antibiotic-resistance (accessed on 11 November 2019).
2. Tackling Antimicrobial Resistance 2019–2024. The UK's Five-Year National Action Plan. HM Government. 2019. Available online: https://assets.publishing.service.gov.uk/government/uploads/system/uploads/attachment_data/file/784894/UK_AMR_5_year_national_action_plan.pdf (accessed on 11 November 2019).
3. Robertsen, H.L.; Musiol-Kroll, E.M. Actinomycete-Derived Polyketides as a Source of Antibiotics and Lead Structures for the Development of New Antimicrobial Drugs. *Antibiotics* **2019**, *8*, 157. [CrossRef] [PubMed]
4. Romero-Calle, D.; Guimarães Benevides, R.; Góes-Neto, A.; Billington, C. Bacteriophages as Alternatives to Antibiotics in Clinical Care. *Antibiotics* **2019**, *8*, 138. [CrossRef] [PubMed]

5. Fernández, L.; Gutiérrez, D.; García, P.; Rodríguez, A. The Perfect Bacteriophage for Therapeutic Applications—A Quick Guide. *Antibiotics* **2019**, *8*, 126. [CrossRef] [PubMed]
6. Mgbeahuruike, E.E.; Stålnacke, M.; Vuorela, H.; Holm, Y. Antimicrobial and Synergistic Effects of Commercial Piperine and Piperlongumine in Combination with Conventional Antimicrobials. *Antibiotics* **2019**, *8*, 55. [CrossRef] [PubMed]
7. Suay-García, B.; Pérez-Gracia, M.T. Present and Future of Carbapenem-resistant Enterobacteriaceae (CRE) Infections. *Antibiotics* **2019**, *8*, 122. [CrossRef] [PubMed]
8. Hood, G.; Hand, K.S.; Cramp, E.; Howard, P.; Hopkins, S.; Ashiru-Oredope, D. Measuring Appropriate Antibiotic Prescribing in Acute Hospitals: Development of a National Audit Tool Through a Delphi Consensus. *Antibiotics* **2019**, *8*, 49. [CrossRef] [PubMed]
9. James, R.; Upjohn, L.; Cotta, M.; Luu, S.; Marshall, C.; Buising, K.; Thursky, K. Measuring antimicrobial prescribing quality in Australian hospitals: Development and evaluation of a national antimicrobial prescribing survey tool. *J. Antimicrob. Chemother.* **2015**, *70*, 1912–1918. [PubMed]
10. Spivak, E.S.; Cosgrove, S.E.; Srinivasan, A. Measuring Appropriate Antimicrobial Use: Attempts at Opening the Black Box. *Clin. Infect. Dis.* **2016**, *63*, 1639–1644. [PubMed]
11. Al-Hasan, M.N.; Winders, H.R.; Bookstaver, P.B.; Justo, J.A. Direct Measurement of Performance: A New Era in Antimicrobial Stewardship. *Antibiotics* **2019**, *8*, 127. [CrossRef] [PubMed]
12. Colliers, A.; Adriaenssens, N.; Anthierens, S.; Bartholomeeusen, S.; Philips, H.; Remmen, R.; Coenen, S. Antibiotic Prescribing Quality in Out-of-Hours Primary Care and Critical Appraisal of Disease-Specific Quality Indicators. *Antibiotics* **2019**, *8*, 79. [CrossRef] [PubMed]
13. Sunde, M.; Nygaard, M.M.; Høye, S. General Practitioners' Attitudes toward Municipal Initiatives to Improve Antibiotic Prescribing—A Mixed-Methods Study. *Antibiotics* **2019**, *8*, 120. [CrossRef] [PubMed]
14. Grigoryan, L.; Nash, S.; Zoorob, R.; Germanos, G.J.; Horsfield, M.S.; Khan, F.M.; Martin, L.; Trautner, B.W. Qualitative Analysis of Primary Care Provider Prescribing Decisions for Urinary Tract Infections. *Antibiotics* **2019**, *8*, 84. [CrossRef] [PubMed]
15. Borek, A.J.; Wanat, M.; Sallis, A.; Ashiru-Oredope, D.; Atkins, L.; Beech, E.; Hopkins, S.; Jones, L.; McNulty, C.; Shaw, K.; et al. How Can National Antimicrobial Stewardship Interventions in Primary Care Be Improved? A Stakeholder Consultation. *Antibiotics* **2019**, *8*, 207. [CrossRef] [PubMed]
16. Holmes, E.A.F.; Hughes, D.A. Challenges for Economic Evaluation of Health Care Strategies to Contain Antimicrobial Resistance. *Antibiotics* **2019**, *8*, 166. [CrossRef] [PubMed]
17. Singh, S.R.; Chua, A.Q.; Tan, S.T.; Tam, C.C.; Hsu, L.Y.; Legido-Quigley, H. Combating Antimicrobial Resistance in Singapore: A Qualitative Study Exploring the Policy Context, Challenges, Facilitators, and Proposed Strategies. *Antibiotics* **2019**, *8*, 201. [CrossRef] [PubMed]
18. Vianna, J.S.; Machado, D.; Ramis, I.B.; Silva, F.P.; Bierhals, D.V.; Abril, M.A.; von Groll, A.; Ramos, D.; Lourenço, M.C.S.; Viveiros, M.; et al. The Contribution of Efflux Pumps in Mycobacterium abscessus Complex Resistance to Clarithromycin. *Antibiotics* **2019**, *8*, 153. [CrossRef] [PubMed]
19. Costa, J.P.; Pinheiro, M.J.F.; Sousa, S.A.; Botelho do Rego, A.M.; Marques, F.; Oliveira, M.C.; Leitão, J.H.; P Mira, N.; Carvalho, N.N.; Fernanda, M.; et al. Antimicrobial Activity of Silver Camphorimine Complexes against Candida Strains. *Antibiotics* **2019**, *8*, 144. [CrossRef] [PubMed]
20. Gavilán, R.E.; Nebot, C.; Patyra, E.; Vazquez, B.; Miranda, J.M.; Cepeda, A. Determination of Florfenicol, Thiamfenicol and Chloramfenicol at Trace Levels in Animal Feed by HPLC–MS/MS. *Antibiotics* **2019**, *8*, 59. [CrossRef] [PubMed]

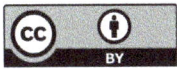

© 2019 by the authors. Licensee MDPI, Basel, Switzerland. This article is an open access article distributed under the terms and conditions of the Creative Commons Attribution (CC BY) license (http://creativecommons.org/licenses/by/4.0/).

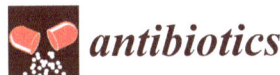

Article

How Can National Antimicrobial Stewardship Interventions in Primary Care Be Improved? A Stakeholder Consultation

Aleksandra J. Borek [1,*], Marta Wanat [1], Anna Sallis [2], Diane Ashiru-Oredope [3], Lou Atkins [4], Elizabeth Beech [5], Susan Hopkins [3,6], Leah Jones [3], Cliodna McNulty [3], Karen Shaw [3,7], Esther Taborn [5,8], Christopher Butler [1], Tim Chadborn [2] and Sarah Tonkin-Crine [1,6]

[1] Nuffield Department of Primary Care Health Sciences, University of Oxford, Radcliffe Observatory Quarter, Oxford OX2 6GG, UK; marta.wanat@phc.ox.ac.uk (M.W.); christopher.butler@phc.ox.ac.uk (C.B.); sarah.tonkin-crine@phc.ox.ac.uk (S.T.-C.)
[2] Public Health England Behavioural Insights, London SE1 8UG, UK; Anna.Sallis@phe.gov.uk (A.S.); Tim.Chadborn@phe.gov.uk (T.C.)
[3] Public Health England, London SE1 8UG, UK; Diane.Ashiru-Oredope@phe.gov.uk (D.A.-O.); Susan.Hopkins@phe.gov.uk (S.H.); Leah.Jones@phe.gov.uk (L.J.); Cliodna.McNulty@phe.gov.uk (C.M.); k.shaw7@nhs.net (K.S.)
[4] Centre for Behavioural Change, University College London, London WC1E 6BT, UK; l.atkins@ucl.ac.uk
[5] NHS England and NHS Improvement, London SE1 6LH, UK; elizabeth.beech@nhs.net (E.B.); esther.taborn@nhs.net (E.T.)
[6] NIHR Health Protection Research Unit in Healthcare Associated Infections and Antimicrobial Resistance, University of Oxford in Partnership with Public Health England, Wellington Square, Oxford OX1 2JD, UK
[7] University College London Hospitals, London NW1 2PG, UK
[8] NHS East Kent Clinical Commissioning Groups, Canterbury CT1 1YW, UK
* Correspondence: aleksandra.borek@phc.ox.ac.uk; Tel.: +44-186-528-9337

Received: 1 October 2019; Accepted: 22 October 2019; Published: 31 October 2019

Abstract: Many antimicrobial stewardship (AMS) interventions have been implemented in England, facilitating decreases in antibiotic prescribing. Nevertheless, there is substantial variation in antibiotic prescribing across England and some healthcare organizations remain high prescribers of antibiotics. This study aimed to identify ways to improve AMS interventions to further optimize antibiotic prescribing in primary care in England. Stakeholders representing different primary care settings were invited to, and 15 participated in, a focus group or telephone interview to identify ways to improve existing AMS interventions. Forty-five intervention suggestions were generated and 31 were prioritized for inclusion in an online survey. Fifteen stakeholders completed the survey appraising each proposed intervention using the pre-defined APEASE (i.e., Affordability, Practicability, Effectiveness, Acceptability, Safety, and Equity) criteria. The highest-rated nine interventions were prioritized as most promising and feasible, including: quality improvement, multidisciplinary peer learning, appointing AMS leads, auditing individual-level prescribing, developing tools for prescribing audits, improving inductions for new prescribers, ensuring consistent local approaches to antibiotic prescribing, providing online AMS training to all patient-facing staff, and increasing staff time available for AMS work with standardizing AMS-related roles. These prioritized interventions could be incorporated into existing national interventions or developed as stand-alone interventions to help further optimize antibiotic prescribing in primary care in England.

Keywords: antimicrobial stewardship; antibiotic prescribing; primary care; implementation; behavior change; stakeholder consultation

1. Introduction

Conserving antibiotics by optimizing antibiotic prescribing to reduce the spread of antimicrobial resistance is a key public health priority both globally and nationally in the UK [1–3]. In England, 81% of antibiotics were prescribed in primary care in 2017 [4], and up to 23% of these are estimated to be prescribed inappropriately, mostly (unnecessarily) for self-limiting respiratory tract infections (RTIs) [5]. While antibiotic prescribing in primary care in England reduced by 13.2% between 2013 and 2017 [4], antibiotic use in the community is still higher than in several other European countries [6]. There is also a considerable variation in antibiotic prescribing between general practices, with many practices remaining high prescribers [7], and between practices and other types of healthcare providers in the community (e.g., out-of-hours, urgent care) [4]. The variations in antibiotic use are not (fully) explained by differences in patient characteristics, such as clinical presentation or prevalence of comorbidities [7,8].

Changing healthcare professionals' (HCP) prescribing behaviors can help reduce antibiotic use and many factors influencing antibiotic prescribing for RTIs in primary care have been identified [9–13]. A range of antimicrobial stewardship (AMS) interventions targeting HCPs have been developed, with many shown effective in trials [14–16]. However, despite the recent decrease in antibiotic prescribing and availability of AMS interventions, further optimizing and reducing inappropriate antibiotic use in English primary care remains critical, especially among the higher prescribers. Further progress has been included in the recent National Health Service (NHS) long-term plan [17] and is required to meet the UK five-year target to reduce antibiotic prescribing in community by 25% by 2024 [2]. Behavioral science evidence shows that to be effective, behavior change interventions need to target relevant determinants of behavior and needs of the targeted population, and fit within the contexts where they are implemented [18,19]. Thus, further improving antibiotic prescribing might involve adapting and implementing effective AMS interventions that have not been yet widely used in England [14], and/or addressing contextual and implementation-specific influences experienced by those using AMS interventions [11].

A recent study aimed to explore nationally implemented AMS interventions in the UK and the extent to which they target behaviors related to antibiotic use. Twenty-two interventions for primary care prescribers and eight for community pharmacy staff were identified, targeting on average 5.8 HCPs' behaviors [10]. A follow-up study identified barriers and facilitators to appropriate antibiotic prescribing in primary care and found nine interventions evaluated in the UK and shown effective at reducing antibiotic prescribing [11]; these included five research-only interventions [20–24] and four nationally available interventions: communication skills training [25], FeverPAIN clinical score [26], the TARGET toolkit [27], and the Chief Medical Officer's letters with prescribing feedback to the highest-prescribing practices [28]. Analyzing the behavioral content of the identified AMS interventions and comparing the extent to which they address relevant behaviors and key barriers and facilitators led to identification of potential changes to, or gaps to be addressed by, AMS interventions. However, such theoretical analysis lacks the insight from the targeted population and intervention users, and does not address factors related to context and implementation of interventions. Therefore, we aimed to build on this recent research by consulting stakeholders (i.e., HCPs from general practices, out-of-hours, community pharmacies and commissioning organizations in England) to: (a) identify barriers and facilitators to optimizing antibiotic prescribing and implementing AMS interventions specific to their settings, (b) generate suggestions for improvements of AMS interventions in their specific, primary care settings in England, and (c) prioritize interventions (using pre-specified feasibility and acceptability criteria). This paper reports the findings of this stakeholder consultation.

2. Results

2.1. Stakeholder Focus Group and Telephone Interviews

Twelve stakeholders attended the focus group and three participated individually by telephone. Seven were representatives from Clinical Commissioning Groups (CCGs, i.e., organizations responsible for planning and commissioning of health care services for their local areas in England), three were from NHS England, two from out-of-hours (OOH) organizations, one from a chain of community pharmacies, and two were general practitioners (GPs).

In the first part, the stakeholders discussed barriers and facilitators to optimizing antibiotic prescribing in primary care settings. These are summarized in Table 1 and reported in more detail in Supplementary Materials (Boxes S1–S4). In brief, as key facilitators to optimizing antibiotic prescribing, the stakeholders reported the availability of many AMS interventions, and awareness of healthcare professionals of the need for appropriate and prudent antibiotic prescribing. As one of the key challenges they reported a variation in use (and sometimes low uptake) of interventions between organizations and HCPs. This was exacerbated by barriers including: limited dissemination of information about specific interventions; insufficient time to engage with interventions (related to large workloads and multiple competing priorities); lack of clarity on which interventions to engage with (influenced by a perceived large number of interventions); insufficient initiatives with professionals collaborating across networks (e.g., involving GPs, pharmacists, nurses) which fueled perceptions of 'working in silos'.

In the second part of the consultation, the stakeholders identified challenges to implementing specific current AMS interventions and made suggestions for improvements. These suggestions were compiled, separately for each primary care setting, and are summarized in Table 1 (and reported in more detail in Supplementary Materials, Boxes S1–S4). Key suggestions included: offering financial incentives; mandating certain target behaviors (e.g., making AMS training a mandatory part of professional development or appraisal); regularly auditing prescribing in all practices and of individual prescribers and, based on this, providing interventions tailored to local contexts and individual needs and addressing specific reasons for suboptimal prescribing; developing multi-professional networks and learning groups to promote communication, collaboration and learning between different professions (e.g., GPs, nurses, pharmacists); incorporating interventions nationally within existing clinical systems; and using point-of-care (POC) diagnostics, such as C-Reactive Protein (CRP) tests or throat swabs (although stakeholders expressed ambivalent views on these). No suggestions were identified for walk-in/urgent care centers as no stakeholders were from this specific setting. However, it was agreed that some of the suggested interventions may be relevant to this setting.

Table 1. Summary findings from stakeholder focus group and interviews.

Examples of Identified Facilitators (F) and Barriers (B)	Examples of Suggestions for Intervention Improvements or New Interventions
Relevant to all settings	
<ul><li>F: Availability of many AMS interventions and guidelines.</li><li>F: Consistency of AMS/antibiotic-related messages and advice across HCPs and organizations.</li><li>F: Knowing practice and prescribers' prescribing rates and resistance rates.</li><li>B: Feeling of guideline 'overload' and lack of time to read them.</li><li>B: Lack of clarity on which AMS interventions should be used; variation in use of interventions across HCPs and organizations.</li><li>B: Insufficient time, high workloads, and related decision-making fatigue.</li><li>B: Insufficient collaboration between professional networks and organizations.</li></ul>	<ul><li>Incentivizing or mandating engagement with AMS training and other interventions.</li><li>Making tools/interventions easy to use by incorporating them into clinical systems.</li><li>Making professional networks more multi-professional and promoting multi-professional collaborations and learning.</li><li>Providing better/easier access to data on prescribing data linked with resistance data.</li><li>Addressing primary care HCPs' concerns about sepsis.</li></ul>
Relevant to general practice	
<ul><li>B: Prescribing antibiotics remaining to be seen as easier and quicker than not prescribing (especially under time pressure).</li><li>B: Prescribing antibiotics 'just in case' prior to limited access to healthcare (e.g., before a weekend).</li><li>B: Prescribers (e.g., locums) not using unique prescriber codes, making it difficult to audit prescribing.</li></ul>	<ul><li>Financial incentives for practices with antibiotic prescribing targets.</li><li>POC CRP testing (but mixed views due to concerns about costs and unintended consequences).</li><li>Auditing prescribing in all practices and by all prescribers, with feedback and tailored approaches to address specific issues.</li><li>Peer review of prescribing in practices.</li><li>Training patient-facing practice staff in signposting patients and self-care advice.</li></ul>

Table 1. Cont.

Examples of Identified Facilitators (F) and Barriers (B)	Examples of Suggestions for Intervention Improvements or New Interventions
Relevant to out of hours (OOH)	
<ul><li>B: Lack of stable patient population.</li><li>B: Prescribers not using unique prescriber codes.</li><li>B: Lack of accountability for prescribing.</li><li>B: Variation in awareness of local guidelines.</li><li>B: Lack of/limited support from commissioners.</li><li>B: Different clinical systems limiting access to patient records.</li></ul>	<ul><li>Developing tools/system to enable/ automate prescribing audits in OOH.</li><li>Making AMS interventions (e.g., training) provided by commissioners available and improving dissemination of information about them to OOH staff.</li><li>Improving induction of new prescribers in OOH to ensure awareness of local guidelines.</li></ul>
Relevant to community pharmacy	
<ul><li>B: Variation in skills and experience between pharmacy staff, with some having low confidence in providing self-care advice.</li><li>B: Limited access to POC diagnostics across pharmacies and concern about using them for financial benefit.</li><li>B: Different computer systems limiting access to, and use of, patient records.</li></ul>	<ul><li>Providing training in giving self-care advice to improve skills and confidence of staff.</li><li>Providing access to POC diagnostics and training to help pharmacy staff distinguish between serious and less serious illness (thus improving confidence in giving self-care advice).</li><li>Promoting use of patient records to identify potentially inappropriate use of antibiotics.</li></ul>

2.2. Revising and Selecting Intervention Suggestions

Additional intervention components were identified based on available evidence on AMS interventions shown to be effective in the UK [11]. In addition, steering group members and the research team provided additional suggestions based on their experience and knowledge of current national AMS policy. These were added to the list of suggestions made by the stakeholders. Altogether, 45 intervention suggestions were identified. Some involved modifications of existing interventions or their implementation (e.g., relating to dissemination of information), whereas others involved new intervention components (e.g., that could form a part of an existing intervention or be implemented as a stand-alone intervention).

In order to identify which influences on antibiotic-related prescribing behaviors the suggested interventions aimed to address, the interventions were mapped onto barriers and facilitators to appropriate antibiotic prescribing. These influences were identified in the literature review [11] and by the stakeholders. After revising and selecting intervention suggestions, 31 interventions were included in an online survey comprising: seven suggestions potentially applicable to all settings, ten suggestions specifically for general practice, nine for OOH, and five for community pharmacy. The full list of the 45 identified interventions is available in Supplementary Materials (Table S1), together with barriers and facilitators that they addressed, source of how each intervention was identified, and indicating which interventions were included in or excluded (with reasons) from the survey.

2.3. Stakeholder Survey and Prioritized Intervention Suggestions

Out of 40 stakeholders invited to complete the survey, 15 (38%) completed it. Seven respondents indicated that they worked (or had expertise) in general practice, five in CCGs, four in OOH, three in walk-in/urgent care centers, one in community pharmacy, and four in other settings (i.e., two working across settings; one in community hospital; one in e-learning for healthcare professionals). The respondents reported between 4 and 23 (mean 10.7) years of relevant experience. The APEASE scores for each intervention and setting are reported in full in Supplementary Materials (Tables S2–S5).

Nine unique interventions were prioritized (Table 2). Three interventions were prioritized for OOH and community pharmacy, and four were prioritized for general practice and walk-in/urgent care centers (as two of the highest-scoring interventions for these two settings had even scores). As some interventions were assessed for multiple settings, four interventions were prioritized for multiple settings: '(2) Multi-disciplinary small group learning' was prioritized for general practice, walk-in/urgent care centers, and community pharmacy; '(3) Appointing AMS leaders' for general practice and OOH; '(7) Agreeing on a consistent local approach to antibiotics' for walk-in/urgent care centers and community pharmacy; '(8) Providing online AMS training to all patient-facing staff' for walk-in/urgent care centers and community pharmacy.

The lowest scoring intervention (with 22.7% of the maximum APEASE score) was 'providing diagnostic point-of-care CRP testing, including training in using it, interpreting the results and maintaining the equipment' in community pharmacy setting, which was assessed by only five out of 11 respondents as relevant to the setting, by two as practical and acceptable and by none as affordable. This intervention was also rated as the second lowest for general practice (44% of the maximum APEASE score), walk-in/urgent care centers (48.7%) and OOH (50%). Participants' comments provided as free text in the survey indicated that cost and funding, time to do the tests, and concern about over-use of the tests by patients and clinicians were considered the main barriers to using this intervention; for example:

"Would need to have clear guidance and uptake would depend on who was funding [POC CRP tests]. Barriers to GP practices are cost of equipment and cost of tests, as well as time it takes to perform the test when only have 5–10 min consultation and test takes a few minutes to perform so practical and affordability issues are the main barriers."

"Concerns [that POC CRP tests] may increase attendance to 'get a test'. May involve clinicians overly relying on a test which is not always accurate or there may be a time lag in the increase in CRP. Time taken in consultation to administer test is a barrier and test strips are costly."

The two second lowest scoring (with 33.3% of maximum APEASE score) interventions were also in community pharmacy setting; although both were assessed by only three participants. One was 'providing training and resources to structure the way(s) of asking patients the right questions about self-limiting infections and identifying red flags to help decide what to advise patients'. In comments, the participants suggested that: *"this sort of training is available* via CPPE, *however uptake is voluntary"* and *"this should already be done as part of the core community pharmacy contract."* The other intervention was 'promoting the use of patient records by pharmacists (e.g., by digital prompts) to review whether antibiotics were prescribed appropriately'. Participants' comments suggested that:

"At present community pharmacists do not have access to enough information to be able to do this effectively. There may need to be specialist clinical training for community pharmacists to do this."

"The relevance will depend on where the community pharmacist is in the patient pathway. If contractual levers remain as is the community pharmacist may require remuneration."

Other lowest scoring interventions (see a full list in Supplementary Materials) were: 'providing information on opening hours of all local healthcare services' for general practice (31.8% of maximum APEASE score) which was scored particularly low on 'effectiveness', and 'co-organizing national AMS events together with different professional networks' for OOH and walk-in/urgent care centers (50% and 38.5%, respectively) which was rated low on 'affordability'.

Table 2. Interventions prioritized by stakeholders.

Prioritized Interventions (Short Title with Detailed Description)	Setting(s) for Which Interventions Were Prioritized (% of Max. APEASE Score)	Facilitators (F)/Barriers (B) Addressed by Interventions
1. Standardized quality improvement with tailored advice and action planning Prescribing advisors or practice prescribing/AMS leads to carry out standardized quality improvement (e.g., supported by IT system functionality) and use prescribing data to identify underlying reasons for high/inappropriate antibiotic prescribers, provide tailored advice to prescribers and agree practice action plans (e.g., practice plan to reduce immediate antibiotic prescribing for acute cough).	General practice (84.9)	F: Advice from colleagues when uncertain or to reinforce appropriate prescribing decisions; perceptions of own prescribing compared to others.
2. Multi-disciplinary small group learning Multi-disciplinary small group learning (e.g., including local GPs, nurses, pharmacists, CCG staff) to identify ways to improve implementation of AMS initiatives and share local examples of good practice and actions taken by others as part of AMS.	General practice (84.5), Walk-in/urgent care centers (61.5), Community pharmacy (56.1)	F: Learning from peers on whether they can improve and how, and about alternative prescribing techniques.
3. Appointing AMS leaders Appoint AMS lead prescribers in all practices/OOH sites to lead on AMS-related issues, e.g., by organizing practice meetings about AMS, disseminating information about new guidelines, encouraging peers to implement interventions.	General practice (83.3), OOH (91.7)	B: Lack of a leader to lead on, and encourage engagement with, AMS-related issues.
4. Auditing individual prescribing Audit prescribing of individual prescribers in general practices, to be done by local prescribing advisors, practice prescribing/AMS leads or practice pharmacists, and provide individual feedback on prescribing, identify underlying reasons for high/inappropriate antibiotic prescribing, provide tailored advice and agree individual action plans (e.g., individual prescriber's plan to reduce immediate antibiotic prescribing for acute cough).	General practice (83.3)	F: Having prescribing monitored and audited, receiving feedback on prescribing. B: Lack of accountability for prescribing.
5. Developing tools/system for auditing prescribing Develop tools/system to enable (automated) audit of prescribing in OOH and provision of personalized feedback and advice.	OOH (77.8)	B: Auditing prescribing in OOH impossible or difficult due to not being linked to population or area.
6. Improving inductions for new prescribers Improve induction for new prescribers in OOH to ensure knowledge of relevant local guidelines (e.g., indications for antibiotic prescribing, first-line antibiotics) and organization-agreed approaches to prescribing antibiotics.	OOH (77.8)	B: Lack of awareness/knowledge of local guidelines by new/locum GPs in OOH.
7. Agreeing on a consistent local approach to antibiotics Agree on a consistent local approach to antibiotic prescribing within an organization, such as a general practice, out-of-hours, walk-in center or community pharmacy, for example, by agreeing an AMS-related action plan, a practice protocol on treating certain infections and/or following national or local guidelines.	Walk-in/urgent care centers (65.4), Community pharmacy (59.1)	B: Inconsistent approaches to antibiotic prescribing. F: Adopting guidelines or evidence as a standard practice (with intention to follow them).
8. Providing online AMS training to all patient-facing staff Provide online AMS training to all patient-facing staff within an organization to improve (and minimize variation in) skills to ensure a consistent approach to providing advice to patients and antibiotic prescribing for respiratory tract infections.	Walk-in/urgent care centers (62.8), Community pharmacy (59.1)	B: Variation in the skills and experience among staff.
9. Increasing staff time for AMS work and standardizing AMS roles Increase staff time available to work on AMS (within relevant organizations) and standardize the AMS-related roles; for example, all organizations to have adequate number of prescribing advisors and/or pharmacists to work more closely with practices, OOH, walk-in centers and community pharmacies (e.g., by auditing prescribing, disseminating information, providing training and advice).	Walk-in/urgent care centers (61.5)	F: Advice from and influence of relevant experts.

3. Discussion

The stakeholder consultation identified setting-specific barriers and facilitators to current antibiotic optimization, and generated and prioritized suggestions for improvements of AMS interventions in primary care in England. Stakeholders' appraisal of relevance, feasibility and acceptability of 31 intervention suggestions led to nine interventions being prioritized across settings. These prioritized interventions address some of the identified influences on antibiotic prescribing. They could be incorporated as part of existing AMS interventions or further developed and implemented as stand-alone interventions.

3.1. Implications within the Context of Current AMS Research and Practice

The interventions assessed and prioritized (or not) by the stakeholders build on AMS interventions currently implemented in England [10] and effective interventions tested in UK-based research studies [11]. How the 31 interventions fit with current research and practice, and how those prioritized may be implemented, is discussed below and summarized in Table 3. Interventions are grouped by intervention 'type', for ease of reference.

Improving engagement with AMS training and resources: There are many AMS interventions available, including AMS training and resources tested and shown effective in trials [21,25,27]. For example, the TARGET antibiotic toolkit (with training and resources primarily targeted at GPs) is available online [29] and practice workshops promoting the TARGET resources were shown effective [27]. Similarly, the STAR online communication skills training (with a practice seminar) was shown effective in a trial [25] and is now available online on the clinical professional development website [30]. CCG professionals report that HCPs are aware of, and promote or engage with, different AMS training and resources (such as the TARGET toolkit), but time, reaching the correct people and lack of clarity on which online training to promote were reported as the main issues with AMS education [31]. Similarly, the stakeholders in our study identified improving engagement with AMS interventions as a challenge, influenced by lack of time and priority, clarity on which interventions to use, incentives, and opportunities (e.g., protected time, training for HCPs in organizations other than general practice). Current AMS interventions may, at least in theory and research trials, facilitate change but improving the uptake of and engagement with AMS interventions in the real world is critical to further optimizing antibiotic use. This may be facilitated by the 'train the trainers' opportunities provided by the TARGET team [29] and by increasing numbers of pharmacists appointed in primary care settings with AMS as part of their roles. The importance of improving engagement with AMS training and resources was reflected by suggestions prioritized by the stakeholders, such as organizing '(2) multi-disciplinary small group learning' (that could be delivered face-to-face, in addition to online resources, and focus on identifying challenges and solutions specific to local contexts), '(8) providing online AMS training to all patient-facing staff' (rather than, as currently, targeting primarily GPs), and '(9) increasing staff time available for AMS work and standardizing AMS roles'. Another suggestion to improve engagement with AMS training that was made by the stakeholders but received medium APEASE score was to make the AMS training mandatory in general practices.

Table 3. Proposed AMS interventions and how they fit with current research and practice.

Types of AMS Intervention	Effective Intervention Trialed in the UK? [1]	Intervention Implemented Nationally? [2]	Interventions Suggested and Prioritized by Stakeholders (Green—Prioritized Interventions, Indicated by Numbers, e.g., (1); Orange—Lowest Scoring, White—Mid Scoring or No Suggestions) [3]
AMS training and resources	Yes [21,25,27]	Yes (e.g., TARGET [29], STAR [30])—but: online only, targeted mainly at prescribers, varied uptake/engagement	(2) Multi-disciplinary small group learning (8) Providing online AMS training to all patient-facing staff (9) Increasing staff time for AMS work and standardizing AMS roles - Online training promoting increased use of delayed/back-up antibiotic prescriptions - Making AMS training mandatory
Antibiotic prescribing data monitoring and feedback	Yes [24,28]	Yes—data publicly available but: varied provision of feedback; lack of national data/feedback on individual prescribing; varied use of prescriber codes	(1) Standardized quality improvement with tailored advice and action planning (4) Auditing individual prescribing with tailored advice and action planning (5) Developing tools/system to enable (automated) audit of prescribing in OOH - Promoting/regulating use of unique prescriber codes to enable individual prescribing feedback - Improving dissemination of data on local antimicrobial resistance patterns - Encouraging GPs to peer review each other's antibiotic prescribing - Making antibiotic prescribing/infection audit in OOH mandatory
Patient leaflets	Yes [2,22]	Yes—but in general practice and OOH only	Promoting routine interactive use of patient leaflets (in community pharmacy)
Clinical decision support tools	Yes [20,26]	Yes—but uptake varies	[No interventions/suggestions for improvements were identified.]
Agreeing a consistent approach to antibiotics	Yes [23]	No	(7) Agreeing on a consistent local approach to antibiotics, e.g., AMS-related action plan, protocol (2) Multi-disciplinary small group learning (8) Providing online AMS training to all patient-facing staff (so that they give consistent messages to patients) Co-organizing national AMS events with different professional networks
POC CRP testing	Yes [21]	No	Providing point-of-care CRP tests
Prescribing guidelines	No trial evidence for specific guidelines	Yes—but guidelines vary locally	(6) Improving inductions for new prescribers in OOH to ensure knowledge of local guidelines and organization-agreed approaches to prescribing antibiotics
AMS leadership	No trial evidence	Yes—but roles vary, little available time	(3) Appointing AMS leaders in all practices to lead on AMS-related issues (9) Increasing staff time for AMS work and standardizing AMS roles - Using respected and trusted, national and local experts to promote AMS
AMS campaigns	No trial evidence	Yes	[No interventions/suggestions for improvements were identified.]
Other interventions for general practice and OOH	No	No	- Incorporating interventions into clinical systems nationally - Making patient information and history available on OOH IT system, and OOH information on GP IT system to enable follow up - Providing information on opening hours of local healthcare services to prevent higher prescribing on Fridays

Table 3. *Cont.*

Types of AMS Intervention	Effective Intervention Trialed in the UK? [1]	Intervention Implemented Nationally? [2]	Interventions Suggested and Prioritized by Stakeholders (Green—Prioritized Interventions, Indicated by Numbers, e.g., (1); Orange—Lowest Scoring, White—Mid Scoring or No Suggestions) [3]
Other interventions for community pharmacy	No	No	- Pharmacy staff to prompt GPs to review long-term and repeat antibiotic prescriptions - Encourage pharmacists to feedback to GPs where antibiotics were not prescribed according to guidelines - Promote the use of patient records by pharmacists to review whether antibiotics were prescribed appropriately - Provide training and resources to structure the way(s) of asking patients the right questions about self-limiting infections and identifying red-flags to help decide what to advise patients

Notes: [1] Nine UK-based studies of effective AMS interventions [8,20–24,26–28] were identified and are reported elsewhere [10]. [2] Twenty six nationally implemented AMS interventions were identified previously and are reported elsewhere [11]. [3] The nine prioritized interventions are numbered as in Table 2 and include the highest-scoring interventions (3–4 per setting) (green rows). Lowest-scoring interventions (3 per setting) are in orange rows; the remaining interventions with the APEASE scores in the middle are in white rows. All APEASE scores for each intervention and setting are reported in the Supplementary Materials (Tables S2–S5).

Enhancing prescribing data monitoring and feedback: Antibiotic prescribing data has been publicly available and fed back to prescribers by a vast majority of CCGs for many years and interventions involving prescribing feedback have been shown effective [24,28]. In contrast, detailed action planning is rarely used (reported for only 16% of CCGs [31], often due to insufficient time for it [32]), as is feedback on individual prescribing—both of these strategies were prioritized. Including them may enhance the impact of monitoring of and feedback on prescribing by specifying and tailoring actions (setting goals and/or 'if-then' plans) to address specific reasons for inappropriate antibiotic prescribing and by activating individual accountability for prescribing. Based on available evidence from lifestyle-related interventions, such behavioral regulation strategies (i.e., self-monitoring, especially when combined with other 'regulatory' techniques such as goal-setting, problem solving or 'if-then' plans) and individual tailoring can be effective behavior change techniques (e.g., [33,34]). Moreover, while monitoring/auditing of, and feedback on, prescribing have likely contributed to reduced antibiotic prescribing in general practice, the stakeholders reported barriers to using these strategies in OOH, such as lack of stable patient population and different computer systems. Developing tools to enable and automate prescribing audit and provision of individualized feedback might further optimize antibiotic prescribing in OOH.

Ensuring consistency in AMS approaches: The suggestion to '(7) agree on a consistent local approach to antibiotics' (prioritized for walk-in/urgent care centers and community pharmacies and also highly scored for general practice and OOH) highlights the importance of consistency in managing infections and reinforcing consistent messages to patients by different HCPs and across organizations. It could be implemented by developing and agreeing within-and between-organization action plans or protocols, for example, on using patient leaflets and other resources promoting messages about infection prevention and self-care. The importance of consistency between HCPs in antibiotic prescribing and the messages given to patients was also reflected in the following interventions prioritized by the stakeholders: '(2) multidisciplinary small group learning' and '(8) providing online AMS training to all patient-facing staff'. Moreover, four interventions were prioritized for multiple settings (i.e., '(7) agreeing on a consistent local approach to antibiotics'; '(2) multi-disciplinary small group learning'; '(8) providing online AMS training to all patient-facing staff'; '(3) appointing AMS leaders') and could be considered for implementation across settings and by involving HCPs from different professional networks. This could help promote a more integrated, system-wide approach to AMS [17]. Respondents in a recent survey representing 99% of Clinical Commissioning Groups (CCGs) reported that AMS training was targeted primarily at GPs, compared to 67% of CCG professionals reporting focus on other prescribers, 42% on all practice staff and only 28% on OOH staff; consequently, a system and practice-wide approach was one of the top suggestions for AMS training by the CCG professionals [31].

Finally, it may also be important to consider interventions that have not been prioritized by stakeholders. Providing POC CRP tests was among the lowest-scoring suggestions in all settings. The stakeholders considered it not affordable or practical to deliver. While POC CRP testing is supported by examples of countries with low prescribing rates that routinely use it (e.g., Netherlands) and trial evidence showing it as an effective and safe strategy to reduce antibiotic prescribing for RTIs in general practice [14,35], it may not have sustained effects on prescribing behavior [36] and is often met with mixed views on its usefulness and feasibility from HCPs [37,38]. Moreover, 'co-organizing national AMS events for participants from different professional networks to facilitate multi-disciplinary AMS work' and 'promoting the use of patient records by pharmacists to review whether antibiotics were prescribed appropriately' seemed to be considered by stakeholders as unaffordable; 'providing information on opening hours of local healthcare services' (to reduce prescribing when concerned about limited access to healthcare) was considered unlikely to be effective; and 'providing training and resources to structure the ways of asking patients the right questions about self-limiting infections and identifying red flags to help decide what to advise patients' in community pharmacy was seen as of low relevance. Our findings suggest that these interventions might be less promising ways to optimize antibiotic use for RTIs, at least as seen by the small number of stakeholders consulted in this study. Further research may need to explore and identify ways to address barriers related to these interventions with a larger group of stakeholders and intervention users. In addition to the nine prioritized interventions and five lowest-scoring interventions, there were also 17 other interventions included in the survey and another 14 suggestions that were not prioritized for inclusion in the survey (all available in the Supplementary Materials) that could potentially be considered and refined.

3.2. Strengths and Limitations

This study was based on expert input from stakeholders and the study steering group, who had practical experience and knowledge about national AMS interventions and policy. Views of stakeholders and intervention users are critical, yet at times under-represented, in theoretical approaches to developing and refining AMS interventions. Our study, focused on views of commissioners and other key stakeholders, may help address this gap and provide some indication for future research on implementation of AMS interventions. However, our findings need to be interpreted with caution. The stakeholders were identified by the steering group members from their own professional networks, and out of 40 stakeholders invited to the focus group and survey, only 15 responded. It is possible that a larger number of stakeholders or intervention users might have generated suggestions for, and prioritized, different interventions. The stakeholders had varied levels of experience and knowledge of AMS interventions and different settings (with less experience specific to OOH, walk-in centers and community pharmacies). This made it difficult to identify very specific improvements to current AMS interventions and to capture a wider range of views from different organizations and settings. As the study focused on stakeholders and interventions in England, the generalizability of the findings may be limited beyond England.

4. Materials and Methods

The following steps were taken: (1) a stakeholder focus group and telephone interviews to identify barriers and facilitators to appropriate antibiotic prescribing and to generate intervention suggestions; (2) revision and selection of intervention suggestions; (3) a stakeholder survey to assess and prioritize interventions according to pre-specified criteria of relevance, feasibility and acceptability. We focused on interventions targeting HCPs' antibiotic prescribing for RTIs in the following settings: general practice, out-of-hours (OOH), walk-in/urgent care center, and community pharmacy. The study was reviewed by the University of Oxford Clinical Trials and Research Governance team and classified as service development, and as such it did not require research ethics review. Participants were free to participate in any stage of the consultation and withdraw at any point without any consequences. They were offered reimbursement of travel expenses but no payment for participation.

4.1. Stakeholder Focus Group and Telephone Interviews

Relevant stakeholders (including HCPs with expertise in and/or experience of antibiotic prescribing in relevant settings) were identified by the study steering group members. The steering group included experts in AMS with expertise in, and experience of, designing and implementing AMS interventions and influencing national AMS policy in the UK. Identified stakeholders were invited by email to attend a 3-hour face-to-face focus group held at Public Health England premises in London. They were followed up once in cases of non-response. Those who could not attend the focus group in person were invited to a telephone interview.

The aims of the focus group were (a) to identify barriers and facilitators to appropriate antibiotic prescribing and to implementing AMS interventions in relevant settings; and (b) to generate suggestions for improvements of current AMS interventions and/or their implementation or for new interventions addressing the identified barriers and facilitators. In the first part of the focus group, the stakeholders were presented with barriers and facilitators identified from a literature review [11]. This was followed by a discussion of stakeholders' experiences and examples of these, and of any other influences on antibiotic prescribing (especially in settings under-represented in the literature, such as community pharmacy, OOH and walk-in centers). In the second part of the focus group, the stakeholders were presented with examples of nationally available AMS interventions and/or interventions trialed in research studies in the UK. This was followed by a discussion about stakeholders' experiences of using these interventions, any challenges to their use or implementation, and suggestions for improvements and/or any new interventions.

The focus group discussions were facilitated by two researchers in a semi-structured way, which included short presentations and general discussion, followed by more specific questions about participants' views, experiences and examples. A third researcher took detailed notes. The focus group was audio-recorded and the recording was subsequently used to check the notes and add more detail. Additionally, participants were provided with handouts including the information on barriers and facilitators and AMS interventions identified in the literature, and with questions for discussion. They could provide additional comments on the handouts and return them to the researchers. The stakeholders interviewed by telephone were given information and asked questions in a similar format to the focus group. Detailed notes were made on each telephone interview. All suggestions made during the focus group, telephone interviews and on the handouts were collated and summarized. The summary of notes was used to generate a list of barriers and facilitators and a list of intervention suggestions.

4.2. Revision and Selection of Intervention Suggestions for a Survey

Barriers and facilitators to appropriate antibiotic prescribing and effective research interventions were identified in a literature review [11]); these were used to generate additional suggestions which were added to the list of interventions identified by the stakeholders. The intervention suggestions were divided into those potentially applicable to all settings or specific to each relevant setting. They were mapped onto barriers and facilitators identified by the stakeholders and in a preceding literature review [11].

The list of suggested interventions was reviewed by the researchers (AB, MW, STC, AS) and steering group members (remaining authors) who provided feedback on and suggestions for rephrasing the suggested interventions, and made additional suggestions that were added to the list of interventions. To reduce a relatively large number of identified suggestions, the comments from the steering group members (who have knowledge of existing AMS interventions and those currently in development) were used to prioritize selection of interventions for the survey; suggestions were excluded if they were considered unfeasible, already implemented, already under development, or insufficiently specific.

4.3. Stakeholder Survey and Prioritization of Interventions

An online survey was used for the stakeholders to assess intervention suggestions using the APEASE criteria [39]: Affordability (is an intervention affordable?), Practicability (can it be delivered easily?), Effectiveness (is it likely to be effective?), Acceptability (is it acceptable to staff?), Side effects and safety (is it safe to implement?), and Equity (can it avoid inequalities in patient care?). The survey was designed and delivered using online Survey Monkey software (www.surveymonkey.com). Stakeholders identified by the steering group (those invited to the focus group) were invited by email, including a brief description about the survey and a link to complete it online. Participants were sent one reminder; responses were anonymous.

The survey asked about participants' roles, work setting or expertise, and years of relevant experience. Participants were then presented with interventions that could be potentially applicable to all settings (i.e., general practice, OOH, walk-in/urgent care center, community pharmacy) and suggestions specific to each setting: general practice, OOH, and community pharmacy. For each suggestion, participants were asked to: (a) assess whether the intervention was relevant to the setting, and, if yes, then (b) to assess it, for that setting, using the APEASE criteria.

Participants could skip questions and whole sections so the numbers of respondents that assessed each intervention for each setting varied. We calculated the number of responses for each intervention in each setting, the maximum possible APEASE score for each intervention/setting, and the actual APEASE score for each intervention/setting. The percentage of the maximum possible APEASE score obtained for each intervention/setting was calculated to allow comparison between interventions.

In order to identify interventions which were rated highly, the following criteria were used to prioritize interventions in each setting: (a) at least 50% of respondents for that question assessed the intervention as relevant to that setting; and (b) intervention was scored as one of the top three (or four in cases of equal scores) based on the percentage of the maximum APEASE score.

5. Conclusions

The study identified a number of barriers and facilitators to optimizing antibiotics and engaging with AMS interventions, and possible ways in which current AMS interventions in primary care in England could be optimized. Nine interventions were prioritized by stakeholders as relevant, acceptable, affordable and feasible to implement in English primary care. They involve suggestions to help improve engagement with existing AMS training and resources (e.g., by face-to-face small group learning, tailoring AMS training to all patient-facing staff rather than prescribers only), enhancing data monitoring and feedback (e.g., audit and feedback on individual's prescribing, or developing tools to automate prescribing audits), and promoting consistency in AMS approaches across healthcare professionals and services (e.g., by agreeing consistent local approaches, upskilling all patient-facing staff). These can be adapted and further developed as part of current AMS initiatives. Additionally, stakeholders prioritized suggestions to incorporate AMS interventions into clinical systems at a national level and enable sharing of patient information between general practice and OOH clinical systems. Future work needs to also focus more on addressing particular barriers to engagement with specific AMS interventions.

Supplementary Materials: The following Supplementary Materials and Data are available online at http://www.mdpi.com/2079-6382/8/4/207/s1: Box S1. Summary findings from stakeholder consultation: relevant to all settings. Box S2. Summary findings from stakeholder consultation: relevant to general practice. Box S3. Summary findings from stakeholder consultation: relevant to out-of-hours. Box S4. Summary findings from stakeholder consultation: relevant to community pharmacy. Table S1. All identified intervention suggestions. Table S2. Stakeholder ratings of interventions for general practice. Table S3. Stakeholder ratings of interventions for out-of-hours. Table S4. Stakeholder ratings of interventions for walk-in/urgent care centers. Table S5. Stakeholder ratings of interventions for community pharmacy.

Author Contributions: Conceptualization: S.T.-C., A.J.B., M.W., A.S., T.C.; methodology: all authors; formal analysis: A.J.B., M.W., S.T.-C.; interpretation of results: all authors; writing—original draft preparation: A.J.B.; writing—review and editing: all authors; study administration: A.J.B.; funding acquisition: S.T.-C., T.C. The study steering group members included: D.A.-O., E.B., S.H., L.J., C.M., K.S., E.T., C.B., and T.C.

Funding: This study was a part of a consultation commissioned and funded by Public Health England Behavioural Insights, and was carried out as a collaboration between the University of Oxford and Public Health England. S.T.-C. was supported by funding from the National Institute for Health Research (NIHR) Health Protection Research Unit in Healthcare Associated Infections and Antimicrobial Resistance at University of Oxford in partnership with Public Health England [HPRU-2012-10041]. The views and opinions expressed in this paper are those of the authors and not necessarily those of the NHS, NIHR, the Department of Health and Social Care or Public Health England.

Acknowledgments: We thank the participants in this study for their helpful contributions.

Conflicts of Interest: C.B. reports receiving advisory board fees from Pfizer and Roche Molecular Systems, and grant support from Roche Molecular Diagnostics. Other authors declare no conflict of interest.

Abbreviations

AMS: Antimicrobial Stewardship; CCG: Clinical Commissioning Group; CRP: C-Reactive Protein; GP: General Practitioner; HCP: Healthcare professional; NHS: National Health Service; NIHR: National Institute of Health Research; OOH: Out-of-hours; POC: Point-of-care; RTI: Respiratory tract infection.

References

1. Davies, S.; Gibbens, N. *UK Five Year Antimicrobial Resistance Strategy 2013 to 2018*; Department of Health: London, UK, 2013.
2. Department of Health and Social Care. *UK Five Year Action Plan for Antimicrobial Resistance 2019 to 2024*; Department of Health and Social Care: London, UK, 2019.

3. World Health Organization. *Global Action Plan to Control the Spread and Impact of Antimicrobial Resistance in Neisseria Gonorrhoeae*; World Health Organization: Geneva, Switzerland, 2015.
4. Public Health England. *English Surveillance Programme for Antimicrobial Utilisation and Resistance (ESPAUR). Report 2018*; Public Health England: London, UK, 2018.
5. Smieszek, T.; Pouwels, K.B.; Dolk, F.C.K.; Smith, D.R.; Hopkins, S.; Sharland, M.; Hay, A.D.; Moore, M.V.; Robotham, J.V. Potential for reducing inappropriate antibiotic prescribing in English primary care. *J. Antimicrob. Chemother.* **2018**, *73*, ii36–ii43. [CrossRef] [PubMed]
6. European Centre for Disease Prevention and Control. *Summary of the Latest Data on Antibiotic Consumption in EU: 2017*; European Centre for Disease Prevention and Control: Stockholm, Sweden, 2017.
7. Pouwels, K.B.; Dolk, F.C.K.; Smith, D.R.M.; Smieszek, T.; Robotham, J.V. Explaining variation in antibiotic prescribing between general practices in the UK. *J. Antimicrob. Chemother.* **2018**, *73*, ii27–ii35. [CrossRef] [PubMed]
8. Butler, C.C.; Hood, K.; Verheij, T.; Little, P.; Melbye, H.; Nuttall, J.; Kelly, M.J.; Molstad, S.; Godycki-Cwirko, M.; Almirall, J.; et al. Variation in antibiotic prescribing and its impact on recovery in patients with acute cough in primary care: Prospective study in 13 countries. *BMJ* **2009**, *338*, b2242. [CrossRef]
9. Pinder, R.J.; Berry, D.; Sallis, A.; Chadborn, T. *Antibiotic Prescribing and Behaviour Change in Healthcare Settings: Literature Review and Behavioural Analysis*; Department of Health & Public Health England: London, UK, 2015.
10. Atkins, L.C.; Tim; Bondaronek, P.; Ashiru-Oredope, D.; Beech, E.; Herd, N.; Lyon, V.; González-Iraizoz, M.; Hopkins, S.; McNulty, C.; et al. Which behaviours and mechanisms of action are targeted by national antimicrobial stewardship interventions for patients, community pharmacy staff, primary care prescribers, providers and commissioners and what is their content? Unpublished work.
11. Borek, A.J.; Nia, W.M.R.; Atkins, L.; Sallis, A.; Tonkin-Crine, S. *Exploring the Implementation of Interventions to Reduce Antibiotic Use (ENACT Study): Report*; Public Health England: London, UK, 2019.
12. Tonkin-Crine, S.; Yardley, L.; Little, P. Antibiotic prescribing for acute respiratory tract infections in primary care: A systematic review and meta-ethnography. *J. Antimicrob. Chemother.* **2011**, *66*, 2215–2223. [CrossRef] [PubMed]
13. Germeni, E.; Frost, J.; Garside, R.; Rogers, M.; Valderas, J.M.; Britten, N. Antibiotic prescribing for acute respiratory tract infections in primary care: An updated and expanded meta-ethnography. *Br. J. Gen. Pr.* **2018**, *68*, e633–e645. [CrossRef]
14. Tonkin-Crine, S.K.; San Tan, P.; van Hecke, O.; Wang, K.; Roberts, N.W.; McCullough, A.; Hansen, M.P.; Butler, C.C.; Del Mar, C.B. Clinician-targeted interventions to influence antibiotic prescribing behaviour for acute respiratory infections in primary care: An overview of systematic reviews. *Cochrane Database Syst. Rev.* **2017**, *9*, CD012252. [CrossRef]
15. Köchling, A.; Löffler, C.; Reinsch, S.; Hornung, A.; Böhmer, F.; Altiner, A.; Chenot, J.F. Reduction of antibiotic prescriptions for acute respiratory tract infections in primary care: A systematic review. *Implement. Sci.* **2018**, *13*, 47. [CrossRef]
16. McDonagh, M.S.; Peterson, K.; Winthrop, K.; Cantor, A.; Lazur, B.H.; Buckley, D.I. Interventions to reduce inappropriate prescribing of antibiotics for acute respiratory tract infections: Summary and update of a systematic review. *J. Int. Med. Res.* **2018**, *46*, 3337–3357. [CrossRef]
17. National Health Service. *The NHS Long Term Plan*. 2019. Available online: https://www.longtermplan.nhs.uk/wp-content/uploads/2019/08/nhs-long-term-plan-version-1.2.pdf (accessed on 30 October 2019).
18. Michie, S.; Johnston, M.; Francis, J.; Hardeman, W.; Eccles, M. From theory to intervention: Mapping theoretically derived behavioural determinants to behaviour change techniques. *Appl. Psychol.* **2008**, *57*, 660–680. [CrossRef]
19. Yardley, L.; Morrison, L.; Bradbury, K.; Muller, I. The person-based approach to intervention development: Application to digital health-related behavior change interventions. *J. Med. Internet Res.* **2015**, *17*, e30. [CrossRef]
20. Gulliford, M.C.; van Staa, T.; Dregan, A.; McDermott, L.; McCann, G.; Ashworth, M.; Charlton, J.; Little, P.; Moore, M.V.; Yardley, L. Electronic health records for intervention research: A cluster randomized trial to reduce antibiotic prescribing in primary care (eCRT study). *Ann. Fam. Med.* **2014**, *12*, 344–351. [CrossRef]
21. Little, P.; Stuart, B.; Francis, N.; Douglas, E.; Tonkin-Crine, S.; Anthierens, S.; Cals, J.W.; Melbye, H.; Santer, M.; Moore, M.; et al. Effects of internet-based training on antibiotic prescribing rates for acute respiratory-tract infections: A multinational, cluster, randomised, factorial, controlled trial. *Lancet* **2013**, *382*, 1175–1182. [CrossRef]
22. Francis, N.A.; Butler, C.C.; Hood, K.; Simpson, S.; Wood, F.; Nuttall, J. Effect of using an interactive booklet about childhood respiratory tract infections in primary care consultations on reconsulting and antibiotic prescribing: A cluster randomised controlled trial. *BMJ* **2009**, *339*, b2885. [CrossRef] [PubMed]

23. Cox, C.M.; Jones, M. Is it possible to decrease antibiotic prescribing in primary care? An analysis of outcomes in the management of patients with sore throats. *Fam. Pract.* **2001**, *18*, 9–13. [CrossRef] [PubMed]
24. McNulty, C.A.; Kane, A.; Foy, C.J.; Sykes, J.; Saunders, P.; Cartwright, K.A. Primary care workshops can reduce and rationalize antibiotic prescribing. *J. Antimicrob. Chemother.* **2000**, *46*, 493–499. [CrossRef] [PubMed]
25. Butler, C.C.; Simpson, S.A.; Dunstan, F.; Rollnick, S.; Cohen, D.; Gillespie, D.; Evans, M.R.; Alam, M.F.; Bekkers, M.J.; Evans, J.; et al. Effectiveness of multifaceted educational programme to reduce antibiotic dispensing in primary care: Practice based randomised controlled trial. *BMJ* **2012**, *344*, d8173. [CrossRef]
26. Little, P.; Hobbs, F.R.; Moore, M.; Mant, D.; Williamson, I.; McNulty, C.; Cheng, Y.E.; Leydon, G.; McManus, R.; Kelly, J.; et al. Clinical score and rapid antigen detection test to guide antibiotic use for sore throats: Randomised controlled trial of PRISM (primary care streptococcal management). *BMJ* **2013**, *347*, f5806. [CrossRef]
27. McNulty, C.; Hawking, M.; Lecky, D.; Jones, L.; Owens, R.; Charlett, A.; Butler, C.; Moore, P.; Francis, N. Effects of primary care antimicrobial stewardship outreach on antibiotic use by general practice staff: Pragmatic randomized controlled trial of the TARGET antibiotics workshop. *J. Antimicrob. Chemother.* **2018**, *73*, 1423–1432. [CrossRef]
28. Hallsworth, M.; Chadborn, T.; Sallis, A.; Sanders, M.; Berry, D.; Greaves, F.; Clements, L.; Davies, S.C. Provision of social norm feedback to high prescribers of antibiotics in general practice: A pragmatic national randomised controlled trial. *Lancet* **2016**, *387*, 1743–1752. [CrossRef]
29. TARGET (Treat Antibiotics Responsibly, Guidance, Education, Tools) Antibiotic Toolkit. Available online: https://www.rcgp.org.uk/clinical-and-research/resources/toolkits/target-antibiotic-toolkit.aspx (accessed on 30 October 2019).
30. STAR: Stemming the Tide of Antibiotic Resistance. Available online: https://www.healthcarecpd.com/course/star-stemming-the-tide-of-antibiotic-resistance (accessed on 30 October 2019).
31. Alison, R.L.D.M.; Beech, E.; Ashiru-Oredope, D.; Costelloe, C.; Owens, R.; McNulty, C.A.M. What resources do NHS commissioning organisations use to support antimicrobial stewardship in primary care in England? Unpublished work.
32. Jones, L.F.; Hawking, M.K.; Owens, R.; Lecky, D.; Francis, N.A.; Butler, C.; Gal, M.; McNulty, C.A.M. An evaluation of the TARGET (Treat Antibiotics Responsibly; Guidance, Education, Tools) Antibiotics Toolkit to improve antimicrobial stewardship in primary care—Is it fit for purpose? *Fam. Pract.* **2017**, *35*, 461–467. [CrossRef]
33. Greaves, C.; Sheppard, K.E.; Abraham, C.; Hardeman, W.; Roden, M.; Evans, P.H.; Schwarz, P. Systematic review of reviews of intervention components associated with increased effectiveness in dietary and physical activity interventions. *BMC Public Health* **2011**, *11*, 119. [CrossRef]
34. Michie, S.; Abraham, C.; Whittington, C.; McAteer, J.; Gupta, S. Effective techniques in healthy eating and physical activity interventions: A meta-regression. *Health Psychol.* **2009**, *28*, 690–701. [CrossRef] [PubMed]
35. Cooke, J.; Butler, C.; Hopstaken, R.; Dryden, M.S.; McNulty, C.; Hurding, S.; Moore, M.; Livermore, D.M. Narrative review of primary care point-of-care testing (POCT) and antibacterial use in respiratory tract infection (RTI). *BMJ Open Respir. Res.* **2015**, *2*, e000086. [CrossRef] [PubMed]
36. Little, P.; Stuart, B.; Francis, N.; Douglas, E.; Tonkin-Crine, S.; Anthierens, S.; Cals, J.W.; Melbye, H.; Santer, M.; Moore, M. Antibiotic Prescribing for Acute Respiratory Tract Infections 12 Months After Communication and CRP Training: A Randomized Trial. *Ann. Fam. Med.* **2019**, *17*, 125–132. [CrossRef] [PubMed]
37. Huddy, J.R.; Ni, M.Z.; Barlow, J.; Majeed, A.; Hanna, G.B. Point-of-care C reactive protein for the diagnosis of lower respiratory tract infection in NHS primary care: A qualitative study of barriers and facilitators to adoption. *BMJ Open* **2016**, *6*. [CrossRef]
38. Eley, C.V.; Sharma, A.; Lecky, D.M.; Lee, H.; McNulty, C.A.M. Qualitative study to explore the views of general practice staff on the use of point-of-care C reactive protein testing for the management of lower respiratory tract infections in routine general practice in England. *BMJ Open* **2018**, *8*. [CrossRef]
39. Michie, S.; Atkins, L.; West, R. The behaviour change wheel. In *A Guide to Designing Interventions*, 1st ed.; Silverback Publishing: Sutton, UK, 2014; pp. 1003–1010.

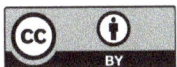

© 2019 by the authors. Licensee MDPI, Basel, Switzerland. This article is an open access article distributed under the terms and conditions of the Creative Commons Attribution (CC BY) license (http://creativecommons.org/licenses/by/4.0/).

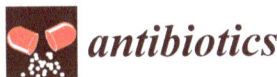

Article

Combating Antimicrobial Resistance in Singapore: A Qualitative Study Exploring the Policy Context, Challenges, Facilitators, and Proposed Strategies

Shweta Rajkumar Singh [1,†], Alvin Qijia Chua [1,†], Sok Teng Tan [1], Clarence C. Tam [1], Li Yang Hsu [1] and Helena Legido-Quigley [1,2,*]

1. Saw Swee Hock School of Public Health, National University of Singapore, Singapore 117549, Singapore; ephshwe@nus.edu.sg (S.R.S.); alvin.chua@nus.edu.sg (A.Q.C.); soktengtan@u.nus.edu (S.T.T.); clarence.tam@nus.edu.sg (C.C.T.); mdchly@nus.edu.sg (L.Y.H.)
2. London School of Hygiene and Tropical Medicine, London WC1H 9SH, UK
* Correspondence: ephhlq@nus.edu.sg
† Authors contributed equally to this paper.

Received: 6 October 2019; Accepted: 27 October 2019; Published: 29 October 2019

Abstract: Antimicrobial resistance (AMR) is a global public health threat that warrants urgent attention. However, the multifaceted nature of AMR often complicates the development and implementation of comprehensive policies. In this study, we describe the policy context and explore experts' perspectives on the challenges, facilitators, and strategies for combating AMR in Singapore. We conducted semi-structured interviews with 21 participants. Interviews were transcribed verbatim and were analyzed thematically, adopting an interpretative approach. Participants reported that the Ministry of Health (MOH) has effectively funded AMR control programs and research in all public hospitals. In addition, a preexisting One Health platform, among MOH, Agri-Food & Veterinary Authority (restructured to form the Singapore Food Agency and the Animal & Veterinary Service under NParks in April 2019), National Environment Agency, and Singapore's National Water Agency, was perceived to have facilitated the coordination and formulation of Singapore's AMR strategies. Nonetheless, participants highlighted that the success of AMR strategies is compounded by various challenges such as surveillance in private clinics, resource constraints at community-level health facilities, sub-optimal public awareness, patchy regulation on antimicrobial use in animals, and environmental contamination. This study shows that the process of planning and executing AMR policies is complicated even in a well-resourced country such as Singapore. It has also highlighted the increasing need to address the social, political, cultural, and behavioral aspects influencing AMR. Ultimately, it will be difficult to design policy interventions that cater for the needs of individuals, families, and the community, unless we understand how all these aspects interact and shape the AMR response.

Keywords: Antimicrobial resistance; policy analysis; One Health; public health; Singapore

1. Introduction

Antimicrobial resistance (AMR) has gained considerable recognition as a major global public health threat [1–4]. The impact of AMR has been described as a "doomsday scenario" where antibiotics can no longer be relied upon and even minor infections could become untreatable and result in severe morbidity, death and significant economic losses [1,4,5]. The World Health Organization (WHO) released a Global Action Plan for AMR in 2015, setting out five strategic objectives to combat AMR [2]. It also highlighted the importance of a "One Health" approach, requiring collaboration among numerous sectors and actors including human and animal health, agriculture, finance, environment, and well-informed consumers.

Singapore is an island nation with a diverse population of 5.6 million people [6]. Public hospitals cater for 80% of tertiary care services while private sector practitioners account for the majority (80%) of primary care services [7]. There is a large, private animal health sector catering for companion animals, but the agricultural animal health sector is small since Singapore has little local agricultural production [8]. Food requirements are almost entirely supported by imports, which are regulated by food laws focused on ensuring consistent foreign supply of food and agricultural products. Imported food is strictly monitored by the Singapore Food Agency (SFA), while non-food related animal, plant and wildlife management services are provided by National Parks Board (NParks) and Animal & Veterinary Service (AVS) [9]. The National Environment Agency (NEA) and the Public Utilities Board (now known as PUB, Singapore's National Water Agency) overlooks the public health aspects of environment [10,11].

In line with the Global Action Plan for AMR, Singapore launched its own National Strategic Action Plan on AMR in November 2017 [12]. This multisectoral action plan was jointly developed by the Ministry of Health (MOH), Agri-Food & Veterinary Authority (AVA) of Singapore (restructured to form the SFA and the AVS under NParks in April 2019), NEA, and PUB. It sets a national One Health framework to reduce the emergence and spread of drug-resistant microorganisms through five core strategies: (1) Surveillance and risk assessment; (2) Research; (3) Education; (4) Prevention and control of infection; and (5) Optimization of antimicrobial use. Chua et al. recently published a paper on AMR in Singapore, detailing the changes in efforts against AMR in Singapore from 2008 to 2018 [13]. The paper mentioned that although a better understanding of AMR as a One Health issue has developed, with significant efforts in improving antibiotic prescribing and controlling AMR in Singapore, it was largely focused on the public hospital setting. Even then, a recent national point prevalence survey conducted across 13 acute private and public hospitals in Singapore reported that more than half the patients in acute hospitals were on at least one systemic antibiotic, a much higher proportion compared to inpatients in European hospitals [14]. Based on the few published AMR epidemiology papers, the actual impact on the control of AMR has been mixed, with better control of methicillin-resistant *Staphylococcus aureus* (MRSA), coupled with an increase in resistant Gram-negative bacteria in the hospitals and the community [15–18]. It has been suggested that more efforts are required in the various sectors, especially the animal/farming and environment sectors, for better AMR control [13].

The AMR issue has been described as a "wicked problem", where there are many stakeholders involved from the various sectors and several ways to frame the problem [19]. This results in a policy arena where politics and conflict are very evident, and can potentially overwhelm policymakers in devising plans to tackle AMR with a One Health approach. Insights into the policy process for AMR will help to disentangle this complexity and provide a better understanding of support and opposition by key stakeholders for alternative AMR mitigation policies [19]. To date, no qualitative study has been conducted to analyze the factors that can aid in successful implementation of AMR policies in Singapore. Therefore, the aim of our study is to discuss the facilitators and challenges to addressing AMR and the dynamics in the policy process for AMR in Singapore via in-depth interviews. In this study, we interviewed experts in human, animal, and environmental health from both public and private sectors to gain their insights on the policy context, AMR awareness, its emergence in Singapore, and steps taken to mitigate AMR generation and spread. We subsequently identified facilitators and key challenges, and discussed proposed strategies for creating more awareness and combating AMR.

2. Materials and Methods

2.1. Data Collection

This qualitative study was conducted from September 2017 to May 2018. We used a purposive sampling method to recruit informants in key roles across sectors relevant to the issue of AMR in Singapore. Potential participants were identified from experts in the area of AMR in Singapore, and were approached for an in-depth interview via email explaining the purpose of research. A total of 21 participants from within and outside Singapore were recruited in this study (Table 1). The participants held expertise in human, animal, or environmental health and worked at either ministry, healthcare institution, academia, or civil society. Most participants were from the human health sector. We had difficulty recruiting participants from the environmental sector as potential participants showed more reservation in accepting the invitation to be interviewed, perhaps based on less knowledge about AMR. We were eventually able to recruit an academic and public health official from the environmental sector.

Table 1. Participants' characteristics according to profession and organization.

Sector	Profession	Count (n)	Organization	Count (n)
Human				
	Medical Practitioners	4	Government agency	3
	Academics	3	Hospital (public and private)	6
	Managers	6	Primary care	1
Animal				
	Academics	2	University	1
	Laboratory Manager	1	Veterinary Clinic	2
	Private practice	2	Government agency	2
	Government agency manager	1		
Environment				
	Policy maker	1	Government agency	1
	Academic	1	University	1
International				
			WHO, NGOs, etc.	4
	Total	21	Total	21

WHO = World Health Organization; NGOs = Non-governmental organizations.

Face-to-face in-depth interviews were conducted by three of the researchers (S.R.S., S.T.T. and H.L.-Q.) in English. Among the interviewers, two were Research Associates and one was an Associate Professor. All interviewers were trained in qualitative research. The interviews were conducted in a quiet space at the preferred location of the participants. Each interview lasted an hour on average and was audio-recorded. There were no repeat interviews. A semi-structured question guide was used to explore the main areas of concern for the participants, in their fields and areas of interest. The question guide was developed with questions focusing on participants' experiences and perceptions of AMR policy and practice including awareness, key challenges and facilitators in their particular area of expertise, and possible strategies and solutions to address key challenges in the Singaporean context. Participants were not remunerated for the interview.

2.2. Ethics

Ethical approval was obtained from the National University of Singapore Institutional Review Board (NUS-IRB). Each participant was provided an information sheet stating the objectives and methods of the research, at the point of recruitment. The confidentiality and anonymity of participants' responses was also highlighted. Written consent was sought before the beginning of each interview, requesting for permission to be audio-recorded and to be quoted anonymously in research outputs. Participants could refuse any of these options, as well as any questions posed to them during the interview itself. All participants were de-identified to maintain confidentiality.

2.3. Data Analysis

All interviews were transcribed verbatim and identifying data were removed from all research documents to ensure confidentiality. QSR NVivo 11 software was used to organize and share the data among study team members. We used an interpretive approach which focuses on the participants' perceptions and interpretations of the topic of discussion. Thematic analysis was used to inductively identify themes from the data. We drew on techniques from the constant comparative method, such as line by line analysis, naming each line and segment of data, and the use of subsequent interviews to test preliminary assumptions. In addition, deviant cases were explored and examined [20,21]. The conduct of the interviews and coding occurred concurrently to enable the researchers to determine when theme saturation had been reached and to cease recruitment. Thematic saturation was established when the research team discussed and agreed that no new themes were emerging from the data. To improve the credibility of our findings, we conducted a member check at the final stage of manuscript preparation to validate our interpretation of the data and to ensure an accurate representation of participant perspectives. We were unable to contact a few of the participants as they have moved on to another role and their contact information was not readily available. See Supplementary Materials for the Consolidated criteria for Reporting Qualitative research checklist (COREQ form).

3. Results

We present our findings under five main themes identified from analysis of participants' responses. The first theme examines the policy context and discusses whether AMR as a policy issue is a priority in Singapore. The second theme discusses the level of AMR awareness among policymakers, professionals, and the general population. The third and fourth theme discusses the perceived facilitators and challenges to combat AMR in the Singaporean context. Finally, the fifth theme reflects on the reported strategies to increase awareness and combat AMR based on participants' perceptions.

3.1. The Policy Context

Policymakers that participated in the study reflected on the importance of addressing infectious diseases in the Singaporean context, especially after the outbreaks of severe acute respiratory syndrome (SARS) and H1N1 influenza which took place in 2003 and 2009, respectively. As a physician highlighted:

> "A lot of incidents drive behavior in Singapore, like for example SARS drove infection control to the front of everything. If you speak to some people, (they) will say infection control became prominent feature with SARS happening." —I11, Human Health

In 2009, the MOH initiated the National Antimicrobial Taskforce (NAT) that helped lay down the basics of mandatory surveillance, stewardship, and infection prevention principles in public restructured hospitals. The NAT was tasked to formulate hospital programs and policies, as well as to implement measure for monitoring and evaluation of these policies. It was later reorganized into the National Antimicrobial Resistance Control Committee (NARCC) in 2014. Participants highlighted that the strategy adopted to keep efforts sustainable was by working with people on the ground to reinforce the implementation of these programs. The MOH's knack for looking at global health issues and comparing itself to other countries also helped in funding and formulation of AMR strategies. The next quote highlights the ways in which the MOH operates including the dedicated funding for antimicrobial stewardship programs:

> "The Ministry keeps an eye out for how it compares itself to other countries. So that drives their interest in looking at where we stand, how good, how bad (...) They directly fund quite a lot of the manpower in the hospital systems, certainly for antimicrobial stewardship."
> —I02, Human Health

Participants also remarked that the ministry looked at other countries and international organizations, such as the WHO and the European Union, for inspiration and implemented policies relevant to the Singapore context.

> "What WHO or even the EU is recommending, (…) I have been trying to push for that. We follow what others are doing, we don't want to reinvent the wheel, so that we can then compare ourselves." —I07, Human Health

Participants credited the proactive Singaporean government with forming a One Health platform, maintaining effective communication, and coordination between the agencies. One example of this was the formulation of the National Strategic Action Plan on AMR that was released in 2017. Despite establishing a One Health platform, participants suggested that the implementation of programs against AMR would be more challenging. They stressed on the necessity of advocating the importance of AMR to raise awareness.

> "Bringing different people to the table in the first instance in Singapore is easy, for somebody that is in charge (…). But at the end, (…) we need to get every single stakeholder to believe in the topic. There's a lot of sales or advocacy involved." —I12, Human Health

3.2. AMR Awareness

Most participants recounted low awareness of AMR among Singaporeans. Furthermore, AMR was identified as a recently coined term and many professionals including physicians were not familiar with the term even though they were knowledgeable of the topic itself. The next quote is an example of such reports:

> "I guess AMR, this phrase (…) if you were to tell me it's AMR, I would not know it's antimicrobial resistance." —I01, Human Health

Participants also remarked there was low awareness of AMR both as a topic as well a term among other One Health stakeholders including farmers and others within the environmental health sector. When we contacted potential participants from the environment sector, very few agreed to be interviewed since many reported not having conducted sufficient work related to AMR. The next quote highlights the concerns expressed by an environmental health expert who was worried about the lack of awareness among his colleagues at "the ground level":

> "At the ground level, they were saying, "What is AMR?" People don't really know. (…) How do we address it? This is a difficult question." —I09, Environment Health

Awareness was also perceived to be low in the general population as expressed by participants. Timely awareness efforts by the academic sector had not yet reached the general population. Since 2016, Singapore has been actively participating in the annual World Antibiotic Awareness Week every November, reaching out to the public at various public forums, hospitals and national libraries [22,23]. In 2017, the MOH and Health Promotion Board organized a social campaign focusing on the general prevention of infection to fight the spread of infectious diseases such as influenza and hand, foot and mouth disease [24]. This was closely followed by a "Use Antibiotics Right" campaign with the key message that antibiotics do not work on viruses [25]. Despite these efforts many participants voiced the lack of civil society or social groups movements to support the agenda of AMR in contrast to the high HIV awareness in the early 90s. The following quote highlights the need to further develop health promotion campaigns:

> "I think we need people who can inform on public policy in a way that would make our population understand. So we don't have those communication agencies. I think we have think tanks, right? And we have scientific groups. But we don't quite have that translation into a public health campaign." —I02. Human Health

Some participants stated the importance of raising AMR awareness to counter its emergence. It was suggested that by raising awareness of the topic and getting more funds to drive AMR programs for the general population and stakeholders alike, AMR emergence could be tackled better.

> "The community somehow must come to feel that this is an important issue. And once they do, then, you know, naturally, I think all the other pieces will fall into place. The politicians will sing the same song. The private sector will start putting money into the issue." —I06, Animal Health

Most stakeholders considered AMR a significant threat to Singapore and global health, but they also mentioned that it was not given the highest priority in the list of local healthcare challenges until several outbreaks of healthcare-associated infection changed the perception of policymakers and administrators with regards to its risk and standing. Until the early 2010s, issues such as ageing population and chronic diseases were rated much higher in priority compared to infectious diseases.

> "We had this roundtable discussion. Everybody, all the movers and shakers, public health systems ... and they were asked to state these priorities. And believe it or not, infection, the scourge of infection wasn't one of the top five." —I02, Human Health

3.3. Challenges to Addressing AMR

3.3.1. Cultural Aspects Influencing AMR

There were many reports suggesting a lack of awareness of AMR from the public. Many participants reiterated the fact that General Practitioners (GPs) may succumb to the pressure of demanding patients to prescribe antibiotics even when they were not clinically indicated. The next quote highlights how patients are "always asking for antibiotics":

> "Patients will always come in and ask for antibiotics. So I think it's something that we should control and not say that it all is well and then we ignore it. But like I said (...) I think the awareness may not be strong enough for us to continue to pursue." —I01, Human Health

It was also highlighted that there is a need for a firm drilling of infection prevention and control practices right in formative years of training for all healthcare professionals. Healthcare professionals needed to be more aware of and prioritize infection control, as it is not currently under "anyone's radar except for the people who do infection control":

> "As far as infection prevention goes, infection prevention and antimicrobial resistance is like stepchild of everyone. Because it's not in anyone's radar except for people who do infection control. So it's about making it a culture in everyone's mind, which is not an easy task."
> —I11, Human Health

3.3.2. Inadequate Infection Prevention and Control Measures

Inadequate infrastructure to facilitate optimal infection prevention and control measures was the most commonly cited challenge in addressing AMR. Though infection prevention and control efforts were highly regulated in both the public and private hospital settings, certain contextual factors such as lack of sufficient single room facility were highly challenging to overcome. A few participants mentioned that the design of hospital wards with one room having six beds or eight beds was not conducive to prevent infections:

> "It's not really our fault. You are sitting here scolding us, that we have a lot of MRSA but it's because, it's not poor infection control. You are making us take care of patients in overcrowded hospitals. You know, it's very different from the US or Europe where most of their rooms are two-bedders. If you have a six-bedder, even if I wash my hands, the uncle there who has a maid, and the maid is talking to the other maid and they all share, you know ... and it's practically, it's all crowded, all these infrastructure issues." —I04, Human Health

3.3.3. Lax Stewardship Policies in Private Health Sector

Overall, participants reported that guidelines and antimicrobial stewardship policies were better established in public-sector hospitals and clinics than their private counterparts. Participants attributed this to strict adherence to the guidelines in the public sector, as well as regular audits and monitoring of antibiotic prescriptions by public-sector pharmacists. The following quote is an example of the audits conducted in the public sector:

> "If the pharmacy notice that the patient is coming back repeatedly with antibiotics, they will alert the senior doctor to say that they've noticed that the doctor's pattern tends to prescribe a lot of antibiotics. At the same time, we also conduct audits annually on antibiotics usage." —I01, Human Health

In contrast, it was reported that private hospitals gave less priority to funding for infection control and stewardship policies than public hospitals. The stewardship element was not strictly monitored in the private hospitals and clinics, where it was reported that the MOH does not have so much leverage. This was raised as a concern by some physicians and policymakers when discussing the extension of AMR policies to the private sector:

> "I feel, in the restructured setting, you know, it's much more, I wouldn't say easier may not be the word, but maybe less challenging because it's much more homogenous within that institution and you only have to work in your institution whereas we have to work across all these little and then we are spending a lot of time and cracking ourselves in bits and pieces whereas it can all be done, you know, under one, I think, more harmonization, less bickering, less fighting, and then we can get more funding." —I18, Human Health

3.3.4. Defensive Medicine Practices and Expensive Diagnostics

Many participants mentioned that there were practical difficulties in being able to perform adequate tests before dispensing or prescribing antibiotics. Hence physicians and veterinarians tended to practice defensive medicine by prescribing broad-spectrum antibiotics.

> "If you are not following the stories in Singapore, it's not too long ago, you notice that the doctors have been held a lot in, they are being suspended for not diagnosing a certain condition (…) So, if you are going to hide under the umbrella of stewardship, are they going to get bailed out? Is someone going to come and rescue them, you know? Pertinent questions. It's not that people want to practice defense medicine, but that is somehow being construed or misconstrued from what is happening out there." —I18, Human Health

Moreover, veterinarians emphasized that the high diagnostics costs were difficult to justify to pet owners as the next quote exemplifies:

> "Textbook always tells us to do so (diagnostics) before you start on any medication. But, in a practical sense, hard to because how do I explain $60 more on top of what they are already paying, for them to get a culture and sensitivity back before we give antibiotics?" —I17, Animal Health

3.3.5. Disagreements between the Human and Animal Health Sectors

Stakeholders differed on their take as to what contributes more to AMR and ultimately which policy may help in reducing it. Physicians reported being aware of the importance of antimicrobial stewardship policies and infection prevention measures to control AMR, but were unsure if these programs alone could alleviate AMR since they believed that AMR could also be generated by antimicrobial use in animal farming as growth promoters. On the contrary, animal health experts believed the animal food industry did not contribute much to the growing resistance since the volume of antimicrobial used over the lifespan of livestock was very low. As reported by an animal health expert:

"Even though the vets use a huge volume of antibiotic in farming, I think the quantity used per animal over a period of time is way less than what we can get from human clinics. Way, way less." —I17, Animal Health

3.3.6. Need to Address the Prevention of AMR outside the Human Health Sector

Many participants also expressed that AMR in Singapore had so far only been addressed in the hospital sector and not much had been done regarding the prevention of AMR in the animal and environment health domains. It was also mentioned that within NAT most of its members and emphasis was still focused on the hospital sector:

"It was still very much hospital-focused. The membership (in the National Antimicrobial Taskforce) still basically comprised representatives of every public-sector hospital, and the chairman and the members were still very much concerned about preventing the spread of AMR organisms in hospitals." —I07, Human Health

3.3.7. Contamination of Environment Serving as Breeding Sites for AMR

Environmental health stakeholders expressed the potential of AMR emergence from farms, the community, and the environment as a whole. In general, the perception was that Singapore has not established strategies to deal with environmental contamination. Untreated effluents from hospitals was noted to serve as one of the potential threats in case of a sewage leak.

"The primary source for us (...) is, of course, our hospitals, also hospital effluents. We know that there are very high concentrations of all these last resort antibiotics, especially from the ICUs (Intensive Care Units) and all that, and it gets into the wastewater which then goes into the sewerage system, all the way to the wastewater treatment plant." —I14, Environment Health

Also, there was a scope for improving the wastewater treatment standard to treat some antibiotic residues so that they do not harbor AMR.

"Even if you look at the wastewater treatment plants, they're not doing so well in removing all the pharmaceuticals, all the antibiotics. Some can be removed very well, but some cannot. And so, that means they will be discharged and be effluent." —I14, Environment Health

Participants reported that antimicrobial laced water leeching in the environment served as breeding sites for AMR as the next quote emphasizes:

"At the treatment end, there's no problem because their treatment process is rigorous enough to remove all these bugs and all that ... But, of course, I think it's more from the environmental leakage (of antibiotics)." —I09, Environment Health

3.3.8. Vested Interests

In addition to the above factors, participants also hinted on the vested interest of different stakeholders. For example, it was mentioned that private practitioners make substantial profits when dispensing antibiotics as it added to their income.

"And by dispensing (antibiotics) they (GPs) are also getting the profits. So, there is already a misaligned incentive." —I04, Human Health

Also, some participants reflected on the vested interests of pharmaceutical companies in marketing for higher sales of their antibiotics for their own profits.

"There is a conflict of interest already, because, they (pharmaceuticals) are producing, they are just selling to the farmers (...) in a way they are trying to encourage certain resistance." —I17, Animal Health

Animal health stakeholders expressed that the not so strict regulations on the import of newer antibiotics with a broader spectrum of activity served as a leeway for some veterinarians to prescribe them even when not clinically needed. Participants pointed out that the abuse of reserved antibiotics favored acquisition of resistance genes by microorganisms, resulting in loss of antibiotic efficacy.

"There are those not very good ones out in the market that actually goes for the most exotic antibiotics because they distinguish themselves in that sense. Some of them actually use what I call the third-level antibiotic as a first line treatment which I personally don't agree. Of course, they charge exorbitant amount because it's 'special' antibiotics." —I17, Animal Health

In addition, owing to a small farming sector, existing veterinarians had limited expertise in agriculture and aquaculture and hence farmers in Singapore were not mandated to attain prescription for accessing antibiotics independently. Participants alluded that farmers not needing to consult a veterinarian for a prescription for antibiotics served in the farmer's interest.

"Vets were not familiar to treat fish, so farmers didn't trust the vets to treat their fish, and vets then became very unwilling to treat farm fish. That's not changed very much, and there are still issues in Singapore. For example, fish farmers can now buy any antibiotic they want by themselves." —I15, Animal Health

3.4. Facilitators to Addressing AMR

3.4.1. Leading Role of the MOH and Provision of Appropriate Funding

Singapore's MOH was unanimously praised by all participants in its proactive approach towards AMR and making way for changes amid very complex issues. It was mentioned that the MOH was transparent and accountable and was operating an efficient public healthcare system in Singapore. Yet, as a drawback some participants argued that having a system that relies too much on decisions made at the highest political level makes the general population and service providers inert.

"That's why I think in Singapore, unless it comes directly from the Prime Minister's office, it will never move anything." —I11, Human Health

In terms of the resources made available to fund AMR programs, it was reported that MOH had effectively funded AMR control programs and research in all public hospitals.

3.4.2. Trust in the Ability of the Government to Design Policies

Most participants affirmed that the Singaporean population and healthcare professionals bestow trust in government programs and policies. The next quote highlights that whether participants agreed or not with the proposed policy, there was a sense that the government is "trying to do a good thing":

"When the Singaporean government gets into doing something, they tend to do it very thoroughly. (...) You may not always agree with the strategy, but you have to give them full marks for trying." —I04, Human Health

In addition, a preexisting One Health platform among MOH, SFA, AVS, NEA, and PUB was perceived to have facilitated the coordination and formulation of Singapore's AMR strategies.

3.4.3. Stewardship Programs

Laying the foundation of surveillance in public hospitals and making the data transparent was appreciated by all participants. Participants also shared recent advances in the capacity to implement stewardship and infection prevention and control policies among different Singapore institutions including nursing homes.

> "We are looking to reaching out to even nursing homes to provide that kind of bold infection prevention, but also infection control." —I03, Human Health

3.4.4. Setting up a Surveillance System

AMR indicators, segregated mainly into process and outcome indicators, were set up in the public hospital surveillance system. Some of the process indicators were antimicrobial use for human and animal health, and infection prevention and control measures such as hand hygiene in hospitals. It was suggested that the Singapore government played a prime role in mandating the standardization, transparency, and sharing of data with the NAT.

> "We wanted to measure stuff in Singapore, but really to do that you really need the government involved, (...) otherwise if it's a voluntary basis, and there are certain biases about data. Whereas if it's systematic surveillance and it's mandatory you get a more comprehensive and representative sample." —I04, Human Health

Participants mentioned that though the AMR surveillance indicators were defined and well set up in the public hospital domain, surveillance needed to be at a national level, extended to private hospitals, primary care and intermediate/long-term care facilities (GPs, community hospitals and nursing homes), as well as animal and environment sectors.

> "The indicators we sort of have been following is still hospital-based indicators. We don't have country-wide, AMR indicators which internationally people are talking about. For example, we don't know what is the level of antibiotic consumption at the country level, we don't know what, for example, when people are talking about "oh, for this bacterial infection, what proportion of this bacterial infection is resistant to what antibiotics" you know? We haven't gone to measuring that kind of level." —I07, Human Health

3.4.5. Highly Motivated Workforce

The motivation of the workforce was attributed to the competition, prestige, and reputation of the workforce. In the hospital setting, metrics and outcomes of antimicrobial stewardship such as average defined daily dose and percentage of appropriate antibiotics prescribed, and length of hospitalization for each department are often reported and shared among the various departments within the hospital. The transparency of data highly motivated the workforce to perform well in these benchmarking exercises. The following quote is an example of such occurrence:

> "More important I think is the peer pressure and peer standing. And when it's made the department target and communicated by the head of the department, no one wants to be the worst department in the stats when they are shown up. So there's lot of department pride and that's what drives stuff. Doctors are often competitive, some of the nurses too. And no one wants to be the idiot that lets the team down." —I03, Human Health

3.4.6. Research Excellence

Research in Singapore was unanimously considered to be well promoted and funded, albeit it was also rated to be very competitive in terms of securing research funding. There was ongoing AMR research including in the areas of surveillance, prevention of transmission, whole genome sequencing, among others. Of the various arms of AMR research, surveillance was considered to be one of the main pillars in AMR research:

> "One of the key reasons in the national action plan is research. And among the research activities there have been sort of highlighted in terms of priority, is better surveillance. You know, how to better measure the different perspectives and areas that we need to, outside the hospitals: primary care, the community and understanding the sort of pathways of antibiotic resistances, what is driving, the drivers of antibiotic resistance locally ... " —I07, Human Health

3.4.7. Close Connections between Researchers and Policymakers

The researcher and academic participants mentioned that the government and ministry were very tightly knit in Singapore. Leadership was very open and attentive to research findings that could be translated into better health practices in Singapore. As the following quote highlights:

> "There's that translation angle number one. There is the One Health angle number two, and then of course number three we also engage with basic science collaborators, to try to understand the basic science mechanisms of this issue." —I08, Human Health

3.4.8. Role of Singapore in Regional AMR

As AMR is a global health issue, participants remarked that Singapore alone could do very little in controlling AMR as a whole. Despite all policies Singapore will not be untouched by rising AMR in the region which can be ultimately transmitted via large imports of agricultural products and humans travelling for trade and tourism. However, most participants mentioned that Singapore could play a role by coordinating and sharing expertise with neighboring member states of the Association of Southeast Asian Nations (ASEAN).

Many participants proposed the idea that Singapore can serve as a research hub owing to its unique positioning and research capacity. Sharing innovative findings both on science, clinical practice and exemplary policy implementation strategies could prove helpful to neighboring countries that share some contextual factors with Singapore.

> "It is an ideal geographic position as well as possibly a good political one with the recognition by the west that Singapore is a high-income country as well as intellectually advanced. That bridge between the west and low- and middle-income countries especially in the Asia Pacific region could really be bridged by your university and your researchers." —I20, Human Health

A few ministerial participants affirmed Singapore's role of coordinating regional efforts on AMR.

> "What Singapore is trying to do is trying to harmonize efforts in the agriculture sector and the livestock sector because these are under different ASEAN stream workgroups. So we also work with FAO to coordinate these." —I13, Animal Health

3.5. Strategies to Raise AMR Awareness and Combat AMR

3.5.1. Projecting AMR Costs

Participants articulated that highlighting the increasing cost of managing patients infected with resistant organisms and the economic loss from AMR could be a potential way of drawing attention to the topic and getting funds to drive programs. As specific examples, participants illustrated not just the costs of treating resistant infections, but also the costs associated with implementing stricter infection control measures.

Some participants believed that healthcare costs would increase due to AMR. These were attributed to many reasons, one of which was the cost of more effective antibiotics required to treat infections with resistant organisms. Another prominent reason mentioned was the costs towards infection prevention and control in healthcare settings. This was considered a necessary step to reduce the risk of healthcare-associated infections, especially in the face of worsening AMR. The following factors were suggested by one participant to prevent the spread of resistant pathogens and to cater to patients harboring resistant or infectious organisms:

> "That is going to jack up costs in all kinds of ways. Number 1, you are going to have to pay for all those gowns, gloves, single rooms, for isolation, etc. Number 2 you need more manpower, because suddenly a nurse is going to be slowed down right? Or a doctor. You have to put on all this gear, you are going to be seeing fewer patients in the same amount of time, just because of ... it's a bother." —I04, Human Health

3.5.2. Push Forward AMR Agenda by Fear of no Treatment

Many participants believed that unless AMR's potential damage to the population and the economy is projected, people are not going to take AMR seriously. Some participants mentioned that only a grave incident such as an AMR outbreak would be able to catch the attention of the general public and extend the prevention efforts of AMR.

3.5.3. Building Communities of Practice

A few participants articulated that rather than forcing a top-down policy approach, AMR could be better tackled by the sharing of best practices through communities of practitioners and creating social movements to encourage and sustain behavior change.

> "Practitioners come together to share best practices, through the ID networks, through the hospital networks, through the volunteer networks, you know, build communities of practice until this becomes a culture. And people are learning from each other (...) But whether it gets done is a question of culture, a culture needs strategy every day (...) so you want to do change, and you want to do large scale change and you want to sustain the change you need to create a movement not a directive ... I think it's more important to you to create the social movement around what that is, because if you are going to achieve this style change of behavior you need a more behavioral approach to this problem not a clinical approach." —I05, Human Health

3.5.4. Engaging the Community and Public Campaigns on the Drivers of AMR

Participants reflected on the need to develop public campaigns to sensitize people to become aware of and understand the fundamentals of programs and strategies against AMR. These include stewardship, adherence to vaccination guidelines, better infection prevention and control practices in hospitals as well as programs in the community. All these programs needed to take into account social, behavioral, and cultural aspects to accommodate the needs and perceptions of the community.

> "There is always a need to build a culture and to build a system for people to do the right thing. And the same applies outside the hospitals. So I think you know the schools have hand washing to teach the next generation." —I05, Human Health

3.5.5. Increase Vaccination

Most participants asserted that one of the probable strategies to counter AMR was to increase vaccination rates in children and adult population. However, increasing vaccination uptake will uncover another set of issues including population awareness, behavior changes, funding for regular vaccination, workforce to administer vaccination, and availability of vaccines.

4. Discussion

This paper has discussed the challenges and facilitators to addressing AMR in a well-resourced setting such as Singapore. Despite Singapore having an established One Health platform representing all the different stakeholders; appropriate funding to address the response; existence of stewardship and surveillance programs in public hospitals; an active program in research; and a motivated workforce; most participants raised several challenges to address AMR efficiently. These included, among other, vested interests among some stakeholders; disagreements between the human and animal health sectors; low public awareness; the need to address prevention of AMR in the animal and environmental sector; political and cultural aspects influencing AMR; and lax stewardship policies in the private sector.

Therefore, the results of this paper highlight how difficult it can be to address AMR, especially when considering that Singapore has well-functioning stewardship programs, comprehensive hospital surveillance systems, and some of the latest technologies and innovations to address it. The example of AMR in Singapore brings to light the increasing need to address the social, economic, political, cultural, and behavioral aspects influencing AMR rather than just focusing on the technical solutions. Unless we understand how all these aspects operate and drive the response, it will be difficult to design appropriate policy interventions. In the next paragraphs we provide an example of each of these aspects to highlight their importance in the Singaporean setting. We address "the social" by analyzing how AMR has been socially constructed in Singapore; we discuss the influence of "politics" by considering power relations and governance approaches for the successful control of AMR; we address "behavioral aspects" by analyzing vested interests; and we consider "cultural components" by exploring how patients' cultural beliefs influence antibiotic consumption.

First, it is important to understand how AMR has been socially constructed in Singapore and how power relations operate between the different stakeholders. Wernli et al. distinguished five different frames that map the global policy discourse on AMR [26]. These are: a One Health approach combining in one paradigm human, animal, and environment health; a health security threat giving rise to the global health security agenda; a healthcare policy issue with the dominance of the medical profession; a development issue where it is considered that low-and-middle income countries drive AMR; and an innovation issue with a focus on new diagnostics and antibiotics. Wernli et al. also distinguish a set of actors and policies for each of the frames described. In the Singaporean context, it is interesting to note that several frames coexist with their respective actors leading the selected frame. First, it was reported that there is a One Health platform where all stakeholders meet. Second, there is a strong healthcare policy frame as it was reported that Singapore's AMR policies were largely driven by a group of infectious disease clinicians. Third, AMR is also seen as an innovation issue where researchers are working to identify novel solutions on all fronts. The results of this study suggest that a deeper understanding is needed of the different power relations between these distinct groups to ensure the successful implementation of policies designed to respond to the threat of resistance. However, from our participants' responses we can tentatively conclude that AMR is predominantly seen as a biomedical problem within the context of healthcare facilities and within the pursuit of clinicians controlling infectious diseases even when they still participate in the One Health platform. It could also be argued that historically the emphasis on AMR has been biomedical because this is where the health burden was seen and therefore where the expertise developed. This, however, does not mean that other areas are not seen as important.

Second, considering governance approaches for the successful control of AMR requires a focus on both whole of society and sector specific approaches [19]. This was detailed in a previous paper where we proposed a new governance framework to investigate power relations and responses for diverse stakeholders addressing AMR [19]. As Kickbusch mentioned, and further discussed in our paper, recently there has been a diffusion of governance moving from a model dominated by the state to a model co-produced by a wide range of actors [27]. As a result, Kickbusch has identified five types of governance present in whole-of-government approaches. These include: (1) governing among others by mixing regulation and persuasion; (2) by collaborating; (3) by engaging citizens;

(4) through independent agencies and expert bodies; (5) and by adaptive policies, resilient structures, and foresight.

In the Singapore setting, many participants highlighted the leading role of the MOH in regulating the health sector, but acknowledged challenges in regulating the private and animal health sector. These challenges present examples where governance structures will need to weigh up the balance between regulation and persuasion as policy approaches. In the Singaporean context, differential policies in the public and private human healthcare sectors, whether by design or practice, are likely to be counterproductive, as patients use both sectors and the occurrence of resistant infections in one sector has implications for the other. On the other hand, the agricultural sector in Singapore is small and the availability of adequate veterinary expertise limited; imposing tight regulations on antibiotic access in the absence of qualified prescribers is therefore challenging, and persuasive strategies to reduce antibiotic use in this sector are likely to be more realistic, at least in the short term. On their collaborative approach towards governance, many participants highlighted the One Health platform as a good way of bringing stakeholders together. The good relationship between researchers and policymakers was also emphasized via the many avenues for researchers to discuss and share their research findings and discuss policy implications with policymakers. However, there were also conflicts reported specifically between human and animal health experts. This was crystalized on their different takes on what contributes more to AMR. Most physicians believed that antimicrobial use in animal farming as growth promoters might be a more significant driver of AMR, as has been explained by studies [28]. In contrast, animal health experts believed the animal food industry did not contribute much to the growing resistance when compared to AMR infection rates in the health sector. Finally, governing AMR through the engagement of citizens and civil society was not reported as a strategy in Singapore. However, this is not unique to Singapore, as it is well recognized that globally there has been a lack of engagement of civil society organizations in addressing AMR, especially when comparing and contrasting to the high HIV involvement in the early 90s.

Third, the AMR policy context represents a policy arena where certain groups engage in "behaviors" that might conflict with the overall goal of controlling AMR. Vested interests are more noticeable than in other health policy areas since different professional groups coexist in the AMR policy arena and there is substantial profit to be made from selling antibiotics [29,30]. In Singapore, vested interests were mentioned among pharmaceutical companies in marketing for higher sales of their antibiotics for their own profits; among private practitioners as they make substantial profits when dispensing antibiotics; and among some veterinarians who prescribed antibiotics even when not clinically needed. Our previous research in other settings (i.e., Pakistan and Cambodia) also suggested several considerations and vested interests around antibiotic use which can hinder the control of AMR in the human and animal health sectors [29,30]. For example, it was reported that among doctors there are monetary incentives to prescribe certain antibiotics as these are often negotiated with pharmaceutical companies. It was also recounted that a large proportion of the income at hospital level and in pharmacies comes from prescribing antibiotics and as a result it might be difficult to introduce stewardship programs to curb their prescription. While these reports were present in Cambodia and Pakistan, they were absent in Singapore. Monetary incentives were not mentioned that often by our participants and were absent at hospital level.

Fourth, many participants reported that "cultural aspects" and perception regarding medication influenced patients' requests for antibiotics, with patients requesting them, and GPs recognizing feeling the pressure to prescribe them. Other research has found similar findings, with Lam et al. observing that primary healthcare physicians over-prescribed antibiotics in order to satisfy their patients [31]. There were also reports suggesting a lack of awareness of AMR from the public and as a result, patients continued demanding antibiotics even when they were not clinically indicated. This was also reported in a Singaporean study that surveyed patients and found that most patients seeking primary health care in Singapore were misinformed about the role of antibiotics, with poor knowledge being associated with wanting antibiotics [32].

To our knowledge, this is one of the first studies to explore the social, political, behavioral, and cultural aspects influencing AMR in a well-resourced setting. A key strength of this study is that we were able to gather the perspectives of multiple stakeholders in the human, animal, and environmental sector. However, we had difficulty in recruiting participants from the environmental sector, and we were only able to interview two participants. A limitation of this study is that participants could have downplayed some of the challenges and some strategies that are considered key to address AMR could have been missed. For example, the fact that Singapore has a well-functioning system for dispensing antibiotics in the human sector, with antibiotics only available with a physician's prescription, was not mentioned as often as a facilitator as one might expect. This could be the case because it was already taken for granted as it has been in existence for several years.

Finally, participants in this study were asked to describe the most important strategies to combat AMR and to raise awareness among the population. The most often mentioned responses were: the need to project AMR costs to draw more attention to the topic; pushing forward the AMR agenda by fear of no treatment; creating a community of practice; considering the social aspects of AMR in order to develop prevention efforts against AMR; engaging the community and public campaigns on the drivers of AMR; and increasing vaccination rates in children and adult population. One important step to realizing these strategies would be to have good quality data obtained from standardized surveillance platforms at the national level. This will allow the conduct of outcome research, which can eventually be translated into messages to increase awareness and to push forward the AMR agenda. For example, Naylor et al. used a national mandatory surveillance database in England to quantify the cost and mortality burden of *Escherichia coli* bacteremia, as well as the influence different resistances have on them. Such findings will be useful for understanding the health and economic impact of future trends in resistance, and for prioritization of funding and strategies to tackle the problem [33]. In addition, future research could focus on exploring further how the current Singapore National Strategic Action Plan is being implemented; exploring in more detail the social, political, behavioral and cultural components affecting AMR; and analyzing at greater length what type of AMR awareness campaigns could be developed to reach the community and engage civil society organizations.

5. Conclusions

The process of designing and implementing AMR policies is complicated even in a country such as Singapore, which has dedicated funding and has developed a multisectoral approach to address AMR. This paper has highlighted the increasing need to address the social, political, cultural, and behavioral aspects influencing AMR rather than just focusing on the technical solutions. Unless we understand how all these aspects operate and drive the response, it will be difficult to design policy interventions that produce the desired results and that cater for the needs of individuals, families, and the community as a whole.

Supplementary Materials: The following are available online at http://www.mdpi.com/2079-6382/8/4/201/s1, COREQ (COnsolidated criteria for REporting Qualitative research) Checklist.

Author Contributions: Conceptualization, H.L.-Q.; methodology and conducting interviews, H.L.-Q., S.R.S., S.T.T.; formal analysis, S.R.S., A.Q.C. and H.L.-Q.; writing—original draft preparation, S.R.S., A.Q.C. and H.L.-Q.; writing—review and editing, all authors; supervision, H.L.-Q.; funding acquisition, L.Y.H. and H.L.-Q.

Funding: This research is funded through the CoSTAR-HS and SPHERiC Collaborative Center Grants from the National Medical Research Council, Singapore.

Acknowledgments: We would like to thank the participants of this study for their time and for sharing their experiences and insights on the topic.

Conflicts of Interest: The authors declare no conflict of interest.

References

1. World Health Organization. Antimicrobial Resistance Global Report on Surveillance. Available online: http://www.who.int/iris/bitstream/10665/112642/1/9789241564748_eng.pdf?ua=1 (accessed on 20 September 2019).

2. World Health Organization. Global Action Plan on Antimicrobial Resistance. Available online: http://www.wpro.who.int/entity/drug_resistance/resources/global_action_plan_eng.pdf (accessed on 20 September 2019).
3. United Nations. Political Declaration of the High-Level Meeting of the General Assembly on Antimicrobial Resistance. Available online: https://digitallibrary.un.org/record/842813?ln=en (accessed on 20 September 2019).
4. O'Neill, J. Tackling Drug-Resistant Infections Globally: Final Report and Recommendations. Available online: https://amr-review.org/sites/default/files/160518_Final%20paper_with%20cover.pdf (accessed on 20 September 2019).
5. Adeyi, O.O.; Baris, E.; Jonas, O.B.; Irwin, A.; Berthe, F.C.J.; Le Gall, F.G.; Marquez, P.V.; Nikolic, I.A.; Plante, C.A.; Schneidman, M.; et al. Drug-resistant Infections: A Threat to Our Economic Future (Final Report). Available online: http://documents.worldbank.org/curated/en/323311493396993758/final-report (accessed on 20 September 2019).
6. Department of Statistics Singapore. Singapore Population. Available online: https://www.singstat.gov.sg/modules/infographics/population (accessed on 20 September 2019).
7. U.S. Commercial Service. Singapore: Healthcare Overview. Available online: http://files.export.gov/x_5985.pdf (accessed on 20 September 2019).
8. Export.gov. Singapore—Agriculture Sectors. Available online: https://www.export.gov/article?id=Singapore-Agricultural-Sectors (accessed on 20 September 2019).
9. Singapore Food Agency. Agri-Food & Veterinary Authority of Singapore (AVA). Available online: https://www.sfa.gov.sg/ava (accessed on 20 September 2019).
10. PUB. PUB Singapore's National Water Agency: About Us. Available online: https://www.pub.gov.sg/about (accessed on 20 September 2019).
11. National Environment Agency. National Environment Agency: About Us. Available online: https://www.nea.gov.sg/corporate-functions/who-we-are/about-us (accessed on 20 September 2019).
12. Agri-Food & Veterinary Authority of Singapore; Ministry of Health; National Environment Agency; National Water Agency. The National Strategic Action Plan on Antimicrobial Resistance, Singapore. Available online: http://extwprlegs1.fao.org/docs/pdf/sin171511.pdf (accessed on 20 September 2019).
13. Chua, A.Q.; Kwa, A.L.; Tan, T.Y.; Legido-Quigley, H.; Hsu, L.Y. Ten-year narrative review on antimicrobial resistance in Singapore. *Singap. Med. J.* **2019**, *60*, 387–396. [CrossRef] [PubMed]
14. Cai, Y.; Venkatachalam, I.; Tee, N.W.; Tan, T.Y.; Kurup, A.; Wong, S.Y.; Low, C.Y.; Wang, Y.; Lee, W.; Liew, Y.X.; et al. Prevalence of healthcare-associated infections and antimicrobial use among adult inpatients in Singapore acute-care hospitals: Results from the first national point prevalence survey. *Clin. Infect Dis.* **2017**, *64*, S61–S67. [CrossRef] [PubMed]
15. Chow, A.; Lim, V.W.; Khan, A.; Pettigrew, K.; Lye, D.C.B.; Kanagasabai, K.; Phua, K.; Krishnan, P.; Ang, B.; Marimuthu, K.; et al. MRSA transmission dynamics among interconnected acute, intermediate-term, and long-term healthcare facilities in Singapore. *Clin. Infect Dis.* **2017**, *64*, S76–S81. [CrossRef] [PubMed]
16. Philomin, L. Hospitals Step up Measures to Curb 'Superbug' that Spreads via Touch. Available online: https://www.todayonline.com/singapore/hospitals-step-measures-curb-superbug-spreads-touch (accessed on 20 September 2019).
17. Teo, J.Q.; Cai, Y.; Lim, T.P.; Tan, T.T.; Kwa, A.L. Carbapenem resistance in gram-negative bacteria: The not-so-little problem in the little red dot. *Microorganisms* **2016**, *4*, 13. [CrossRef]
18. Teo, J.W.P.; Tan, P.; La, M.-V.; Krishnan, P.; Tee, N.; Koh, T.H.; Deepak, R.N.; Tan, T.Y.; Jureen, R.; Lin, R.T.P. Surveillance trends of carbapenem-resistant Enterobacteriaceae from Singapore, 2010–2013. *J. Glob. Antimicrob. Resist.* **2014**, *2*, 99–102. [CrossRef]
19. Legido-Quigley, H.; Khan, M.S.; Durrance-Bagale, A.; Hanefeld, J. Something borrowed, something new: A governance and social construction framework to investigate power relations and responses of diverse stakeholders to policies addressing antimicrobial resistance. *Antibiotics* **2018**, *8*, 3. [CrossRef]
20. Strauss, A.L. *Qualitative Analysis for Social Scientists*; Cambridge University Press: New York, NY, USA, 1987.
21. Charmaz, K. *Constructing Grounded Theory: A Practical Guide through Qualitative Analysis*; Sage: London, UK, 2006.
22. Choy, C.Y.; Hsu, L.Y. World Antibiotic Awareness Week. *Ann. Acad. Med. Singap.* **2017**, *46*, 413–414.
23. Hsu, L.Y. The Campaign for Global Antibiotic Awareness. Available online: https://www.todayonline.com/daily-focus/health/campaign-global-antibiotic-awareness (accessed on 5 October 2018).
24. Health Promotion Board. FIGHT The Spread of Infectious Diseases. Available online: https://www.healthhub.sg/programmes/52/Fight_The_Spread (accessed on 5 October 2018).

25. Health Promotion Board. Use Antibiotics Right. Available online: https://www.healthhub.sg/programmes/146/use-antibiotics-right (accessed on 5 October 2019).
26. Wernli, D.; Jorgensen, P.S.; Morel, C.M.; Carroll, S.; Harbarth, S.; Levrat, N.; Pittet, D. Mapping global policy discourse on antimicrobial resistance. *BMJ Glob. Health* **2017**, *2*, e000378. [CrossRef]
27. Kickbusch, I.; Gleicher, D. Governance for Health in the 21st Century. Available online: http://www.euro.who.int/__data/assets/pdf_file/0019/171334/RC62BD01-Governance-for-Health-Web.pdf (accessed on 4 October 2019).
28. Pires, S.M.; Vieira, A.R.; Hald, T.; Cole, D. Source attribution of human salmonellosis: An overview of methods and estimates. *Foodborne Pathog. Dis.* **2014**, *11*, 667–676. [CrossRef] [PubMed]
29. Khan, M.S.; Durrance-Bagale, A.; Legido-Quigley, H.; Mateus, A.; Hasan, R.; Spencer, J.; Hanefeld, J. 'LMICs as reservoirs of AMR': A comparative analysis of policy discourse on antimicrobial resistance with reference to Pakistan. *Health Policy Plan.* **2019**, *34*, 178–187. [CrossRef]
30. Suy, S.; Rego, S.; Bory, S.; Chhorn, S.; Phou, S.; Prien, C.; Heng, S.; Wu, S.; Legido-Quigley, H.; Hanefeld, J.; et al. Invisible medicine sellers and their use of antibiotics: A qualitative study in Cambodia. *BMJ Glob. Health* **2019**, *4*, e001787. [CrossRef]
31. Lam, T.P.; Lam, K.F. What are the non-biomedical reasons which make family doctors over-prescribe antibiotics for upper respiratory tract infection in a mixed private/public Asian setting? *J. Clin. Pharm. Ther.* **2003**, *28*, 197–201. [CrossRef]
32. Pan, D.S.; Huang, J.H.; Lee, M.H.; Yu, Y.; Chen, M.I.; Goh, E.H.; Jiang, L.; Chong, J.W.; Leo, Y.S.; Lee, T.H.; et al. Knowledge, attitudes and practices towards antibiotic use in upper respiratory tract infections among patients seeking primary health care in Singapore. *BMC Fam. Pract.* **2016**, *17*, 148. [CrossRef]
33. Naylor, N.R.; Pouwels, K.B.; Hope, R.; Green, N.; Henderson, K.L.; Knight, G.M.; Atun, R.; Robotham, J.V.; Deeny, S.R. The health and cost burden of antibiotic resistant and susceptible Escherichia coli bacteraemia in the English hospital setting: A national retrospective cohort study. *PLoS ONE* **2019**, *14*, e0221944. [CrossRef] [PubMed]

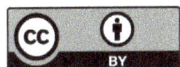

© 2019 by the authors. Licensee MDPI, Basel, Switzerland. This article is an open access article distributed under the terms and conditions of the Creative Commons Attribution (CC BY) license (http://creativecommons.org/licenses/by/4.0/).

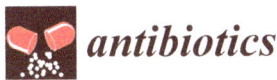

Article

The Contribution of Efflux Pumps in *Mycobacterium abscessus* Complex Resistance to Clarithromycin

Júlia S. Vianna [1,†], Diana Machado [2,†], Ivy B. Ramis [1], Fábia P. Silva [1], Dienefer V. Bierhals [1], Michael Andrés Abril [1], Andrea von Groll [1], Daniela F. Ramos [1], Maria Cristina S. Lourenço [3], Miguel Viveiros [2,*,‡] and Pedro E. Almeida da Silva [1,‡]

1. Núcleo de Pesquisas em Microbiologia Médica, Universidade Federal de Rio Grande, Rua Visconde de Paranaguá, 102, Rio Grande 96200-190, RS, Brazil; jusvianna@hotmaiL.com (J.S.V.); ivybramis@gmail.com (I.B.R.); fabiapeixoto@gmail.com (F.P.S.); dienefer_bierhals@hotmail.com (D.V.B.); andresabrilg94@gmail.com (M.A.A.); avongrol@hotmail.com (A.v.G.); daniferamos@gmail.com (D.F.R.); pedrefurg@gmail.com (P.E.A.d.S)
2. Unidade de Microbiologia Médica, Global Health and Tropical Medicine, Instituto de Higiene e Medicina Tropical, Universidade NOVA de Lisboa, 1349-008 Lisboa, Portugal; diana@ihmt.unl.pt
3. Instituto Nacional de Infectologia Evandro Chagas, Fundação Oswaldo Cruz, Campus Manguinhos, Rio de Janeiro 21040-360, Brazil; cristina.lourenco@ini.fiocruz.br
* Correspondence: mviveiros@ihmt.unl.pt; Tel.: +351-213-652-653
† Shared first co-authorship.
‡ Shared senior co-authorship.

Received: 5 September 2019; Accepted: 16 September 2019; Published: 18 September 2019

Abstract: The basis of drug resistance in *Mycobacterium abscessus* is still poorly understood. Nevertheless, as seen in other microorganisms, the efflux of antimicrobials may also play a role in *M. abscessus* drug resistance. Here, we investigated the role of efflux pumps in clarithromycin resistance using nine clinical isolates of *M. abscessus* complex belonging to the T28 *erm*(41) sequevar responsible for the inducible resistance to clarithromycin. The strains were characterized by drug susceptibility testing in the presence/absence of the efflux inhibitor verapamil and by genetic analysis of drug-resistance-associated genes. Efflux activity was quantified by real-time fluorometry. Efflux pump gene expression was studied by RT-qPCR upon exposure to clarithromycin. Verapamil increased the susceptibility to clarithromycin from 4- to ≥64-fold. The efflux pump genes *MAB_3142* and *MAB_1409* were found consistently overexpressed. The results obtained demonstrate that the T28 *erm*(41) polymorphism is not the sole cause of the inducible clarithromycin resistance in *M. abscessus* subsp. *abscessus* or *bolletii* with efflux activity providing a strong contribution to clarithromycin resistance. These data highlight the need for further studies on *M. abscessus* efflux response to antimicrobial stress in order to implement more effective therapeutic regimens and guidance in the development of new drugs against these bacteria.

Keywords: efflux inhibitors; efflux pumps; *erm*(41); mutations; mycobacteria; verapamil

1. Introduction

Species belonging to the *Mycobacterium abscessus* complex are responsible for pulmonary and extrapulmonary infections affecting mostly the skin and soft-tissues [1,2]. These species are estimated to account for 5–20% of all nontuberculous mycobacteria (NTM) infections worldwide [3]. Nevertheless, the incidence is likely underestimated due to the absence of compulsory notification in most countries. The occurrence of outbreaks of *M. abscessus* (*sensu lato*) infections has been related to healthcare settings and occurs mainly in immunocompromised patients [3,4].

M. abscessus complex comprises three subspecies: *M. abscessus* subsp. *abscessus*, *M. abscessus* subsp. *massiliense* and *M. abscessus* subsp. *bolletii* [1,5]. The pattern of drug susceptibility differs according to the subspecies stressing the importance of their differentiation among the complex, as they will respond differently to the therapeutic regimen [1,6–8]. Therapeutic regimens are based on a macrolide, usually clarithromycin, an aminoglycoside, generally amikacin, and a β-lactam, imipenem or cefoxitin [9,10]. *M. abscessus* subspecies differ on their antimicrobial susceptibilities, particularly to macrolides, the first-line antibiotic for the treatment of these infections [10].

Macrolide resistance in *M. abscessus* can be due to mutations in the gene *erm*(41), encoding the erythromycin ribosome methyltransferase Erm(41), and to mutations in the gene *rrl*, encoding the 23S rRNA. *M. abscessus* subsp. *massiliense* has a non-functional Erm(41) [6,11,12]. Consequently, this gene is not associated with clarithromycin resistance in this subspecies. On the contrary, *M. abscessus* subsp. *abscessus* and *M. abscessus* subsp. *bolletii* have a functional Erm(41) protein. Mutations in the *erm*(41) gene are the most common mechanism of resistance to clarithromycin in these subspecies [6,12–14]. Resistance to aminoglycosides is mainly associated with mutations in the *rrs* gene, encoding the 16S rRNA or aminoglycoside-modifying enzymes [15] and resistance to β-lactams occurs due to the production of Bla$_{Mab}$, a chromosome-encoded Ambler class A β-lactamase [16].

Poor treatment outcomes of *M. abscessus* infections have been attributed to innate and acquired drug resistance. Current treatment options are suboptimal and therapeutic options are limited [17,18]. *M. abscessus* is intrinsically resistant to several classes of antibiotics mainly due to the impermeability of its cell membrane. Efflux activity has been proposed as a drug resistance mechanism in mycobacteria where the induction of efflux pumps due to the exposure to non-inhibitory concentrations of antibiotics is proposed as the first step of acquired drug resistance that leads to high-level chromosomal-mutation-related resistance that may hamper the activity of several antibiotics [19,20]. Recently, efflux activity has been correlated with clinical resistance to macrolides, aminoglycosides, bedaquiline, and clofazimine also in *M. abscessus* [21–23]. Therefore, an alternative approach to overcome *M. abscessus* drug resistance driven by efflux activity is the inhibition of efflux of antibiotics with the aid of efflux inhibitors, compounds that are able to reduce the intrinsic resistance of the bacteria by increasing the intracellular concentration of antimicrobial compounds [23]. Real-time fluorometric assays have been used to detect and quantify increased efflux activity using fluorescent substrates, such as ethidium bromide, which is capable of accumulating inside the bacteria in the presence of an efflux inhibitor and this increased efflux activity has been correlated with clinically relevant antibiotic resistance [20,24–27].

The increasing number of infections caused by *M. abscessus*, together with the reduced therapeutic options available, highlights the need to increase our knowledge on the mechanisms of drug resistance in *M. abscessus*. Previous studies have shown that the inhibition of efflux activity by verapamil in *M. tuberculosis* and *M. avium* complex can improve the activity of antimicrobial compounds [20,28–30]. In this study, we have evaluated the contribution of efflux to *M. abscessus* clarithromycin resistance correlating the levels of resistance, in the presence and absence of verapamil, with the presence of mutations in the clarithromycin resistance-associated genes, *erm*(41) and *rrl*. Furthermore, we have investigated the role of increased efflux pump gene mRNA levels and the consequently increased efflux activity in six *M. abscessus* strains when exposed to sub-inhibitory concentrations of clarithromycin as one of the mechanisms contributing to inducible macrolide resistance.

2. Results

2.1. Phenotypic and Genotypic Characterization of the M. abscessus Strains

In this work, we studied four *M. abscessus* subsp. *abscessus* strains (three clinical isolates and the ATCC19977^T reference strain) plus three *M. abscessus* subsp. *bolletii* and three *M. abscessus* subsp. *massiliense* clinical isolates from two geographically distinct origins, Brazil and Portugal. We used the GenoType NTM-DR assay to determine the *erm*(41) sequevars and search for mutations in the *rrl* and *rrs* genes (Table 1). We found that all the strains belong to the *erm*(41) T28 sequevar.

Table 1. Phenotypic and genotypic characterization of the *M. abscessus* strains studied.

Strain	Species/Subspecies	Genetic Background			MICs (µg/mL), Day 3 *			
		CLA	AMK		Compounds			
		erm(41)	rrl	rs	CLA	AMK	VP	EtBr
MabATCC19977[T]	*M. abscessus* subsp. *abscessus*	T28	wt	wt	2 (S)	16 (S)	1024	128
MabBR1	*M. abscessus* subsp. *abscessus*	T28	wt	wt	2 (S)	8 (S)	4096	256
MabBR2	*M. abscessus* subsp. *bolletii*	T28	wt	wt	1 (S)	4 (S)	1024	64
MabBR3	*M. abscessus* subsp. *massiliense*	T28	A2059C	wt	256 (R)	16 (S)	1024	32
MabPT1	*M. abscessus* subsp. *abscessus*	T28	wt	wt	0.25 (S)	4 (S)	1024	64
MabPT2	*M. abscessus* subsp. *bolletii*	T28	wt	wt	2 (S)	4 (S)	2048	128
MabPT3	*M. abscessus* subsp. *massiliense*	T28	wt	wt	0.5 (S)	4 (S)	1024	256
MabPT4	*M. abscessus* subsp. *bolletii*	T28	wt	wt	2 (S)	4 (S)	1024	128
MabPT5	*M. abscessus* subsp. *massiliense*	T28	wt	wt	1 (S)	4 (S)	1024	256
MabPT6	*M. abscessus* subsp. *abscessus*	T28	wt	wt	1 (S)	4 (S)	2048	64

* Ref [10]. AMK, amikacin; CLA, clarithromycin; EtBr, ethidium bromide; MIC, minimum inhibitory concentration; R, resistant; S, susceptible; VP, verapamil; wt, wild-type sequence.

Clarithromycin and amikacin MICs are presented in Table 1. None of the strains presented a multidrug-resistant phenotype, i.e., simultaneous resistance to clarithromycin and amikacin [14]. With regard to amikacin, all strains were susceptible to this antibiotic (breakpoint for resistance: MIC ≥ 64 µg/mL) [10]. The susceptibility results were 100% concordant with those obtained with the GenoType NTM-DR, i.e., no mutation was detected in the *rrs* gene associated with amikacin resistance. Concerning clarithromycin, the results matched 100% with the results obtained with the GenoType NTM-DR. Nine strains were susceptible to clarithromycin and one was resistant. The latter presented an MIC of 256 µg/mL consistent with the presence of a mutation in the *rrl* gene (MIC ≥ 256 µg/mL) [10].

Next, we evaluated the presence of inducible clarithromycin resistance since all strains belong to the *erm*(41) T28 sequevar (Table 2). According to the CLSI guidelines, macrolide inducible resistance is defined as an increase in the MIC of clarithromycin from ≤2 µg/mL at day 5 to ≥8 µg/mL at day 14 of incubation [10]. Of the 10 strains tested, only three presented an inducible resistance phenotype to clarithromycin, namely two *M. abscessus* subsp. *abscessus* strains (ATCC19977[T] and MabPT6) and one *M. abscessus* subsp. *bolletii* (MabPT2). No inducible resistance was found in the *M. abscessus* subsp. *massiliense* isolates, as expected, since this subspecies harbors a non-functional Erm(41) protein.

Table 2. Analysis of inducible vs. non-inducible clarithromycin resistance in the *M. abscessus* strains studied.

Strain	Mutations		CLA MICs (µg/mL)		CLA Susceptibility Profile at Day 14 *	
	erm(41)	rrl	Day 5	Day 14		
MabATCC19977[T]	T28	wt	4 (I)	16 (R)	Resistant	Inducible
MabBR1	T28	wt	2 (S)	4 (I)	Intermediate	Non-inducible
MabBR2	T28	wt	16 (R)	256 (R)	Resistant	Non-inducible
MabBR3	T28	A2059C	256 (R)	256 (R)	Resistant	Non-inducible
MabPT1	T28	wt	0.25 (S)	2 (S)	Susceptible	Non-inducible
MabPT2	T28	wt	4 (I)	16 (R)	Resistant	Inducible
MabPT3	T28	wt	0.5 (S)	0.5 (S)	Susceptible	Non-inducible
MabPT4	T28	wt	16 (R)	64 (R)	Resistant	Non-inducible
MabPT5	T28	wt	1 (S)	1 (S)	Susceptible	Non-inducible
MabPT6	T28	wt	2 (S)	16 (R)	Resistant	Inducible

CLA, clarithromycin; I, intermediate; MIC, minimum inhibitory concentration; R, resistant; S, susceptible; wt, wild-type sequence. * Ref. [10].

Of the 10 strains studied, two *M. abscessus* subsp. *bolletii* strains (MabBR2 and MabPT4) presented increased resistance to clarithromycin after five days of incubation (Table 2) that, according to the CLSI guidelines, could not be attributed to the presence of T28 nucleotide change, a finding indicating the existence of another mechanism of resistance to clarithromycin. Since no mutations were found in the *rrl* gene and active efflux has been associated with clarithromycin resistance in several microorganisms including mycobacteria and *M. abscessus* [19–23,30,31], we continued the work with the evaluation of the presence of increased active efflux systems despite the presence of the T28 polymorphism. For this purpose, we studied all strains to assess the contribution of active efflux to their macrolide susceptibility phenotype.

2.2. Evaluation of the Synergistic Effect between Efflux Inhibitors and Clarithromycin

For these assays, we selected verapamil as reference efflux inhibitor since several works have already shown that this is the most efficient efflux inhibitor for several mycobacterial species [20,23,28,29]. The MICs of verapamil are given in Table 1. The synergistic effect between verapamil and clarithromycin and the modulation factor (MF) obtained for each combination are listed in Table 3.

Table 3. Minimum inhibitory concentration and modulation factor of clarithromycin in the presence of verapamil for the *M. abscessus* strains in study.

Strain	MIC (µg/mL) (MF)					
	Day 3		Day 5		Day 14	
	CLA	CLA+VP	CLA	CLA+VP	CLA	CLA+VP
MabATCC19977^T	2 (S)	0.5 (S) (↓4)	4 (I)	1 (S) (↓4)	16 (R)	16 (R)
MabBR1	2 (S)	1 (S) (↓2)	2 (S)	2 (S)	4 (I)	4 (I)
MabBR2	1 (S)	0.25 (S) (↓4)	16 (R)	2 (S) (↓8)	256 (R)	128 (R) (↓2)
MabBR3	256 (R)	256 (R)	256 (R)	256 (R)	256 (R)	256 (R)
MabPT1	0.25 (S)	0.0625 (S) (↓4)	0.25 (S)	0.0625 (S) (↓4)	2 (S)	0.5 (S) (↓4)
MabPT2	2 (S)	≤0.0625 (S) (≥↓32)	4 (I)	≤0.0625 (S) (≥↓64)	16 (R)	16 (R)
MabPT3	0.5 (S)	0.0625 (S) (↓4)	0.5 (S)	0.25 (S) (↓2)	0.5 (S)	0.5 (S)
MabPT4	2 (S)	0.5 (S) (↓4)	16 (R)	4 (I) (↓4)	64 (R)	32 (R) (↓2)
MabPT5	1 (S)	0.5 (S) (↓2)	1 (S)	0.5 (S) (↓2)	1 (S)	0.5 (S) (↓2)
MabPT6	1 (S)	≤0.03125 (S) (≥↓32)	2 (S)	0.125 (S) (↓16)	16 (R)	8 (R) (↓2)

CLA, clarithromycin; I, intermediate; MIC, minimum inhibitory concentration; MF, modulation factor; R, resistant; S, susceptible; VP, verapamil. In red are denoted the reductions of the MICs of clarithromycin in the presence of verapamil corresponding to a MF ≥ 4.

As can be observed, the MIC of clarithromycin at day 3 and day 5 was significantly reduced in seven of the 10 strains studied. Among the three remaining strains, MabBR1 and MabPT5 were susceptible to clarithromycin and they do not present inducible clarithromycin resistance. Their MICs decreased only two-fold in the presence of verapamil, which was not considered significant, and this phenotype was maintained until day 14 of incubation. The third strain, MabBR3, harbors a mutation in the *rrl* gene, which confers high-level resistance to clarithromycin and as expected no effect was observed on the MIC of clarithromycin in the presence of verapamil. For the remaining seven strains, the MICs of clarithromycin decreased in the presence of $\frac{1}{2}$ the MIC of verapamil (determined for each strain and presented in Table 1) by four-fold to ≥32-fold at day 3 and by four-fold to ≥64-fold at day 5 (Table 3). At day 14, MabPT1 was the only strain for which the MIC of clarithromycin was reduced by four-fold in the presence of verapamil. Moreover, the lack of effect of the efflux inhibitor verapamil at day 14 is interpreted as the result of the emergence of other resistance mechanisms during clarithromycin exposure, e.g., the development of mutations in target genes associated with clarithromycin resistance such as the *rrl*, *rplV* or *rplD*, which will be analyzed in further studies. These results showed that the synergistic effect of verapamil does not depend on the *M. abscessus* subspecies studied nor by the presence of the T28 polymorphism in *erm*(41). This data demonstrates the existence of efflux activity in these strains that can be reduced by verapamil. Altogether, these results reveal, for the first time, that the inducible clarithromycin resistance in the strains assayed is also due to increased efflux activity in spite of the inducible resistance via *erm*(41).

2.3. Assessment of Efflux Activity by Real-Time Fluorometry

After the demonstration of the synergistic effect between the efflux inhibitor verapamil and clarithromycin, indirectly correlating efflux with resistance via the inhibitory effect of verapamil, we studied the presence of active efflux activity in these strains by real-time fluorometry using the broad efflux substrate ethidium bromide in the presence of glucose as a source of metabolic energy and in the presence and absence of verapamil. First, was determined the lowest concentration that causes minimal accumulation of ethidium bromide, i.e., the concentration for which there is an equilibrium between influx and efflux of the substrate (Figure 1A, Table 4).

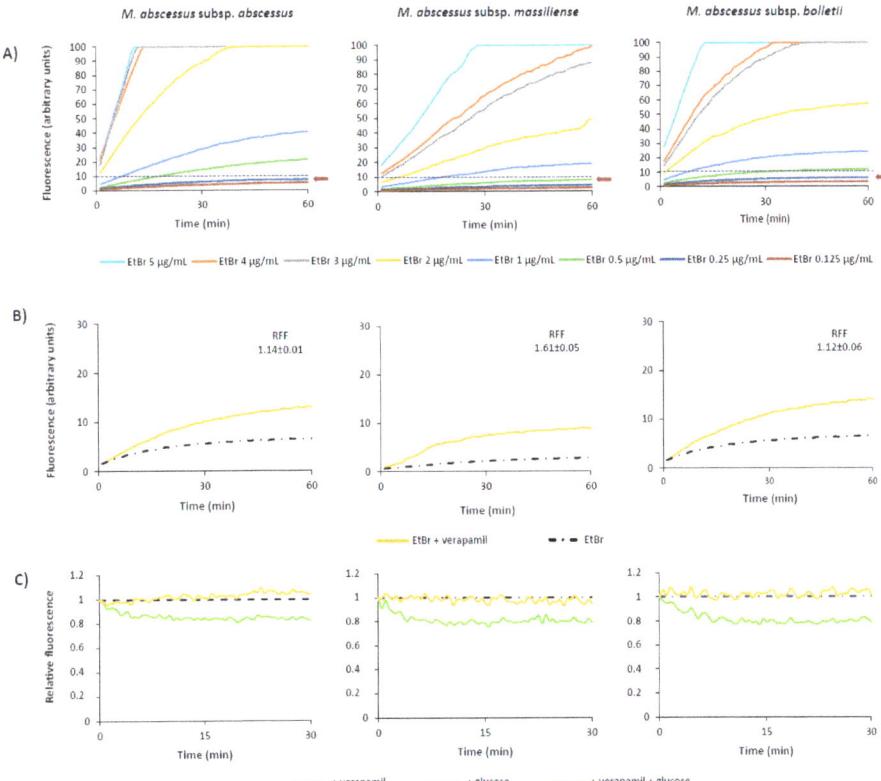

Figure 1. Accumulation and efflux of *M. abscessus*. The figure shows one representative assay for each subspecies, as follows: *M. abscessus* subsp. *abscessus*—MabPT1, *M. abscessus* subsp. *massiliense*—MabPT3, and *M. abscessus* subsp. *bolletii*—MabBR2. (**A**) Accumulation of increasing concentrations of ethidium bromide. The equilibrium concentration was determined for each strain as the concentration that promoted a plateau of no more than 10% of relative fluorescence units during the 60 min of the assay (black broken line) and is indicated in each graph by an arrow. The assays were performed in the presence of 0.4% of glucose. (**B**) Accumulation of ethidium bromide in the presence of verapamil. Each strain was tested at its equilibrium concentration (Table 4) in the presence and absence of $\frac{1}{2}$ MIC of verapamil (see Table 1 for MICs). The assays were performed in the presence of glucose. RFF, relative final fluorescence. (**C**) Efflux of ethidium bromide. The strains were loaded with ethidium bromide at the equilibrium concentration and efflux took place in the presence of glucose, which was inhibited by verapamil at $\frac{1}{2}$ MIC.

The lowest concentration that resulted in an equilibrium between the influx and efflux of ethidium bromide (Ceq) for all the strains varied between 0.125 µg/mL to 0.5 µg/mL (Table 4).

Table 4. Characterization of the *M. abscessus* strains according to their efflux capacity.

Strains	C_{Eq} (µg/mL)	RFF_{VP}
MabATCC19977^T	0.25	1.15 ± 0.03
MabBR1	0.125	0.78 ± 0.01
MabBR2	0.25	1.12 ± 0.06
MabBR3	0.125	0.19 ± 0.05
MabPT1	0.25	1.14 ± 0.01
MabPT2	0.25	0.63 ± 0.01
MabPT3	0.5	1.61 ± 0.05
MabPT4	0.125	1.61 ± 0.01
MabPT5	0.5	0.26 ± 0.00
MabPT6	0.25	1.64 ± 0.11

C_{Eq}, equilibrium concentration; RFF, relative final fluorescence; VP, verapamil

Next, we performed ethidium bromide accumulation assays in the presence of verapamil as a proof of concept (Figure 1B) and determined the RFF indexes (Table 4). The RFF index reflects how efficient verapamil is in promoting intracellular accumulation of ethidium bromide, in this case, in *M. abscessus*. The results showed that verapamil is able to increase the ethidium bromide accumulation in all the tested strains (Table 4) and at highly significant levels in six of the 10 strains studied. The RFF values of these strains are in the same range varying between 1.12 to 1.64. Comparing the different subspecies, no relevant differences were observed on the levels of ethidium bromide accumulation. These results demonstrate that verapamil is able to promote intracellular accumulation of ethidium bromide on *M. abscessus* evidencing that real-time active efflux is present in this species and can be inhibited by verapamil.

To confirm that the efflux activity of these strains could be inhibited in the presence of verapamil we performed efflux assays (Figure 1C). Analyzing the results of each strain and comparing the curves corresponding to the strain in the presence of verapamil and glucose (orange) with the curve of the strain in the presence of glucose but without verapamil (green), we conclude that ethidium bromide efflux is inhibited by verapamil in the *M. abscessus* strains studied, strengthening the correlation between active efflux and drug resistance in these strains.

2.4. Quantification of Efflux Pump mRNA Levels by RT-qPCR

To analyze the contribution of the overexpression of efflux pumps to clarithromycin resistance, we selected three main efflux pump genes correlated with antibiotic-resistant phenotypes, including macrolides, in mycobacteria and in particular in *M. tuberculosis*, as proof of concept [20,23,32], namely *MAB_3142* (homologue of *M. tuberculosis p55*), *MAB_1409* (*Rv1258c* or *tap-like*) and *MAB_2807* (*efpA*). We chose two strains of each *M. abscessus* subspecies to analyze the changes in the mRNA transcriptional levels after exposure to $\frac{1}{2}$ of the respective MIC of clarithromycin. The relative mRNA transcription levels were determined against the respective non-exposed strain (Figure 2).

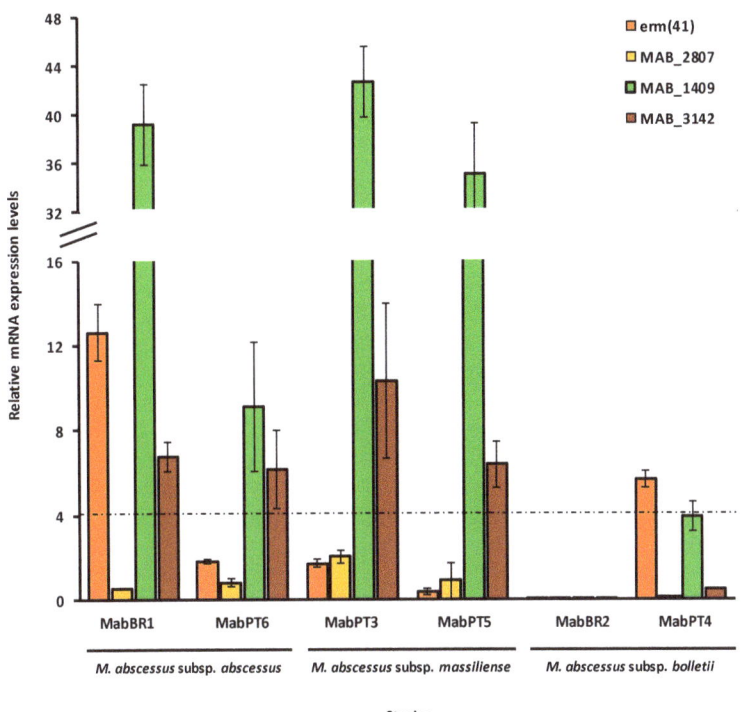

Figure 2. Relative quantification of efflux pump gene mRNA levels in the *M. abscessus* strains exposed to clarithromycin. Strains were grown in MGIT medium for the MGIT 960 system in the presence of half MIC of clarithromycin (see Table 1 for MICs). The relative expression of the efflux pump genes was evaluated comparing the relative quantity of the respective mRNA in the presence of clarithromycin to the respective unexposed strain. A level of relative expression equal to 1 indicates that the expression level is identical to the non-exposed parental strain. Genes showing expression levels above four were considered overexpressed (black dashed line in the graph).

Increased mRNA levels were detected in all strains with the sole exception of MabBR2. This strain does not present overexpression of any of the three efflux pump genes studied nor *erm*(41). Comparing these results with those obtained in the MICs assays, we noticed that MabBR2 was susceptible to clarithromycin at day 3, with an MIC of 2 µg/mL. The concentration used for the analysis of efflux pump mRNA levels was 1 µg/mL. Although there was a four-fold decrease in the MIC of clarithromycin in the presence of verapamil at day 3, this effect may be attributed to a combined effect between the two compounds and not exclusively to efflux pump overexpression at this time point. Moreover, MabBR2 does not have inducible clarithromycin resistance which is consistent with a non-expressed *erm*(41) gene. Notably, at day 5 we noted a reversion of the phenotype from resistant to susceptible in the presence of verapamil that may be attributed to the efflux activity due to the prolonged exposure to clarithromycin. At day 14, no effect was seen in the presence of the efflux inhibitor, indicating that the *M. abscessus* subsp. *bolletii* BR2 may have acquired other resistance mechanisms as a mutation in the *rrl* gene that is associated with high-level clarithromycin resistance (MIC ≥ 256 µg/mL) [10]. Therefore, we studied another *M. abscessus* subsp. *bolletii* strain (MabPT4) to assess the contribution of the subspecies to the response to clarithromycin exposure. In terms of antibiotic susceptibility in the presence and absence of verapamil, the results are entirely equivalent between both strains (Table 3), however, MabPT4 has the *erm*(41) gene overexpressed despite having a non-inducible phenotype and shows borderline overexpression of the *MAB_1409* (*tap-like*) gene (Figure 2). This result shows that *erm*(41) gene expression is not the sole cause of clarithromycin resistance in this strain. Efflux activity is present in this strain (Table 4) representing a late stress response to clarithromycin exposure. Concerning *M. abscessus* subsp. *massiliense*, we analyzed MabPT3 and MabPT5, both susceptible to clarithromycin without inducible resistance consistent with the lack of expression of *erm*(41) encoding a non-functional Erm(41) protein. Although susceptible, the MICs of clarithromycin decreased in the presence of verapamil by four-fold in MabPT3 and two-fold in MabPT5 (Table 3). Both strains showed overexpression of *MAB_3142* and *MAB_1409* (Figure 2). Comparing to the real-time efflux assays, MabPT3 has increased efflux activity although MabPT5 showed lower efflux activity than MabPT3. This result shows that efflux activity acts also as a first-line response in these *M. abscessus* subsp. *massiliense* strains. Finally, we studied two strains of *M. abscessus* subsp. *abscessus*, namely MabBR1 and MabPT6. MabBR1 showed intermediate resistance at day 14, and consequently, non-inducible resistance to clarithromycin, whereas MabPT6 was resistant at day 14 through an inducible resistant phenotype to this antibiotic. Comparing this data with the RT-qPCR assays, MabBR1 exhibited overexpression of *MAB_3142* and *MAB_1409* efflux pump genes and, somehow unexpected, also *erm*(41). On the contrary, MabPT6 that presents inducible resistance to clarithromycin, although at low levels (16 µg/mL), showed no expression of *erm*(41). However, this strain shows overexpression of *MAB_3142* and *MAB_1409* efflux pump genes. Comparing with the real-time efflux assays, MabBR1 showed lower levels of efflux than MabPT6, probably due to the presence of an overexpressed *erm*(41). No overexpression was observed concerning the gene *MAB_2807* for any of the six strains analyzed.

3. Discussion

Members of the *M. abscessus* complex are clinically important pathogens. At present, only few antibiotics showed antimicrobial activity with clinical significance against this species, namely, clarithromycin and amikacin, and either cefoxitin or imipenem. The main reasons commonly accepted for this scarce therapeutic panel is the low permeability of *M. abscessus* complex cell wall, the presence of mutations in the drug target genes and, in the case of clarithromycin, the presence of an inducible *erm*(41) gene [14]. Recently, the hypothesis of efflux-mediated drug resistance has been appointed as a putative contributor to drug resistance in *M. abscessus* [21,22].

All bacteria express efflux pumps. Efflux transporters are transmembrane proteins involved in the extrusion of harmful compounds and cellular metabolites from the cells into the external environment [33]. Indirectly, they are also involved in drug resistance by expelling antimicrobials, reducing their intracellular concentration. Treatment failure has been mainly attributed to *M. abscessus* belonging to the T28 sequevar [12,34,35]. Similar to what is observed in *M. avium* complex infections, acquired resistance to clarithromycin also evolves rapidly during therapy in *M. abscessus* [36]. Therefore, it is legitimate to raise the hypothesis of whether the overexpression of efflux pumps is also involved in the resistance to clarithromycin even in the *M. abscessus* sequevar T28? Ongoing work showed that resistance towards clarithromycin in *M. avium* results from the balance between the presence of drug resistance-associated mutations and increased efflux activity. We also noticed that this increased efflux activity was accompanied by the overexpression of several efflux pump genes upon exposure to clarithromycin. Therefore, to answer this question, we investigated the contribution of efflux transporters to the induced clarithromycin resistance in *M. abscessus* complex belonging to the *erm*(41) T28 sequevar.

The strains were blindly selected in relation to their clarithromycin susceptibility status and included a panel of nine clinical strains, comprising three isolates of each *M. abscessus* subspecies, namely, subsp. *abscessus*, *bolletii* and *massiliense*. The *M. abscessus* subsp. *abscessus* ATCC19977^T reference strain was included as control. Firstly, we searched for mutations associated with clarithromycin resistance the *M. abscessus* strains. We found that all belong to the *erm*(41) T28 sequevar which, at least theoretically, is responsible for the inducible resistance to clarithromycin in *M. abscessus* [12,14]. One of the strains harbors a mutation in *rrl*, and consequently, displays high-level resistance to clarithromycin, and was used as mutation-driven resistance control. These initial results are in accordance with those described in the literature that states that the majority of the *M. abscessus* strains are susceptible to clarithromycin and resistance is acquired during treatment [1,14]. To test the role of the *erm*(41) T28 polymorphism in the induced resistance of the strains analyzed, we read the MICs at day 5 of incubation and prolonged the incubation until day 14. Surprisingly, of the eight strains, only two clinical strains and the reference strain showed induced resistance to clarithromycin, one *M. abscessus* subsp. *abscessus* and the other *M. abscessus* subsp. *bolletii*. Interestingly, two *M. abscessus* subsp. *bolletii* strains were shown to be already resistant to clarithromycin at day 5 and according to the CLSI guidelines, they do not fit in the category of clarithromycin-inducible resistance. These results demonstrate that the T28 polymorphism in *erm*(41) is not the sole cause of clarithromycin-induced resistance in these *M. abscessus* strains indicating the existence of another mechanism of resistance in this collection of strains.

We then studied the presence of active efflux activity in these strains through the determination of the MICs of clarithromycin in the presence of the efflux inhibitor verapamil. The results obtained supported our hypothesis that efflux is also involved in *M. abscessus* induced resistance to clarithromycin. At day 3 and day 5, all the MICs of clarithromycin for all strains, with the sole exception of the strain with the *rrl* mutation, could be reduced in the presence of the efflux inhibitor verapamil. In particular, it was possible to reverse to clinically significant levels the resistance to clarithromycin at day 5 for four strains, one from resistant to susceptible, one from resistant to intermediate and two from intermediate to susceptible. After 14 days of exposure, no inhibitory effect was noted for these, meaning that these strains may have acquired other mutational mechanisms of resistance, a subject that will be addressed in subsequent studies. Concurrently with real-time fluorometric assays, using verapamil as reference efflux inhibitor and ethidium bromide as substrate, we detected significant efflux activity in the 10 strains, which could be inhibited in the presence of verapamil. It was also demonstrated that this efflux activity does not depend on subspecies of the strains, as it was detected in all the three subspecies, although at different levels, nor due to their phenotype since it was detected in inducible and non-inducible clarithromycin resistance strains. These data demonstrated the presence and importance of active efflux in *M. abscessus* strains resistant to clarithromycin, which could be inhibited by verapamil.

Finally, to further analyze the contribution of the expression of efflux pumps to clarithromycin resistance in these strains, three efflux pump genes, *MAB_3142*, *MAB_1409* and *MAB_2807*, and the *erm*(41) gene, were selected to examine changes in mRNA transcriptional levels after exposure to $\frac{1}{2}$ MIC of clarithromycin determined for each of the six strains selected. We noted increased mRNA expression levels of the efflux pumps *MAB_3142* and *MAB_1409* in four out of six of the strains and found also *erm*(41) overexpression in two strains, one presenting inducible resistance while the other does not have induced resistance to clarithromycin.

This exploratory study consolidates and strengthens the hypothesis that efflux activity plays a role in *M. abscessus* intrinsic resistance to clarithromycin in strains belonging to the T28 sequevar and that the inhibition of this efflux activity by compounds such as verapamil could potentiate the clinical effect of clarithromycin, the most efficient antibiotic to treat *M. abscessus* infections, certainly reducing or preventing the emergence of the, so far almost inexorable, acquired resistance to macrolides during treatment against *M. abscessus* infections.

4. Materials and Methods

4.1. M. abscessus Complex Strains

The strains selected for this study are described in Table 1 and were isolated from Brazilian (BR) and Portuguese (PT) patients. Brazilian clinical strains were granted by Fundação Oswaldo Cruz (Rio de Janeiro, Brazil). The Portuguese clinical strains are part of the strain collection of the Mycobacteriology Laboratory of the Instituto de Higiene e Medicina Tropical, Universidade NOVA de Lisboa (Lisboa, Portugal). The strains were identified using the GenoType NTM-DR assay (Hain Lifescience, GmbH, Nehren, Germany) according to the manufacturer's instructions. Informed consent was not required for the present study since it corresponds to a retrospective study from which all patient identification was unlinked from the results, and no patient information was collected. *M. abscessus* subsp. *abscessus* ATCC19977^T reference strain was obtained from the American Type Culture Collection (Virginia, USA) and was included as a control strain.

4.2. Compounds and Reagents

Amikacin, clarithromycin, verapamil, ethidium bromide, dimethyl sulfoxide (DMSO), and glucose were purchased from Sigma-Aldrich (St. Louis, MO, USA). Clarithromycin was prepared in DMSO, while the remaining drugs were prepared in sterile deionized water. Stock solutions were stored at −20 °C. Working solutions of both antibiotics and ethidium bromide were prepared in Mueller–Hinton broth (MHB; Oxoid, Hampshire, UK) on the day of the experiments. Löwenstein–Jensen medium, Middlebrook 7H9, BBL OADC (oleic acid/albumin/dextrose/catalase) supplement and the mycobacteria growth indicator tubes (MGITs) were purchased from Becton Dickinson (Diagnostic Systems, Sparks, MD, USA).

4.3. Detection of Mutations Associated with Clarithromycin and Amikacin Resistance

Total DNA was extracted from clinical strains and the reference strain using the GenoLyse kit (Hain Lifescience) according to the manufacturer's instructions. The presence of mutations in *rrl*, *erm*(41) and *rrs* were analyzed with the Genotype NTM-DR assay.

4.4. Susceptibility Testing

4.4.1. Growth of the Strains

All strains were maintained in MGITs tubes supplemented with 10% OADC. For minimum inhibitory concentration (MIC) determination and synergism assays, the *M. abscessus* strains were inoculated in Löwenstein–Jensen medium and incubated at 37 °C for three to five days.

4.4.2. MIC Determination of Compounds

For the determination of the MICs of the antibiotics, the efflux inhibitor verapamil and the efflux substrate ethidium bromide, the inoculum of each strain was prepared by diluting the bacterial cultures in MHB to a final density of approximately 10^5 cells/mL [37]. The MICs were determined using a tetrazolium microplate-based assay (TEMA) [38] with small modifications. Briefly, aliquots of 0.1 mL of inoculum were transferred to each well of the plate that contained 0.1 mL of each compound at concentrations prepared from two-fold serial dilutions in MHB medium. Growth controls (only inoculum without drug) and a sterility control (only medium) were included in each plate. Two hundred microliters of sterile deionized water were added to the outer-perimeter wells of the 96-well plates to reduce evaporation of the medium during the incubation. The inoculated plates were sealed in permeable plastic bags and incubated at 37 °C for three days. After this period, 10 μL of a solution of 5× MTT/10%T80 (1:1) was added to each well and the plates incubated for four hours at room temperature. The bacterial growth was registered for each well based on the MTT color change. As the intensity of the color generated is directly proportional to the number of viable cells, a precipitate of cells stained black can be observed in the bottom of the well. The MIC was defined as the lowest concentration of compound that totally inhibited bacterial growth, i.e., no color change [39]. All assays were performed in triplicate. For amikacin, the breakpoints used were: ≤16 μg/mL, susceptible; 32 μg/mL, intermediate; and ≥64 μg/mL, resistant. For clarithromycin at day 3, the breakpoints used were: ≤2 μg/mL, susceptible; 4 μg/mL, intermediate and ≥8 μg/mL, resistant [10].

To evaluate clarithromycin induced resistance, the MIC determination of clarithromycin was extended for 14 days. To do this, plates containing clarithromycin were prepared in quadruplicate to be read at the following time points: 3, 5 and 14 days [14]. After each period of incubation, MTT was added and the results read and interpreted as described above. Susceptible isolates at day 3 (MIC ≤ 2 μg/mL) and resistant at day 5 (MIC ≥ 8 µg/mL), were considered to have an inducible *erm*(41) gene [10]. All assays were carried out in triplicate.

4.4.3. MIC Determination of Antibiotics and Ethidium Bromide in the Presence of Verapamil

The MICs of amikacin, clarithromycin, and ethidium bromide were determined in the presence of verapamil. The assays were performed as described above with the exception that verapamil was added to each well to a final concentration of $\frac{1}{2}$ of the MIC. The results were read and interpreted as described above. The modulation factor (MF) was calculated and used to quantify the inhibitory effect of verapamil on the MICs of clarithromycin through the following formula: MF = MIC antimicrobial / MIC antimicrobial + efflux inhibitor [40]. The MF reflects the reduction of the MIC values of a given antimicrobial in the presence of an efflux inhibitor, being considered significant when MF ≥ 4 (four-fold reduction) [41]. Each assay was carried out in triplicate.

4.4.4. Semi-Automated Fluorometric Method

The evaluation of efflux activity on a real-time basis was performed using a semi-automated fluorometric method [26] with modifications [Machado et al., unpublished]. The *M. abscessus* strains were grown in 10 ml of 7H9/10%OADC with 0.05% tyloxapol at 37 °C until they reached an OD$_{600}$ of 0.8. For the accumulation assays, the cultures were centrifuged at 3500 rpm for three minutes, the supernatant discarded and the pellet washed in 7H9. The OD$_{600}$ was adjusted to 0.8 with 7H9. In order to determine the concentration of ethidium bromide that establishes the equilibrium between efflux and influx, aliquots of 0.05 mL of the bacterial suspension were added to 0.2 mL microtubes containing 0.05 mL different concentrations of ethidium bromide that ranged from 0.625 µg/mL to 5 µg/mL with and without 0.4% glucose. The assays were conducted at 37 °C in a Rotor-Gene 3000 (Corbett Research, Sydney, Australia), using the 530 nm band-pass and the 585 nm high-pass filters as the excitation and detection wavelengths, respectively. Fluorescence data were acquired every 60 seconds for 60 min. The selected concentration of ethidium bromide was further used for the evaluation of the capacity of verapamil to retain ethidium bromide inside the cells. Verapamil was tested at $\frac{1}{2}$ MIC with and without 0.4% glucose and ethidium bromide at the equilibrium concentration determined for each strain and the assays performed as described above. The inhibitory activity of verapamil was determined through the determination of the relative final fluorescence (RFF) value according to the following formula [42]: RFF = (RF$_{treated}$-RF$_{untreated}$)/RF$_{untreated}$. In this formula, the RF$_{treated}$ corresponds to the relative fluorescence at the last time point of ethidium bromide accumulation curve (min 60) in the presence of verapamil, and the RF$_{untreated}$ corresponds to the relative fluorescence at the last time point of the ethidium bromide accumulation curve of the untreated control tube. An index of activity above zero indicate that the cells accumulate more ethidium bromide under the condition used than those of the control (untreated cells). Negative RFF values indicate that the treated cells accumulated less ethidium bromide than those of the control condition [28,32].

For the efflux assays, the strains were exposed to conditions that promote the maximum accumulation of ethidium bromide, i.e., ethidium bromide equilibrium concentration for each strain, no glucose, presence of verapamil at $\frac{1}{4}$ MIC, and incubation at 20 °C for one hour [26]. Before incubation, the cultures were centrifuged at 3500 rpm for three minutes, resuspended in 7H9, centrifuged again and OD$_{600}$ adjusted to 0.4. The suspension was incubated with ethidium bromide and verapamil under the conditions described above. Aliquots of 0.05 mL of cells were transferred to 0.2 mL microtubes containing 0.05 mL of verapamil at $\frac{1}{2}$ MIC without ethidium bromide. Control tubes with only cells and cells with and without 0.4% glucose were included. Fluorescence was measured in a Rotor-Gene™ 3000 and data were acquired every 30 seconds for 30 min. Efflux activity was quantified by comparing the fluorescence data obtained under conditions that promote efflux (presence of glucose and absence of efflux inhibitor) with the data from the control in which the mycobacteria are under conditions of no efflux (presence of an inhibitor and no energy source). Thus, the relative fluorescence corresponds to the ratio of fluorescence that remains per unit of time, relatively to the ethidium bromide-loaded cells [27].

4.5. Efflux Pump Gene Expression

4.5.1. Sample Preparation

For the analysis of efflux pump gene expression, each strain was inoculated into 7H9 containing 10% OADC plus clarithromycin at $\frac{1}{2}$ the MIC (see Table 1 for MIC values). The strains were then incubated at 37 °C within the MGIT system until growth was achieved [20]. At this time point, samples of each culture were taken for RNA extraction and RT-qPCR analysis.

4.5.2. RNA Extraction

Total RNA was isolated from the cells using the RNeasy mini kit (QIAGEN, GmbH, Hilden, Germany) according to the manufacturer's instructions with modifications [20]. Briefly, from a culture with 100–200 GU (about 10^6–10^8 cells/ml), 1 ml aliquot was removed and centrifuged at 13,000 rpm during 10 min. Then, 500 µL supernatant was removed and 1 mL of RNAprotect Bacteria Reagent (QIAGEN) added. An enzymatic lysis step was carried out with lysozyme at 3 mg/mL (Sigma) for 10 min, followed by lysis in an ultrasonic bath at 35 kHz (Gen-Probe, CA, USA) during 15 min. The RNA was purified using the RNeasy kit (QIAGEN) and treated with RNase-free DNase I (QIAGEN) during 2 h and 15 min by on-column digestion at room temperature to reduce the presence of contaminating DNA. All RNA samples were stored at −20 °C until required.

4.5.3. RT-qPCR Assay

The relative expression level of mRNA of genes that code for membrane efflux transporters in *M. abscessus* (*MAB_2807*, *MAB_1409* and *MAB_3142*) and *erm*(41) was analyzed by RT-qPCR. The normalization of the data was done using the *M. abscessus* 16S rDNA. The RT-qPCR procedure was performed in a Rotor-Gene 3000 thermocycler and followed the protocol recommended for use with the One-step NZY RT-qPCR Green kit (Nzytech, Portugal). The determination of the relative mRNA expression level was performed using the comparative quantification cycle (Cq) method [43]. The relative expression of the genes analyzed was assessed by comparison of the relative quantity of the respective mRNA in the presence of clarithromycin to the non-exposed culture, following the same technical approach previously published [20]. Each culture was assayed in triplicate using total RNA obtained from three independent cultures. A level of relative expression equal to 1 indicates that the expression level was identical to the unexposed strain. Genes showing expression levels equal or above four, when compared with the unexposed strain, were considered to be overexpressed [20].

5. Conclusions

The results obtained in this study provide evidence that efflux activity is an intrinsic characteristic of *M. abscessus* clinical strains and is directly involved in clarithromycin resistance. Literature review indicated that *M. abscessus* subsp. *abscessus* T28 and *M. abscessus* subsp. *bolletii* T28 are intrinsically resistant to clarithromycin conferred by an altered Erm(41) methylase [1]. The change of cytosine by thymine at position T28 on Erm(41) causes resistance to clarithromycin due to prolonged exposure leading to treatment failure [12–14]. In our hands, the results obtained pointed out that *erm*(41) expression is not the sole cause of the inducible clarithromycin resistance in *M. abscessus* subsp. *abscessus* and *M. abscessus* subsp. *bolletii* T28 sequevars and that efflux pump overexpression has a strong contribution to clarithromycin resistance acting both as a first-line response or a late response to drug pressure. This study was designed as a proof of concept. Therefore, due to the small number of strains studied, we could not generalize the results obtained here. Future work will include a higher number of strains belonging to the three subspecies. Another limitation of this study, consequence of the random selection of the strains, is the absence of strains from the C28 sequevar, which will be also studied further. Nevertheless, our results point out efflux as an important contributor to the emergence of *M. abscessus* clarithromycin resistance and highlight the need of further studies on *M. abscessus senso lato* efflux response to stress imposed by antimicrobials in order to implement more effective therapeutic regimens and aid in the development of new drugs against these bacteria.

Author Contributions: Conceptualization, J.S.V., D.M., I.B.R., D.F.R., M.V. and P.E.A.d.S.; data curation, J.S.V., D.M., I.B.R. and M.V.; funding acquisition, D.M., M.V. and P.E.A.d.S.; methodology, J.S.V., D.M., I.B.R., F.P.S., D.V.B., M.A.A. and D.F.R.; resources, D.M., I.B.R., M.C.S.L., M.V. and P.E.A.d.S.; supervision, J.S.V., D.M., I.B.R., A.v.G., M.V. and P.E.A.d.S.; writing—original draft, J.S.V. and I.B.R.; writing—review & editing, J.S.V., D.M., I.B.R., M.V. and P.E.A.d.S.

Funding: Coordenação de Aperfeiçoamento de Pessoal de Nível Superior (CAPES, MEC, Brazil) for financial support to Ivy B. Ramis and Miguel Viveiros. through the program "Ciências sem Fronteiras/Professor Visitante Especial" (Projecto 88881.064961/2014-01 - José R. Lapa e Silva/UFRJ coordinator). Diana Machado and Miguel Viveiros work was partially supported by project PTDC/BIA-MIC/30692/2017 and the Global Health and Tropical Medicine (GHTM) Research Center (Grant UID/Multi/04413/2013) from Fundação para a Ciência e a Tecnologia, Portugal.

Acknowledgments: Diana Machado would like to acknowledge Fundação para a Ciência e a Tecnologia, Portugal, for the support under the program "Stimulus of Scientific Employment".

Conflicts of Interest: The authors declare no conflict of interest. The funders had no role in the design of the study; in the collection, analyses, or interpretation of data; in the writing of the manuscript, or in the decision to publish the results.

References

1. Mougari, F.; Guglielmetti, L.; Raskine, L.; Sermet-Gaudelus, I.; Veziris, N.; Cambau, E. Infections caused by *Mycobacterium abscessus*: Epidemiology, diagnostic tools and treatment. *Expert Rev. Anti Infect. Ther.* **2016**, *14*, 1139–1154. [CrossRef] [PubMed]
2. Mukherjee, D.; Wu, M.; Teo, J.; Dick, T. Vancomycin and clarithromycin show synergy against *Mycobacterium abscessus* in vitro. *Antimicrob. Agents Chemother.* **2017**, *61*, e01298–e01317. [CrossRef] [PubMed]
3. Roux, A.-L.; Catherinot, E.; Ripoll, F.; Soismier, N.; Macheras, E.; Ravilly, S.; Bellis, G.; Vibet, M.-A.; Le Roux, E.; Lemonnier, L.; et al. Multicenter study of prevalence of nontuberculous mycobacteria in patients with cystic fibrosis in France. *J. Clin. Microbiol.* **2009**, *47*, 4124–4128. [CrossRef] [PubMed]
4. Mirsaeidi, M.; Farshidpour, M.; Allen, M.; Ebrahimi, G.; Falkinham, J. Highlight on advances in nontuberculous mycobacterial disease in North America. *Biomed. Res. Int.* **2014**, *919474*, 1–10. [CrossRef] [PubMed]
5. Leão, S.; Tortoli, E.; Euzéby, J.; Garcia, M. Proposal that *Mycobacterium massiliense* and *Mycobacterium bolletii* be united and reclassified as *Mycobacterium abscessus* subsp. *bolletii* comb. nov., designation of *Mycobacterium abscessus* subsp. *abscessus* subsp. nov. and emended description of *Mycobacterium abscessus*. *Int. J. Syst. Evol. Microbiol.* **2011**, *61*, 2311–2313. [CrossRef]
6. Kim, H.-Y.; Kim, B.; Kook, Y.; Yun, Y.-J.; Shin, J.; Hwan, J.; Kim, B.-J.; Kook, Y.-H. *Mycobacterium massiliense* is differentiated from *Mycobacterium abscessus* and *Mycobacterium bolletii* by erythromycin ribosome methyltransferase gene (erm) and clarithromycin susceptibility patterns. *Microbiol. Immunol.* **2010**, *54*, 347–353. [CrossRef] [PubMed]
7. Singh, S.; Bouzinbi, N.; Chaturvedi, V.; Godreuil, S.; Kremer, L. In vitro evaluation of a new drug combination against clinical isolates belonging to the *Mycobacterium abscessus* complex. *Clin. Microbiol. Infect.* **2014**, *20*, O1124–O1127. [CrossRef] [PubMed]
8. Zhang, Z.; Lu, J.; Liu, M.; Wang, Y.; Zhao, Y.; Pang, Y. In vitro activity of clarithromycin in combination with other antimicrobial agents against *Mycobacterium abscessus* and *Mycobacterium massiliense*. *Int. J. Antimicrob. Agents* **2017**, *49*, 383–386. [CrossRef]
9. Griffith, D.; Aksamit, T.; Brown-Elliott, B.; Catanzaro, A.; Daley, C.; Gordin, F.; Holland, S.; Horsburgh, R.; Huitt, G.; Iademarco, M.; et al. An official ATS/IDSA statement: Diagnosis, treatment, and prevention of nontuberculous mycobacterial diseases. *Am. J. Respir. Crit. Care Med.* **2007**, *175*, 367–416. [CrossRef]
10. Clinical Laboratory Standards Institute. *Susceptibility Testing of Mycobacteria, Nocardiae, and Other Aerobic Actinomycetes; Approved Standard*; CLSI document M24-A2; Clinical Laboratory Standards Institute (CLSI): Wayne, PA, USA, 2011.

11. Wallace, R.; Meier, A.; Brown, B.; Zhang, Y.; Sander, P.; Onyi, G.; Böttger, E. Genetic basis for clarithromycin resistance among isolates of *Mycobacterium chelonae* and *Mycobacterium abscessus*. *Antimicrob. Agents Chemother.* **1996**, *40*, 1676–1681. [CrossRef]
12. Nash, K.; Brown-Elliott, B.; Wallace, R. A novel gene, erm (41), confers inducible macrolide resistance to clinical isolates of *Mycobacterium abscessus* but is absent from *Mycobacterium chelonae*. *Antimicrob. Agents Chemother.* **2009**, *53*, 1367–1376. [CrossRef] [PubMed]
13. Bastian, S.; Veziris, N.; Roux, A.; Brossier, F.; Gaillard, J.; Jarlier, V.; Cambau, E. Assessment of clarithromycin susceptibility in strains belonging to the *Mycobacterium abscessus* group by erm41 and rrl sequencing. *Antimicrob. Agents Chemother.* **2011**, *55*, 775–781. [CrossRef] [PubMed]
14. Mougari, F.; Amarsy, R.; Veziris, N.; Bastian, S.; Brossier, F.; Berçot, B.; Raskine, L.; Cambau, E. Standardized interpretation of antibiotic susceptibility testing and resistance genotyping for *Mycobacterium abscessus* with regard to subspecies and erm41 sequevar. *J. Antimicrob. Chemother.* **2016**, *71*, 2208–2212. [CrossRef] [PubMed]
15. Maurer, F.; Bruderer, V.; Castelberg, C.; Ritter, C.; Scherbakov, D.; Bloemberg, G.; Böttger, E. Aminoglycoside-Modifying enzymes determine the innate susceptibility to aminoglycoside antibiotics in rapidly growing mycobacteria. *J. Antimicrob. Chemother.* **2015**, *70*, 1412–1419. [CrossRef] [PubMed]
16. Dubée, V.; Bernut, A.; Cortes, M.; Lesne, T.; Dorchene, D.; Lefebvre, A.; Hugonnet, J.-E.; Gutmann, F.; Mainardi, J.-L.; Herrmann, J.-L.; et al. β-Lactamase inhibition by avibactam in *Mycobacterium abscessus*. *J. Antimicrob. Chemother.* **2014**, *70*, 1051–1058. [CrossRef]
17. Oh, W.; Stout, J.; Yew, W. Advances in the management of pulmonary disease due to *Mycobacterium abscessus* complex. *Int. J. Tuberc. Lung Dis.* **2014**, *18*, 1141–1148. [CrossRef]
18. Diel, R.; Ringshausen, F.; Richter, E.; Welker, L.; Schmitz, J.; Nienhaus, A. Microbiological and clinical outcomes of treating non-*Mycobacterium avium* complex nontuberculous mycobacterial pulmonary disease: A systematic review and meta-analysis. *Chest* **2017**, *152*, 120–142. [CrossRef] [PubMed]
19. Schmalstieg, A.; Srivastava, S.; Belkaya, S.; Deshpande, D.; Meek, C.; Leff, R.; van Oers, N.; Gumbo, T. The antibiotic resistance arrow of time: Efflux pump induction is a general first step in the evolution of mycobacterial drug resistance. *Antimicrob. Agents Chemother.* **2012**, *56*, 4806–4815. [CrossRef] [PubMed]
20. Machado, D.; Couto, I.; Perdigão, J.; Rodrigues, L.; Portugal, I.; Baptista, P.; Veigas, B.; Amaral, L.; Viveiros, M. Contribution of efflux to the emergence of isoniazid and multidrug resistance in *Mycobacterium tuberculosis*. *PLoS ONE* **2012**, *7*, e34538. [CrossRef]
21. Ramis, I.; Vianna, J.; Silva, L., Jr.; von Groll, A.; Ramos, D.; Zanatta, N.; Viveiros, M.; da Silva, P.E.A. In silico and in vitro evaluation of tetrahydropyridine compounds as efflux inhibitors in *Mycobacterium abscessus*. *Tuberculosis* **2019**, *118*, 101853. [CrossRef]
22. Gutiérrez, A.; Richard, M.; Roquet-Banères, F.; Viljoen, A.; Kremer, L. The TetR-family transcription factor MAB_2299c regulates the expression of two distinct MmpS-MmpL efflux pumps involved in cross-resistance to clofazimine and bedaquiline in *Mycobacterium abscessus*. *Antimicrob. Agents Chemother.* **2019**, AAC.01000-19. [CrossRef]
23. Da Silva, P.E.A.; Machado, D.; Ramos, D.; Couto, I.; von Groll, A.; Viveiros, M. Efflux pumps in mycobacteria: Antimicrobial resistance, physiological functions, and role in pathogenicity. In *Efflux-Mediated Antimicrobial Resistance in Bacteria*; Li, X.-Z., Elkins, C.A., Zgurskaya, H.I., Eds.; Springer International Publishing: Cham, Switzerland, 2016; pp. 527–559. [CrossRef]
24. Marquez, B. Bacterial efflux systems and efflux pumps inhibitors. *Biochimie* **2005**, *87*, 1137–1147. [CrossRef] [PubMed]
25. Shapiro, H.M. Flow cytometry of bacterial membrane potential and permeability. *Methods Mol. Med.* **2008**, *142*, 175–186. [CrossRef] [PubMed]
26. Viveiros, M.; Rodrigues, L.; Martins, M.; Couto, I.; Spengler, G.; Martins, A.; Amaral, L. Evaluation of efflux activity of bacteria by a semi-automated fluorometric system. *Methods Mol. Biol.* **2010**, *642*, 159–172. [CrossRef] [PubMed]
27. Blair, J.; Piddock, L. How to measure export via bacterial multidrug resistance efflux pumps. *MBio* **2016**, *7*, e00840–e00916. [CrossRef] [PubMed]
28. Machado, D.; Perdigão, J.; Portugal, I.; Pieroni, M.; Silva, P.; Couto, I.; Viveiros, M. Efflux activity differentially modulates the levels of isoniazid and rifampicin resistance among multidrug resistant and monoresistant *Mycobacterium tuberculosis* strains. *Antibiotics* **2018**, *7*, 18. [CrossRef] [PubMed]

29. Gupta, S.; Tyagi, S.; Almeida, D.; Maiga, M.; Ammerman, N.; Bishai, W. Acceleration of tuberculosis treatment by adjunctive therapy with verapamil as an efflux inhibitor. *Am. J. Respir. Crit. Care Med.* **2013**, *188*, 600–607. [CrossRef]
30. Rodrigues, L.; Sampaio, D.; Couto, I.; Machado, D.; Kern, W.; Amaral, L.; Viveiros, M. The role of efflux pumps in macrolide resistance in *Mycobacterium avium* complex. *Int. J. Antimicrob. Agents* **2009**, *34*, 529–533. [CrossRef]
31. Versalovic, J.; Shortridge, D.; Kibler, K.; Griffy, M.; Beyer, J.; Flamm, R.; Tanaka, S.; Graham, D.; Go, M. Mutations in 23S rRNA are associated with clarithromycin resistance in *Helicobacter pylori*. *Antimicrob. Agents Chemother.* **1996**, *40*, 477–480. [CrossRef]
32. Machado, D.; Coelho, T.; Perdigão, J.; Pereira, C.; Couto, I.; Portugal, I.; Maschmann, R.; Ramos, D.; von Groll, A.; Rossetti, M.; et al. Interplay between mutations and efflux in drug resistant clinical isolates of *Mycobacterium tuberculosis*. *Front. Microbiol.* **2017**, *8*, 711. [CrossRef]
33. Piddock, L. Multidrug-resistance efflux pumps? not just for resistance. *Nat. Rev. Microbiol.* **2006**, *4*, 629. [CrossRef] [PubMed]
34. Koh, W.; Jeon, K.; Lee, N.; Kim, B.; Kook, Y.; Lee, S.; Park, Y.; Kim, C.; Shin, S.; Huitt, G.; et al. Clinical significance of differentiation of *Mycobacterium massiliense* from *Mycobacterium abscessus*. *Am. J. Respir. Crit. Care Med.* **2011**, *183*, 405–410. [CrossRef] [PubMed]
35. Harada, T.; Akiyama, Y.; Kurashima, A.; Nagai, H.; Tsuyuguchi, K.; Fujii, T.; Yano, S.; Shigeto, E.; Kuraoka, T.; Kajiki, A.; et al. Clinical and microbiological differences between *Mycobacterium abscessus* and *Mycobacterium massiliense* lung diseases. *J. Clin. Microbiol.* **2012**, *50*, 3556–3561. [CrossRef] [PubMed]
36. Nash, K.; Inderlied, C. Genetic basis of macrolide resistance in *Mycobacterium avium* isolated from patients with disseminated disease. *Antimicrob. Agents Chemother.* **1995**, *29*, 2625–2630. [CrossRef] [PubMed]
37. Eliopoulos, G.; Moellering, R., Jr. Antimicrobial combinations. In *Antibiotics in Laboratory Medicine*, 4th ed.; Lorian, V., Ed.; Lippincott Williams & Wilkins: Philadelphia, PA, USA, 1996; pp. 330–396.
38. Caviedes, L.; Delgado, J.; Gilman, R. Tetrazolium microplate assay as a rapid and inexpensive colorimetric method for determination of antibiotic susceptibility of *Mycobacterium tuberculosis*. *J. Clin. Microbiol.* **2002**, *40*, 1873–1874. [CrossRef] [PubMed]
39. Gomez-Flores, R.; Gupta, S.; Tamez-Guerra, R.; Mehta, R. Determination of MICs for *Mycobacterium avium-M. intracellulare* complex in liquid medium by a colorimetric method. *J. Clin. Microbiol.* **1995**, *33*, 1842–1846. [PubMed]
40. Gröblacher, B.; Kunert, O.; Bucar, F. Compounds of *Alpinia katsumadai* as potential efflux inhibitors in *Mycobacterium smegmatis*. *Bioorg. Med. Chem.* **2012**, *20*, 2701–2706. [CrossRef]
41. Coelho, T.; Machado, D.; Couto, I.; Maschmann, R.; Ramos, D.; von Groll, A.; Rossetti, M.; da Silva, P.A.; Viveiros, M. Enhancement of antibiotic activity by efflux inhibitors against multidrug resistant *Mycobacterium tuberculosis* clinical isolates from Brazil. *Front. Microbiol.* **2015**, *6*, 330. [CrossRef]
42. Machado, L.; Spengler, G.; Evaristo, M.; Handzlik, J.; Molnár, J.; Viveiros, M.; Kiec-Kononowicz, K.; Amaral, L. Biological activity of twenty-three hydantoin derivatives on intrinsic efflux pump system of *Salmonella enterica* serovar Enteritidis NCTC 13349. *In Vivo* **2011**, *25*, 769–772.
43. Livak, K.; Schmittgen, T. Analysis of relative gene expression data using real-time quantitative PCR and the $2^{-\Delta\Delta CT}$ method. *Methods* **2001**, *25*, 402–408. [CrossRef]

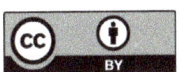

© 2019 by the authors. Licensee MDPI, Basel, Switzerland. This article is an open access article distributed under the terms and conditions of the Creative Commons Attribution (CC BY) license (http://creativecommons.org/licenses/by/4.0/).

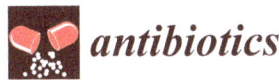

Article

Antimicrobial Activity of Silver Camphorimine Complexes against *Candida* Strains

Joana P. Costa [1], M. Joana F. Pinheiro [1,2], Sílvia A. Sousa [2], Ana M. Botelho do Rego [3], Fernanda Marques [4], M. Conceição Oliveira [1], Jorge H. Leitão [2,*], Nuno P. Mira [2,*] and M. Fernanda N. N. Carvalho [1,*]

[1] Centro de Química Estrutural, Instituto Superior Técnico, Universidade de Lisboa, Av. Rovisco Pais, 1049-001 Lisboa, Portugal
[2] Instituto de Bioengenharia e Biociências, Departamento de Bioengenharia, Instituto Superior Técnico Universidade de Lisboa, Av. Rovisco Pais, 1049-001 Lisboa, Portugal
[3] Centro de Química-Física Molecular e BSIRG, Instituto de Bioengenharia e Biociências, Instituto Superior Técnico Universidade de Lisboa, Av. Rovisco Pais, 1049-001 Lisboa, Portugal
[4] C2TN Centro de Ciências e Tecnologias Nucleares (C2TN), Instituto Superior Técnico, Universidade de Lisboa, Estrada Nacional 10 (km 139,7), 2695-066 Bobadela LRS, Portugal
* Correspondence: jorgeleitao@tecnico.ulisboa.pt (J.H.L.); nuno.mira@tecnico.ulisboa.pt (N.P.M.); fcarvalho@tecnico.ulisboa.pt (M.F.N.N.C.)

Received: 22 August 2019; Accepted: 9 September 2019; Published: 10 September 2019

Abstract: Hydroxide [Ag(OH)L] (L = ^{IV}L, ^{V}L, ^{VI}L, ^{VII}L), oxide [{AgL}$_2$](μ-O) (L = ^{I}L, ^{II}L, ^{III}L, ^{V}L, ^{VI}L) or chloride [Ag^{II}L]Cl, [Ag(^{VI}L)$_2$]Cl complexes were obtained from reactions of mono- or bicamphorimine derivatives with Ag(OAc) or AgCl. The new complexes were characterized by spectroscopic (NMR, FTIR) and elemental analysis. X-ray photoelectron spectroscopy (XPS), ESI mass spectra and conductivity measurements were undertaken to corroborate formulations. The antimicrobial activity of complexes and some ligands were evaluated towards *Candida albicans* and *Candida glabrata*, and strains of the bacterial species *Escherichia coli*, *Burkholderia contaminans*, *Pseudomonas aeruginosa* and *Staphylococcus aureus* based on the Minimum Inhibitory Concentrations (MIC). Complexes displayed very high activity against the *Candida* species studied with the lowest MIC values (3.9 µg/mL) being observed for complexes **9** and **10A** against *C. albicans*. A significant feature of these redesigned complexes is their ability to sensitize *C. albicans*, a trait that was not found for the previously investigated [Ag(NO$_3$)L] complexes. The MIC values of the complexes towards bacteria were in the range of those of [Ag(NO$_3$)L] and well above those of the precursors Ag(OAc) or AgCl. The activity of the complexes towards normal fibroblasts V79 was evaluated by the MTT (3-[4,5-dimethylthiazol-2-yl]-2,5 diphenyl tetrazolium bromide) assay. Results showed that the complexes have a significant cytotoxicity.

Keywords: silver complexes; camphorimine; anti-*Candida* activity; antifungals; antibacterials

1. Introduction

The resistance of microorganisms to conventional antimicrobials is presently a serious threat to public health worldwide, representing a huge financial burden for public health systems. The group of bacterial pathogens known as ESKAPE is of particular concern, which includes *Enterococcus faecium*, *Staphylococcus aureus*, *Klebsiella pneumoniae*, *Acinetobacter baumannii*, *Pseudomonas aeruginosa*, and *Enterobacter* spp. [1]. In addition, fungal infections, and notably candidiasis caused by members of the *Candida* genus, are also of increasing concern worldwide. These infections range from superficial infections to life-threatening disseminated mycoses [2,3]. Although *Candida albicans* remains the major causative agent of candidiasis, there is an increase of the incidence of disseminated infections caused by *C. glabrata*, together with an increased resistance to antifungals among clinical isolates of this species [4,5].

The increasing resistance of pathogenic microorganisms to existing antimicrobials has been accompanied by a scarce increment in the number of alternative compounds commercially available, due to the low interest shown by the pharma industry in the search and development of new antimicrobials [6,7]. The present situation is an explosive combination of increasing resistance to antimicrobials and the lack of investment in novel antimicrobials. Therefore, it is urgent to find novel molecules with chemical characteristics different from those commercially available. Ideally, these molecules should display new modes of action and point to new microbial targets [8]. Aware of such a need, the scientific community has engaged in a search for novel antifungals alternative to azoles, echinocandins, or polyenes [9], as well as for novel antibacterials as alternative to penicillins, cephalosporin, tetracyclines, macrolides, quinolones or sulphonamides [10,11]. Consequently, many new molecules with antimicrobial activity have been described, including peptides from a multitude of species [12,13], natural extracts from plants, herbs, and spices [14], polymers modified with antimicrobial functional groups [15], and metal-based molecules [16].

Complexes are feasible alternatives to the most used organic compounds, since the specific properties of the metal site introduces steric and electronic characteristics relevant to switch distinct mechanisms of action (e.g. electron transfer and redox processes) [17].

The design of complexes to tailor efficient antimicrobial agents requires that the metal and the ligands are chosen according to the antifungal or antibacterial purpose, since the activity towards fungi or bacteria is commonly different [18]. The choice of silver and copper as precursors for the synthesis of complexes is attractive as these metals have been in use for thousands of years. For instance, silver and copper vessels have been used for water and food preservation since the Persian kings due to their antimicrobial properties [16].

Silver-based camphorimine complexes [Ag(NO$_3$)L] emerged among the newly developed molecules with strong antimicrobial potential, having excellent antifungal activity against several pathogenic species of the *Candida* genus [18]. Despite the demonstrated efficacy of the developed camphorimine complexes in inhibiting growth of *C. glabrata*, *C. tropicalis*, and *C. parapsilosis*, there was no inhibition against *C. albicans* by silver nitrate camphorimine complexes [18], a drawback that has now been reported to be surpassed by redesign of the complexes. The characteristics of the camphor ligands to tune the properties, reactivity, and applications of the complexes was evidenced in former work [19–22]. Therefore, a new set of camphorimine complexes was synthesized that exhibits very high activity against *C. albicans*, highlighting the relevance of both the ligands (camphor derivatives) and the co-ligands (NO$_3^-$, OH$^-$ or O^{2-}) to achieve microbial growth inhibition.

2. Results

A new set of camphorimine silver complexes were synthesized using silver acetate (AgOAc) or silver chloride (AgCl) as metal precursors to tune the properties and the antimicrobial activity of the complexes. The objective was to keep the structure of the complexes while replacing the nitrate ion by a less acidic anionic co-ligand (OAc$^-$ or Cl$^-$), aiming to overcome the lack of antifungal activity displayed by the nitrate complexes [Ag(NO$_3$)L] towards *C. albicans*. The absence of antifungal activity was accompanied by formation of silver nanoparticles (AgNPs) [18]. The acidic character of the nitrate ion was hypothesized to favor the reduction processes mediated by a protein existing in *C. albicans*, but not at other *Candida* species. Less acidic co-ligands (OAc$^-$, Cl$^-$) are expected to be less efficient in the activation of AgNPs formation.

The low solubility of silver acetate (AgOAc) in solvents other than water requires that reactions with camphor compounds are carried out in H$_2$O/EtOH since the camphor derivatives used as ligands are not soluble in H$_2$O. Solutions of silver acetate in water have acidic character (pH ca. 4), consistent with release of acetic acid (pKa = 4.76) [23] and formation of silver hydroxide (AgOH) or silver oxide (Ag$_2$O) solutions (Scheme 1).

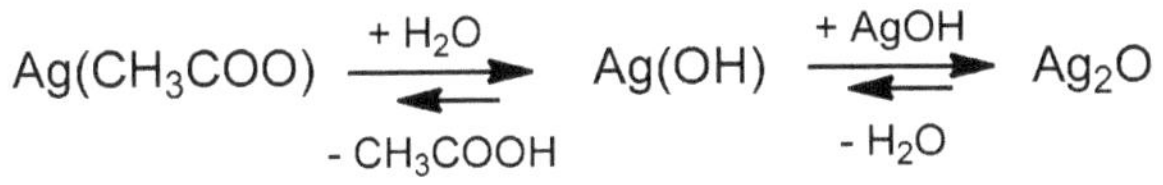

$$\text{Ag(CH}_3\text{COO)} \xrightleftharpoons[-\text{CH}_3\text{COOH}]{+\text{H}_2\text{O}} \text{Ag(OH)} \xrightleftharpoons[-\text{H}_2\text{O}]{+\text{AgOH}} \text{Ag}_2\text{O}$$

Scheme 1. Silver species in aqueous solutions of AgOAc.

Since different forms of silver species co-exist in solution, complexes with different metal cores can be obtained, depending on the characteristics of the camphorimine derivatives (Figure 1) and the experimental conditions.

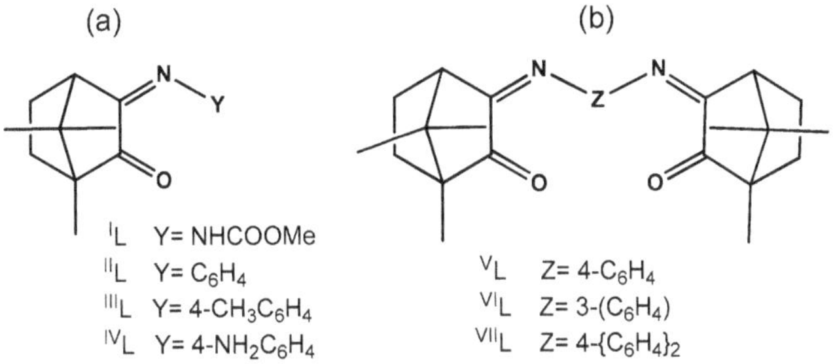

(a)

^{I}L   Y= NHCOOMe
^{II}L Y= C$_6$H$_4$
^{III}L Y= 4-CH$_3$C$_6$H$_4$
^{IV}L Y= 4-NH$_2$C$_6$H$_4$

(b)

^{V}L   Z= 4-C$_6$H$_4$
^{VI}L Z= 3-(C$_6$H$_4$)
^{VII}L Z= 4-{C$_6$H$_4$}$_2$

Figure 1. Camphor derivatives used as ligands: (a) camphorimine and (b) bicamphor type.

Addition of the camphorimine (OC$_{10}$H$_{14}$NY, Figure 1a) or bicamphorimine compounds (OC$_{10}$H$_{14}$N)$_2$Z, Figure 1b) to the silver acetate solution increases the pH value to ca. 7–8, prompting the formation of hydroxide or oxide silver complexes. The camphor mono imine ligands (^{I}L-^{III}L) favor the formation of binuclear complexes with the two silver sites bridged by oxygen [{AgL}$_2$(µ-O)] (1–3), while ^{IV}L and the bicamphor ligands (^{V}L-^{VII}L) prompt the formation of hydroxide type complexes [AgL(OH)] (4–6,10) (Scheme 2).

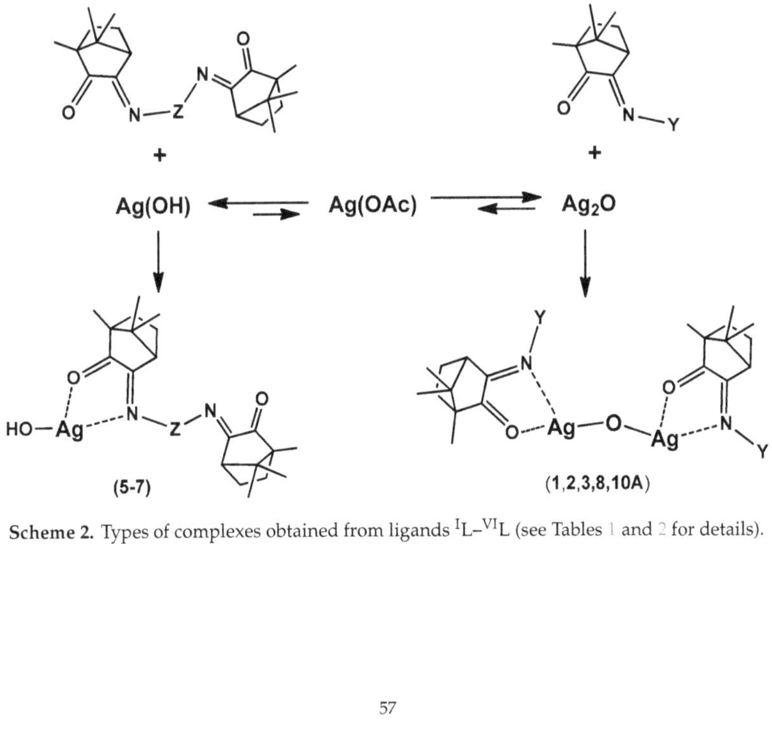

Scheme 2. Types of complexes obtained from ligands ^{I}L-^{VI}L (see Tables 1 and 2 for details).

Table 1. Complexes obtained from reaction of Ag(OAc) with camphor ligands (L).

COMPLEX	LIGAND (L)			IR (cm^{-1}) [a]		^{13}C NMR (δ ppm)	
		Y	Z	$\nu_{C=O}$	$\nu_{C=N}$	C=O	C=N
[{Ag^{I}L}$_2$(μ-O)]	^{I}L (1)	NHCOOMe		1722	1649	(b)	
[{Ag(^{II}L)}$_2$(μ-O)]	^{II}L (2)	C$_6$H$_5$		1745	1652	207.4	173.3 [c]
[{Ag(^{III}L)}$_2$(μ-O)]	^{III}L (3)	4-CH$_3$C$_6$H$_4$		1747	1653	206.8	171.9 [d]
[Ag(OH)(^{IV}L′)] [e]	^{IV}L (4)	4-NH$_2$C$_6$H$_4$		1733	1642 [f]	207.4	169.1 [c]
[{Ag(OH)}(^{V}L)]	^{V}L (5)		4-C$_6$H$_4$	1754	1685	207.3	173.2 [c]
[{Ag(OH)}$_3$(^{VI}L)$_2$]	^{VI}L (6)		3-C$_6$H$_4$	1751	1668	206.6	173.0 [g]
[Ag(OH)(^{VII}L)]	^{VII}L (7)		4-(C$_6$H$_4$)$_2$	1745	1660	206.7	172.5 [g]

[a] In KBr pellets. [b] Not soluble enough. [c] In CD$_3$CN. [d] In MeOH-d$_4$. [e] IVL′ = ^{IV}L·CH$_3$COOH. [f] ν (O=CO), 1593, 1567 cm^{-1}. [g] In CD$_2$Cl$_2$.

The absence of OH stretches in the IR spectra of complexes **1–3** (Table 1) support their formulation as oxide rather than hydroxide complexes. The hydroxide complexes (**4,5,7**) fit in a 1:1 ligand to metal ratio, consistent with a coordination polymer character. At complex **4** ([Ag(^{IV}L′)(OH)]) the ligand (Y=NH$_2$) is protonated (^{IV}L′ = ^{IV}L·HOOCCH$_3$), as confirmed by elemental analysis and FTIR (Table 1) through bands at 3455 and 3340 cm^{-1} (attributed to the OH$^-$ and NH$_4{}^+$ groups) and at 1593, 1567 cm^{-1} (attributed to the acetate (COO$^-$) group). The metal to ligand ratio at **6** (3:2) differs from that of all the other complexes, conceivably due to steric demands of the bicamphorimine ligand. All complexes (**1–7**) were characterized by spectroscopic (FTIR, NMR) and analytical techniques. The relevant spectroscopic characteristics are highlighted in Table 1 (see experimental section for further details). Complex **1** is not sufficiently soluble to obtain NMR data, thus formulation was supported by X-ray photoelectron spectroscopy (XPS).

2.1. Analysis of Complex **1** by XPS

Complex **1** was characterized by XPS. Besides the survey spectrum (not shown), the detailed regions C 1s, N 1s, O 1s, and Ag 3d were analyzed and are shown in Figure 2.

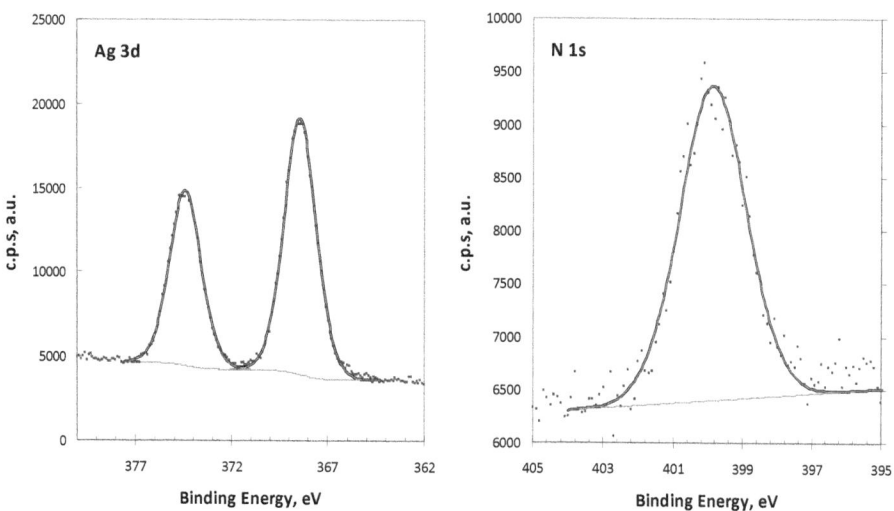

Figure 2. *Cont.*

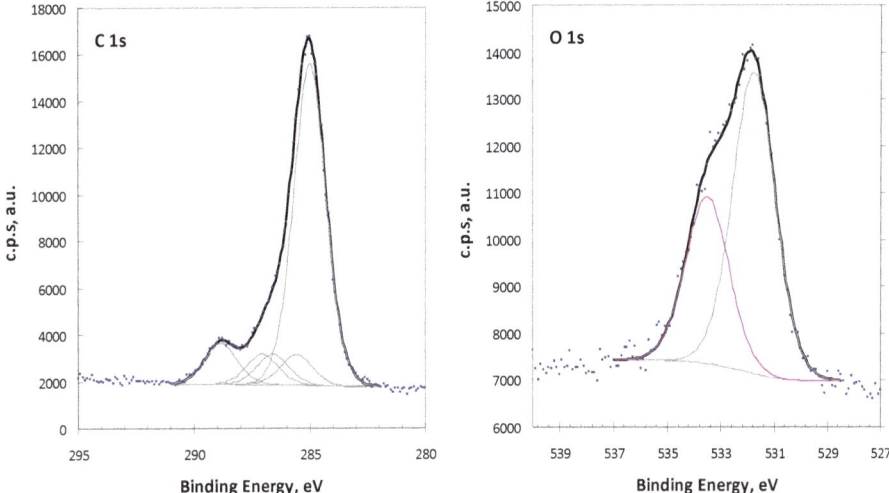

Figure 2. XPS regions Ag 3d, N 1s, C 1s and O 1s for complex **1**.

Ag 3d region displays a doublet with the main component, Ag 3d5/2, centered at 368.4 ± 0.2 eV and the minor component, Ag 3d3/2, at a BE 6 eV higher. N 1s is fittable with a single peak centered at 399.9 ± 0.2 eV. C 1s was fitted with a main peak (used to correct all the binding energies for charge accumulation effects) assigned to all the carbons just bound to other carbon atoms and/or hydrogen atoms set at 285 eV. Other peaks at 285.6 ± 0.2, 286.6 ± 0.2, and 287.1 ± 0.2 eV are assigned to carbon in C–N, in C–O and in C=O bonds, respectively. Finally, a peak at 288.8 ± 0.2 eV is assigned to the urethane group (NHCOOMe) in the ligand and to the acetate group in the precursor. Quantitative results are compatible with the coexistence of the complex and small amounts of the precursor (silver acetate). Discounting the precursor contributions, computed atomic ratios for the complex give the following values: Ag/N = 0.50, Ag/O = 0.29 and O/N = 1.75, fully consistent with the formulation [{Ag^{I}L}2(μ-O)] (L = C$_{10}$H$_{18}$N$_2$O$_3$) proposed for **1**.

2.2. Silver Chloride Derived Complexes

The solubility of silver chloride in common solvents is even lower than that of silver acetate, however it is reasonably soluble in ammonia. Thus, the reactions of AgCl with the camphorimine derivatives (L) were performed in NH$_3$·H$_2$O/EtOH. In such basic medium, silver oxide exists in solution, thus accounting for the formation of the oxide complexes (**3, 9, 10A**). At [{Ag(NH$_3$)}$_2$(μ-^{V}L)(μ-O)] (**9**), ammonia (NH$_3$) further acts as a co-ligand. Complex **3** is either obtained from reaction of ligand ^{III}L with AgCl or Ag(OAc), in agreement with the formation of silver oxides either from silver acetate or silver chloride under the experimental conditions used. By strict control of the order of addition of AgCl to the solutions of ligands ^{II}L and ^{VI}L, non-oxide complexes [Ag(^{II}L)]Cl (**8**) and [Ag(^{VI}L)$_2$]Cl (**10**) were obtained. The cationic character of complex **10** was achieved by ESI-MS analysis. The ESI(+)/MS spectrum for a solution of [Ag(^{VI}L)$_2$]Cl shows a group of peaks at m/z 915/317 (Figure 3), consistent with the ionic complex [Ag(C$_{26}$H$_{32}$N$_2$O$_2$)$_2$]$^+$ formed by two neutral ligands and a silver cation, with the characteristic isotopic distribution of silver-containing species (Figure 3, right upper insert).

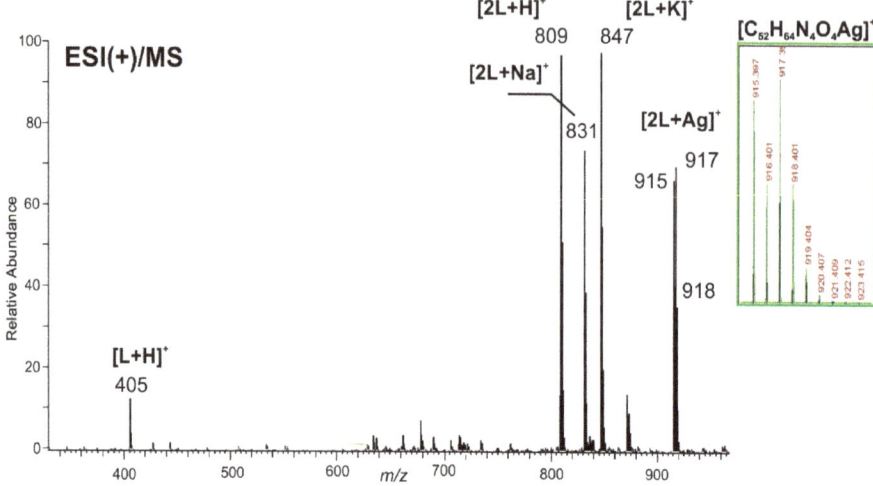

Figure 3. ESI (+) mass spectrum of a solution of [Ag(^{VI}L)$_2$]Cl (**10**) in acetonitrile. The insert shows the theoretical isotopic pattern of the cation [Ag(^{VI}L)$_2$]$^+$ i.e., [Ag(C$_{26}$H$_{32}$N$_2$O$_2$)$_2$]$^+$.

The cationic character of **8** was further confirmed through conductivity measurement (138 Ω^{-1}.cm^2.mole^{-1}) in acetonitrile. The value is within the range (120–160 Ω^{-1}.cm^2.mole^{-1}) expected for a 1:1 electrolyte [24]. Such as for the above complexes **1–7**, the characterization of complexes **8–10A** was achieved by elemental analysis, FTIR and NMR. Some relevant spectroscopic details are displayed in Table 2.

Table 2. Complexes obtained from reaction of silver chloride with camphor ligands (L).

COMPLEX	LIGAND (L)		IR (cm^{-1})		^{13}C NMR (δ ppm)	
	Y	Z	ν$_{C=O}$	ν$_{C=N}$	C=O	C=N
[Ag(^{II}L)]Cl	^{II}L (**8**)	C$_6$H$_5$	1744	1651	207.5	173.2 [a]
[{Ag(^{III}L)}$_2$(μ-O)]	^{III}L (**3**)	4-CH$_3$C$_6$H$_4$	1747	1654	206.8	171.9 [b]
[{Ag(NH$_3$)}$_2$(μ-^{V}L)(μ-O)]	^{V}L (**9**)	4-C$_6$H$_4$	1744	1651	207.5	173.2 [b]
[Ag(^{VI}L)$_2$]Cl	^{VI}L (**10**)	3-C$_6$H$_4$	1750	1661	207.2	173.8 [a]
[Ag$_2$(μ-^{VI}L)(μ-O)]	^{VI}L (**10A**)	3-C$_6$H$_4$	1749	1660	207.3	173.9 [a]

[a] In CD$_3$CN. [b] In CD$_2$Cl$_2$; From reactions of AgCl with ligands ^{I}L and ^{IV}L (Figure 1) no complexes could be obtained. In the case of ^{IV}L, the hydrated ligand was recovered (^{IV}L·H$_2$O) from solution.

2.3. Antimicrobial Activity Assessment

The antimicrobial properties of the above complexes were assessed for *C. albicans* and *C. glabrata*, as well as for the bacterial pathogens *E. coli* ATCC25922, *S. aureus* Newman, *B. contaminans* IST408 and *P. aeruginosa* 477, based on the evaluation of the values of Minimum Inhibitory Concentration (MIC). The selected bacterial strains represent pathogens of medical relevance, difficult to treat and eradicate worldwide, mainly due to their resistance to multiple antibiotics. *B. contaminans* IST408 was isolated from a Portuguese Cystic Fibrosis patient [24]. *P. aeruginosa* and *S. aureus* are members of the ESKAPE group, responsible for many hospital- and community-acquired infections [1]. *E. coli* ATCC25922 is a commonly used reference in antimicrobial activity assays. The antimicrobial activities of complexes **1**, **4**, and **5** were not assessed due to their low solubility (**1**) or stability (**4, 5**).

All the complexes essayed display anti-*Candida* activity that range from 15.6 μg/mL (**1, 2, 6, 9, 10A**) to 125–250 μg/mL (**8, 10**). The antibacterial activity of the complexes (Table 3) ranged from 19 μg/mL (*P. aeruginosa*, **2**) to ≥112 μg/mL (**6, 8, 10**). The MIC values measured for the ligands (^{II}L, ^{III}L, ^{V}L and ^{VI}L) display very high MIC values (≥500 μg/mL) consistent with their lack of antimicrobial activity.

Table 3. Biological values assessed for the camphorimine silver complexes.

Complex.	MIC$_{50}$ (µg/mL)		MIC (µg/mL)				IC$_{50}$ [a] (µg/mL)
	C. albicans	C. glabrata	E. coli ATCC25922	B. contaminans IST408	P. aeruginosa 477	S. aureus Newman	V79 Cells
2	7.8 ± 0.1	15.6 ± 0.1	59.4 ± 0.3	47 ± 7	19 ± 3	125	7 ± 5
3	31.3 ± 0.1	31.3 ± 0.1	56 ± 5	78 ± 2	43 ± 11	58 ± 2	8 ± 5
6	7.8 ± 0.1	15.6 ± 0.1	125	125	60 ± 7	125	3 ± 1
7	15.6 ± 0.1	15.6 ± 0.1	54 ± 3	>125	61 ± 4	>125	12 ± 5
8	125 ± 1	250 ± 1	250	>250	112 ± 14	250	25 ± 14
9	3.9 ± 0.4	7.8 ± 0.1	32 ± 1	125	19 ± 3	125	2 ± 1
10	-	-	>250	>250	>250	>250	-
10A	3.9 ± 0.1	15.6 ± 0.1	52.2 ± 0.2	23 ± 3	43 ± 10	125	1.7 ± 0.9
Ag(OAc)	>500	>500	30.9 ± 0.4	12 ± 2	16 ± 3	29.5 ± 0.1	0.6 ± 0.2
AgCl	500 ± 1	>500	14 ± 2	10 ± 1	12 ± 1	30 ± 2	>30

[a] IC$_{50}$ values for 48 h incubation.

The MIC values (Table 3) show that the complexes are active against bacterial strains *E. coli* ATCC25922, *B. contaminans* IST408, *P. aeruginosa* 477, and *S. aureus* Newman, although at relatively high MIC values. In contrast, the MIC$_{50}$ values obtained for the two *Candida* species are very low, thereby showing that the complexes have higher antifungal than antibacterial activity. Although previous work showed that silver camphorimine complexes [Ag(NO$_3$)L] have high anti *Candida* spp. activity (MIC$_{50}$ 2.0–15.6 µg/mL for *C. parapsilosis*) the complexes **2, 6, 9, 10A**, display values (7.8 µg/mL, **9**) that are even lower than those formerly reported against *C. glabrata* (MIC$_{50}$ ≥15.6 µg/mL) [18]. More important, all complexes (except **8**) are efficient against *C. albicans*, a feature not observed for the nitrate complexes [Ag(NO$_3$)L] [18]. So, by replacing nitrate by hydroxide or oxide co-ligands, we were able to synthesize complexes that inhibit growth of *C. albicans* even more efficiently (MIC$_{50}$ 3.9 µg/mL; **9, 10A**) than *C. glabrata*. The lack of activity of [Ag(^{II}L)]Cl (**8**) towards the two *Candida* species and the bacterial strains under study is attributed to its cationic character. Complex **10**, which is also cationic, displays a relatively low activity (Table 3). These results reinforce those previously obtained for the cationic [Ag(OC$_{10}$H$_{13}$NOH)$_2$]NO$_3$ [19]. The ionic character of the complexes decreases their lipophilicity and conceivably makes it more difficult for their penetration into the intracellular environment of *Candida* spp. or bacterial cells, thereby reducing their activity.

In general, the complexes display both antibacterial and antifungal activities, although they perform better as antifungals than as antibacterials. The MIC values show that some of the complexes have very high antibacterial activity (40–60 µg/mL) and/or excellent antifungal activities (4–8 µg/mL). Overall, the complexes perform better for Gram-negative (MIC 19–61 µg/mL) than for Gram-positive bacteria (*S. aureus* Newman, 58–250 µg/mL). Complexes [{Ag(^{II}L)}$_2$(µ-O)] (**2**) and [{Ag(NH$_3$)}$_2$(µ-^{V}L)(µ-O)] (**9**) display the highest activity against *P. aeruginosa* 477 (MIC, 19 µg/mL) while complex [Ag$_2$(µ-^{VI}L)(µ-O)] (**10A**) displays the highest activity towards *B. contaminans* IST408 (MIC 23 ± 3 µg/mL). These complexes have in common a dinuclear character with the two metals sharing an oxygen atom and camphorimine ligands that may prompt electron delocalization through the aromatic ring. Such characteristics conceivably are not just circumstantial for their antimicrobial activity.

To obtain insights into the toxicity of the complexes towards mammalian cells, the IC$_{50}$ measurements of representative complexes were evaluated towards V79 normal fibroblasts which are cells commonly used to assess the toxicological effects of drugs [25]. Data shows that IC$_{50}$ values of the complexes are low and comparable or even lower than those of the MIC values obtained for fungi (Table 3).

These results were not completely unexpected since fungi and mammalian cells are eukaryotes and therefore some of the mechanisms by which the complexes exert toxicity against the *Candida* spp. may be conserved in the mammalian cells [26]. This difficulty in achieving specificity is a recognized challenge in the design of new compounds selectively targeting fungal cells. Future work will focus on the design of silver camphorimine complexes with both reduced cytotoxicity and enhanced antimicrobial activities.

3. Materials and Methods

3.1. General Procedures

The camphorimines were obtained from camphorquinone by reaction with the appropriate amine or hydrazine in ethanol using reported procedures [18,27–29]. In the case of air sensitive complexes, Schlenk and vacuum techniques were used. Ethanol was purchased from Fisher Scientific, ammonia from Sigma-Aldrich and acetonitrile from Carlo Erba. The amines and hydrazines were purchased from Sigma-Aldrich and silver acetate and silver chloride from Merck.

The IR spectra were obtained from KBr pellets using a JASCO FT/IR 4100 spectrometer. The NMR spectra (^{1}H, ^{13}C, DEPT, HSQC and HMBC) were obtained from MeOH-d4, CD$_3$CN or CD$_2$Cl$_2$ solutions using Bruker Avance II+ spectrometers (300 or 400 MHz). NMR chemical shifts are referred to tetramethylsilane (TMS) (δ = 0 ppm).

The ESI mass spectrum was obtained on a LCQFleet ion trap mass spectrometer equipped with an electrospray source (Thermo Scientific^{TM}, Waltham, MA USA), operating in the positive ion mode. The XPS data was obtained using a Kratos XSAM800 equipment.

Conductivity was measured in acetonitrile (1.0 × 10^{-3} M solution) at 25 °C using a CON 510 bench conductivity meter provided with a Conductivity/TDS electrode (code No. ECCONSEN91W/35608-50, K = 1).

3.2. Synthesis

Complexes 1–7 were obtained from reaction of the suitable ligand with silver acetate (1:1). Air was partially excluded by bubbling of nitrogen (3 minutes). The reaction mixtures were protected from light to preclude reduction of Ag$^+$ to Ag^0. The typical procedure is described for **1**. Complexes 8–10 were obtained from reaction of the suitable ligand with silver chloride (1:1). A typical procedure is described for **8**.

[{Ag^{I}L}$_2$(μ-O)] (**1**)—A solution of the camphorimine OC$_{10}$H$_{14}$NNHCOOMe (^{I}L, 72 mg, 0.35 mmol) in EtOH (5 mL) was added to a suspension of Ag(OAc) (50 mg, 0.35 mmol) in H$_2$O (5 mL) under N$_2$. The whitish suspension was stirred for ca. 1h. The slight suspension still remaining was then removed by filtration and the solution was evaporated to dryness to yield the complex. Yield 55%. Elem. Anal. (%) for Ag$_2$C$_{24}$H$_{36}$N$_4$O$_7$. Found: C, 41.6; N, 7.9; H, 5.1; Calc.: C, 41.4; N, 7.5; H, 5.5. IR (cm^{-1}): 1722 (C=O), 1649 (C=N), 1588 (O=COMe). ^{1}H NMR (400 MHz, MeOH-d4, δ ppm): 4.56 (s, 3H), 3.81 (sbr, 1H), 1.88–1.81 (m, 2H), 1.54–1.44 (m, 2H), 1.18 (s, 3H), 1.04 (s, 3H), 0.85 (s, 3H). ^{13}C NMR Decomposes during acquisition.

[{Ag^{II}L}$_2$(μ-O)] (**2**)—OC$_{10}$H$_{14}$NC$_6$H$_4$ (^{II}L, 72 mg; 0.3 mmol) in ethanol (5 mL) and silver acetate (50 mg; 0.3 mmol) in H$_2$O (5 mL) were stirred for 4 h. Yield 74%. Elem. Anal. (%) for Ag$_2$C$_{32}$H$_{36}$N$_2$O$_3$. Found: C, 54.9 N, 3.5; H, 5.8; Calc.: C, 54.7; N, 3.8; H, 6.2. IR (cm^{-1}): 1745 (C=O), 1652 (C=N), 1567 (CH$_{arom}$). ^{1}H NMR (300 MHz, CD$_3$CN, δ ppm) 7.40 (t, J = 7.8 Hz, 2H), 7.19 (t, J = 7.5 Hz, 1H), 6.90 (d, J = 7.5 Hz, 2H), 2.74 (d, J = 5.1 Hz, 1H), 1.90 (mc, 2H), 1.61 (mc, 2H) 1.04 (s, 3H), 0.97 (s, 3H), 0.86 (s, 3H). ^{13}C NMR (300 MHz, CD$_3$CN, δ ppm): 207.4, 173.3, 130.1, 126.0, 120.9, 59.0, 51.0, 45.3, 30.8, 24.8, 21.16, 17.6, 9.4.

[{Ag^{III}L}$_2$(μ-O)] (**3**)—OC$_{10}$H$_{14}$NC$_6$H$_4$CH$_3$-4 (^{III}L, 76 mg; 0.3 mmol) in ethanol (5 mL) and silver acetate (50 mg; 0.3 mmol) in H$_2$O (5 mL) were stirred for 4 h. Yield 89%. Elem. Anal. (%) for Ag$_2$C$_{34}$H$_{42}$N$_2$O$_3$. Found: C, 55.3 N, 3.5; H, 5.9; Calc.: C, 55.0; N, 3.8; H, 5.7. IR (cm^{-1}): 1747 (C=O), 1653 (C=N), 1565 (CH$_{arom}$). ^{1}H NMR (300 MHz, CD$_2$Cl$_2$, δ ppm): 7.24 (d, J = 7.5 Hz, 2H), 6.97 (d, J = 7.5 Hz, 2H), 2.92 (d, J = 4.8 Hz, 1H), 2.36 (s, 3H), 2.3–1.9 (m, 2H), 1.6–1.5 (m, 2H), 1.61 (s, 3H) 1.07 (s, 3H), 0.98 (s, 3H), 0.87 (s, 3H). ^{13}C NMR (300 MHz, CD$_2$Cl$_2$, δ ppm): 206.9, 174.2, 146.2, 138.6, 130.9, 123.2, 59.1, 52.2, 46.0, 31.3, 24.9, 21.3, 21.0, 17.4, 9.2.

Compound **3** can alternatively be obtained from reaction of AgCl (50 mg; 0.35 mmol in 5 mL of ammonia 33%) with ^{III}L (89 mg; 0.35mmol in 5 mL EtOH) upon stirring overnight, filtration to eliminate residues of silver followed by solvent evaporation until precipitation which is then dried under vacuum to obtain 3. The yield (60%) is lower than that in reaction of ^{III}L with Ag(OAc).

[Ag(^{IV}L)(OH)]·CH$_3$COOH (**4**)—OC$_{10}$H$_{14}$NC$_6$H$_4$NH$_2$-4 (^{IV}L, 46 mg; 0.18 mmol) in ethanol (3 mL) and silver acetate (30 mg; 0.18 mmol) in H$_2$O (3 mL). The solutions were degassed. The mixture was stirred for 4 h under N$_2$. Yield 57%. Elem. Anal. (%) for AgC$_{18}$H$_{25}$N$_2$O$_4$. Found: C, 49.3; N, 6.2; H, 5.4; Calc.: C, 49.0; N, 6.4; H, 5.7; IR (cm^{-1}): 3454 (OH), 3339 (NH$_2$), 1733 (C=O), 1625 (C=N), 1593 (CH$_{arom}$), 1567 (O=CO), 1504 (NH$_2$). ^{1}H NMR (300 MHz, CD$_3$CN, δ ppm): 6.93 (d, J = 8.6 Hz, 2H), 6.70 (d, J = 8.6 Hz, 2H), 4.30 (sbr, 2H) 2.98 (d, J = 4.7 Hz, 1H), 1–91–1.84 (m, 3H), 1.68–1.51 (m, 3H), 1.06 (s, 3H), 1.00 (s, 3H), 0.83 (s, 3H). ^{13}C NMR (300 MHz, CD$_3$CN, δ ppm): 207.0, 169.1, 161.3, 146.1, 139.8, 124.5, 115.3, 58.0, 51.0, 45.3, 30.8, 24.4, 20.9, 17.7, 9.2.

[{Ag(OH)(^{V}L)] (**5**)—A solution of 4-C$_6$H$_4$(OC$_{10}$H$_{14}$N)$_2$ (^{V}L, 117 mg; 0.3 mmol) in ethanol (5 mL) and silver acetate (50 mg; 0.3 mmol) in H$_2$O (5 mL) were stirred for 5 h. The complex precipitates from reaction mixture. Yield 54%. Elem. Anal. (%) for AgC$_{26}$H$_{33}$N$_2$O$_3$·H$_2$O. Found: C, 57.2 N, 4.8; H, 6.1; Calc.: C, 57.0; N, 5.1; H, 6.4. IR (cm^{-1}) 1750 (C=O), 1649 (C=N), 1559 (CH$_{arom}$). ^{1}H NMR(300 MHz, CD$_3$CN, δ ppm) 6.98 (s, 4H), 2.86 (d, J = 4.9 Hz, 2H), 1.9 (mc, 3H), 1.05 (s, 6H), 0.99 (s, 6H), 0.86 (s, 6H). ^{13}C NMR (300 MHz, CD$_3$CN, δ ppm): 207.3, 173.2, 148.0, 122.4, 58.9, 51.2, 45.3, 30.9, 24.9, 21.2, 17.6, 9.4.

[{Ag(OH)}$_3$(^{VI}L)$_2$] (**6**)—3-C$_6$H$_4$(OC$_{10}$H$_{14}$N)$_2$ (^{VI}L, 199 mg; 0.5 mmol) in ethanol (8.5 mL) was added to a solution of silver acetate (95 mg; 0.5 mmol) in H$_2$O (8.5 mL) and the mixture stirred overnight. Yield 62%. Elem. Anal. (%) for Ag$_3$C$_{52}$H$_{67}$N$_4$O$_7$ Found: C, 53.1 N, 4.3; H, 5.6; Calc.: C, 52.8; N, 4.7; H, 5.7. IR (cm^{-1}): 1751 (C=O), 1668 (C=N), 1566 (CH$_{arom}$). ^{1}H NMR (400 MHz, CD$_2$Cl$_2$, δ ppm): 7.34 (t, J = 7.9, Hz,1H), 6.68 (2d, J = 1.9 Hz, 2H), 6.34 (s, 1H), 2.77 (d, J = 4.4 Hz, 2H), 2.16–2.01 (m, 2H), 1.94–1.80 (m, 2H), 1.68–1.54 (m, 4H), 1.03 (s, 6H), 0.94 (s, 6H), 0.85 (s, 6H). ^{13}C NMR(400 MHz, CD$_2$Cl$_2$, δ ppm): 206.6, 173.0, 151.1, 130.1, 117.2, 111.4, 58.5, 50.6, 44.8, 30.5, 24.7, 21.1, 17.6, 9.2.

[Ag(OH)(^{VII}L)] (**7**)—^{VII}L (44 mg; 0.3 mmol) in ethanol (10 mL) was added to Ag(OAc) (100 mg; 0.6 mmol) in H$_2$O (10 mL) and stirred overnight. Yield 88%. Elem. Anal. (%) for AgC$_{32}$H$_{37}$N$_2$O$_3$ Found: C, 64.0; N, 4.3; H, 6.1; Calc.: C, 63.6; N, 4.6; H, 6.2. IR (cm^{-1}): 3421 (OH), 1745 (C=O), 1660 (C=N), 1566 (CH$_{arom}$). ^{1}H NMR (300 MHz, CD$_2$Cl$_2$, δ ppm): 7.65 (d, J = 8.1 Hz, 4H), 7.03 (d, J = 7.9 Hz, 4H), 2.89 (d, J = 4.5 Hz, 2H), 2.21–2.07 (m, 2H), 1.96–1.81 (m, 2H), 1.72–1.60 (m, 4H), 1.10 (s, 6H), 1.01 (s, 6H), 0.92 (s, 6H). ^{13}C NMR (300 MHz, CD$_2$Cl$_2$, δ ppm): 206.7, 172.5, 149.3, 137.9, 127.8, 121.5, 58.4, 50.7, 44.9, 30.6, 24.7, 21.1, 17.7, 9.2.

[{AgCl(^{II}L)] (**8**)—To a solution of AgCl (50 mg; 0.35 mmol) in ammonia (33%,5 mL) a solution of the ligand ^{III}L (84 mg; 0.35 mmol) in EtOH (5 mL) was added. N$_2$ was then bubbled for a few minutes. The mixture was stirred for 3 h at RT. The slight suspension was filtered off and the volume of the solution was reduced until precipitation. Upon filtration the title compound was obtained and dried under vacuum. Yield 59%. Elem. Anal. (%) for AgClC$_{16}$H$_{19}$NO. Found: C, 50.3; N, 3.6; H, 5.1; Calc.: C, 50.0; N, 3.6; H, 5.0. IR (cm^{-1}): 1744 (CO), 1651 (CN), 1589 (CH$_{arom}$). ^{1}H NMR (400 MHzCD$_3$CN, δ ppm): 7.40 (t, J = 7.5 Hz, 2H), 7.19 (t, J = 7.3 Hz 1H), 6.90 (d, J = 7.7 Hz, 2H), 2.74 (d, J = 4.3 Hz, 1H), 1.91–1.84 (m, 2H), 1.66–1.55 (m, 2H) 1.04 (s, 3H), 0.97 (s, 3H), 0.86 (s, 3H). ^{13}C NMR(400 MHz, CD$_3$CN, δ ppm): 207.5, 150.9, 130.1, 126.0, 120.9, 58.9, 51.1, 45.2, 30.8, 24.8, 21.2, 17.6, 9.4.

[{Ag(NH$_3$)}$_2$(μ-^{V}L)(μ-O)] (**9**)—A solution of the ligand ^{V}L (75 mg; 0.19 mmol) in EtOH (2.5 mL) was added to a solution of AgCl (23 mg; 0.16 mmol) in ammonia (33%, 2.5 mL). The mixture was stirred for 4 h at RT. Yield 69%. Anal. (%) for Ag$_2$C$_{26}$H$_{38}$N$_4$O$_3$. Found: C, 46.4 N, 8.0; H, 5.3; Calc.: C, 46.6; N, 8.4; H, 5.7. IR (cm^{-1}): 3341 (NH), 1753 (CO), 1621 (CN), 1595 (CH$_{arom}$), 1505 (NH). ^{1}H NMR (400 MHz, MeOH-d$_4$, δ ppm): 7.06 (s, 4H), 2.92 (d, J = 4.4 Hz, 2H), 2.29–2.17 (m, 2H), 2.02–1.93 (m, 2H), 1.75–1.56 (m, 4H) 1.09 (s, 6H), 1.07 (s, 6H), 0.83 (s, 6H). ^{13}C NMR (400 MHz, MeOH-d$_4$, δ ppm): 190.5, 169.8, 148.8, 125.4, 123.1, 116.2, 58.9, 49.5, 45.7, 31.3, 25.0, 21.3, 17.9, 9.3. There is evidence for two isomers in solution that were not further investigated.

[AgCl(^{VI}L)$_2$] (**10**)—Solid AgCl (50 mg; 0.35 mmol) was added to ^{VI}L (137 mg; 0.35 mmol) in Et$_2$OH (5 mL) followed by addition of ammonia (33%, 5 mL). The mixture was stirred for 3 h. Yield 72%. Anal. (%) AgClC$_{52}$H$_{64}$N$_4$O$_4$. Found: C, 65.9 N, 5.8; H, 6.8; Calc.: C, 65.6; N, 5.9; H, 6.8. IR (cm^{-1}): 1750

(CO), 1661 (CN), 1579 (CH$_{arom}$). ^{1}H NMR (400 MHz, CD$_3$CN, δ ppm): 7.4 (t, J = 7.9 Hz, 1H); 6.7 (2d, J = 7.9 Hz, 2H), 6.34 (m, 1H), 2.77 (d, J = 4.5 Hz, 2H), 1.04 (s, 3H), 0.98 (s, 3H), 0.87 (s, 3H). ^{13}C NMR (400 MHz, CD$_3$CN, δ ppm): 207.2, 173.8, 152.1, 131.1, 111.3, 59.0, 51.2, 45.2, 30.8, 24.9, 21.2, 17.6, 9.4.

[Ag$_2$(μ-^{VI}L)(μ-O)] (**10A**)—Addition of ^{VI}L (137 mg; 0.35 mmol, 5 mL H$_2$O) after complete dissolution of AgCl (50 mg; 0.35 mmol) in ammonia (33%, 5 mL) followed by stirring overnight. Yield 56%. Anal. (%) Ag$_2$C$_{26}$H$_{32}$N$_2$O$_3$·H$_2$O. Found: C, 47.7; N, 4.5; H, 5.0. Calc.: C, 47.7; N, 4.3; H, 5.2. IR (cm^{-1}): 1749 (CO), 1660 (CN), 1579 (CH$_{arom}$). ^{1}H NMR (400 MHz, CD$_3$CN, δ ppm): 7.43 (t, J = 7.9 Hz, 1H), 6.7 (dd, J = 1.7, Hz J = 7.9 Hz, 2H), 6.34 (m, 1H), 2.77 (d, J = 4.9 Hz, 2H), 2.12–2.03 (m, 2H), 1.91–1.75 (m, 2H), 1.64–1.56 (m, 4H), 1.04 (s, 6H), 0.98 (s, 6H), 0.87 (s, 6H). ^{13}C NMR (400 MHz, CD$_3$CN, δ ppm): 207.3, 173.9, 152.0, 130.9, 117.4, 111.3, 59.0, 51.1, 45.1, 30.8, 24.9, 21.2, 17.6, 9.3.

3.3. Antibacterial Activity Determinations

The antibacterial activity of compounds was assessed by determining their Minimal Inhibitory Concentration (MIC) towards the Gram-positive *Staphylococcus aureus* Newman and the Gram-negative *Escherichia coli* ATCC 25922, *Pseudomonas aeruginosa* 477 and *Burkholderia contaminans* IST408. These bacterial strains are clinical isolates and were chosen as representatives of important bacterial pathogens [1,25,30–32]. MICs were determined using Mueller Hinton Broth (MHB; Becton, Dickinson and Company) as growth medium, based on microdilution assays, using previously described methods [20,21]. In brief, a colony from a bacterial culture freshly grown in MHB solid medium was transferred into MHB liquid medium and incubated for 4–5 h with agitation (250 rpm) at 37 °C. Bacterial cultures were then diluted using fresh MHB to obtain ca. 10^6 colony forming units (CFUs) per mL. These cultures were used to inoculate approximately 5×10^5 CFUs per mL in 96-well polystyrene microtiter plates containing 100 μL of MHB supplemented with different concentrations of each compound, obtained by 1:2 serial dilutions ranging 0.5 to 512 μg/mL. Stock solutions of compounds were prepared with DMSO. After inoculation, microtiter plates were incubated at 37 °C for 20 h. Bacterial growth was assessed by measuring the cultures optical density at 640 nm, in a SPECTROstarNano (BMG LABTECH) microplate reader. Experiments were carried out at least four times in duplicates. Wells containing 100 μL of 1× concentrated MHB and 100 μL of 10^6 CFUs per mL were used as positive controls, while wells containing 200 μL of sterile MHB 1 × concentrated were used as negative controls.

3.4. Assessment of Complexes Anti-Candida Activity

The ability of the complexes 1–10A or of the ligands to inhibit growth of *C. albicans* or *C. glabrata* was assessed using the highly standardized microdilution method recommended by EUCAST (European Committee on Antimicrobial Susceptibility Testing). The MIC$_{50}$ values were considered to be the concentration of drug that reduced yeast growth by more than 50% of the growth registered in drug-free medium [33]. The strains used in this work were *C. albicans* SC5314 and *C. glabrata* CBS138, largely used as reference strains. Briefly, cells of the different species were cultivated (at 30 °C and with 250 rpm orbital agitation) for 17 h in Yeast Potato Dextrose (YPD) growth medium and then diluted in fresh Roswell Park Memorial Institute (RPMI) growth medium (Sigma) to obtain a cell suspension having an OD$_{530nm}$ of 0.05. From these cell suspensions, 100 μL aliquots were mixed in the 96-multiwell polystyrene plates with 100 μL of fresh RPMI medium (control) or with 100 μL of this same medium supplemented with 0.98–500 μg/mL of the different compounds. As a control we also examined the inhibitory effect of Ag(OAc) or of AgCl. After inoculation, the 96-multiwell plates were incubated without agitation at 37 °C for 24 h. After that time, cells were re-suspended and the OD$_{530nm}$ of the cultures was measured in a SPECTROstarNano (BMG LABTECH) microplate reader. The MIC$_{50}$ value was taken as being the highest concentration tested at which the growth of the strains was 50% of the value registered in the control lane.

3.5. Toxicity Assessment

The toxicity of the compounds was evaluated towards normal fibroblasts V79, obtained from the American Type Culture Collection (ATCC). The cell lines were grown in Dulbeco's Modified Eagle Medium (DMEM) + Glutamax® medium supplemented with 10% Fetal Bovine serum (FBS) and maintained in a humidified atmosphere at 37 °C using an incubator (Heraeus, Germany) with 5% CO_2. Cell viability was measured by the MTT (3-[4,5-dimethylthiazol-2-yl]-2,5 diphenyl tetrazolium bromide) assay, based on the conversion of the tetrazolium bromide into formazan crystals by living cells which determines mitochondria activity [34]. For the assay, cells were seeded in 96-well plates at a density of 10^4 cells per well in 200 µL medium and allowed to attach overnight. Complexes were first diluted in DMSO to solubilize and then in medium to prepare the serial dilutions in the range 10^{-7}–10^{-4} M. The maximum concentration of DMSO in the medium (1%) had no toxicity effect. After careful removal of the medium, 200 µL of each dilution were added to the cells, and incubated for another 48 h at 37 °C. At the end of the treatment, the medium was aspirated and 200 µL of MTT solution (1.5 mM in PBS) was applied to each well. After 3 h at 37 °C, the medium was discarded and 200 µL of DMSO was added to solubilize the formazan crystals. The cellular viability was assessed by measuring the absorbance at 570 nm using a plate spectrophotometer (Power Wave Xs, Bio-Tek). The IC_{50} values were calculated using the GraphPad Prism software (version 5.0). Results are mean ± SD of at least two independent experiments done with six replicates each and represent the percentage of cellular viability related to the controls (no treatment).

3.6. X-ray Photoelectron Spectroscopy

For X-ray photoelectron spectroscopy characterization (XPS), a XSAM800 XPS dual anode spectrometer from KRATOS was used. The unmonochromatic Mg Kα radiation (main line at hν = 1256.6 eV) was used. Operating conditions, data acquisition and data treatment are described elsewhere [35]. For charge correction purposes, carbon bound to carbon and hydrogen in C 1s peak was set to a binding energy (BE) of 285 eV. For quantification purposes, the following sensitivity factors were used: 0.318 for C 1s, 0.736 for O 1s, 0.505 for N 1s, and 6.345 for Ag3d.

4. Conclusions

Silver hydroxide [Ag(OH)L] (L = ^{IV}L, ^{V}L, ^{VI}L, ^{VII}L), oxide [{AgL}$_2$}(µ-O)] (L = ^{I}L, ^{II}L, ^{III}L, ^{V}L, ^{VI}L) and homoleptic [Ag^{II}L]Cl, [Ag(^{VI}L)$_2$]Cl camphorimine complexes were synthesized using Ag(OAc) or AgCl as metal sources. The basic characteristics of the reaction medium prompted the formation of hydroxide or oxide rather than acetate or chloride complexes. The selection of the camphorimine ligands (L) that encompass mono- and bi-camphors, allowed the design of complexes with considerable distinct electronic and steric properties and thus different biological activities.

In summary, the most relevant achievement of this study is that the new oxo and hydroxo silver camphorimine complexes overreach the resistance of *C. albicans*. Additionally, the complexes reach MIC_{50} values for *C. glabrata* even lower than those previously reported for the camphorimine nitrate complexes [Ag(NO$_3$)L]. In fact, the antifungal activity of the oxo and hydroxo silver camphorimine complexes is even higher towards *C. albicans* than *C. glabrata*.

Author Contributions: Conceptualization, M.F.N.N.C., N.P.M., and J.H.L.; Experimental data acquisition, J.P.C., M.J.F.P., S.A.S., M.C.O., A.M.B.R., F.M., M.F.N.N.C.; methodology and data curation: all authors; writing—original draft preparation, M.F.N.N.C., J.H.L., N.P.M., A.M.B.R., F.M.; writing—review and editing, all authors; funding acquisition, M.F.N.N.C., N.P.M., J.H.L., F.M.

Funding: This research received no external funding.

Acknowledgments: Financial support by FCT-Fundação para a Ciência e Tecnologia through projects ID/QUI/00100/2019, UID/BIO/04565/2019, UID/MULTI/04349/2019, Grant BL-CQE/2018-013, contract PTDC/BIA-MIC/31515/2017 and Programa Operacional Regional de Lisboa 2020 (Project No. 007317) is gratefully acknowledged as well as facilities from the NMR and Mass Spectra Networks (IST-UTL Nodes).

Conflicts of Interest: The authors declare no conflict of interest. The funders had no role in the design of the study; in the collection, analyses, or interpretation of data; in the writing of the manuscript, or in the decision to publish the results.

References

1. Boucher, H.W.; Talbot, G.H.; Bradley, J.S.; Edwards, J.E., Jr.; Gilbert, D.; Rice, L.B.; Scheld, M.; Spellberg, B.; Bartlett, J. Bad bugs, no drugs: No ESKAPE! An update from the Infectious Diseases Society of America. *Clin. Infect. Dis.* **2009**, *48*, 1–12. [CrossRef] [PubMed]
2. Lim, C.S.; Rosli, R.; Seow, H.F.; Chong, P.P. *Candida* and invasive candidiasis: Back to basics. *Eur. J. Clin. Microbiol. Infect. Dis.* **2012**, *31*, 21–31. [CrossRef] [PubMed]
3. Witherden, E.A.; Shoaie, S.; Hall, R.A.; Moyes, D.L. The Human Mucosal Mycobiome and Fungal Community Interactions. *J. Fungi* **2017**, *3*, 56. [CrossRef] [PubMed]
4. Pfaller, M.A.; Diekema, D.J.; Gibbs, D.L.; Newell, V.A.; Ellis, D.; Tullio, V.; Rodloff, A.; Fu, W.; Ling, T.A.; Global Antifungal Surveillance Group. Results from the ARTEMIS DISK Global Antifungal Surveillance Study, 1997 to 2007: A 10.5-year analysis of susceptibilities of *Candida* Species to fluconazole and voriconazole as determined by CLSI standardized disk diffusion. *J. Clin. Microbiol.* **2010**, *48*, 1366–1377. [PubMed]
5. Pfaller, M.A.; Diekema, D.J.; Turnidge, J.D.; Castanheira, M.; Jones, R.N. Twenty Years of the SENTRY Antifungal Surveillance Program: Results for *Candida* Species From 1997–2016. *Open Forum Infect. Dis.* **2019**, *15*, S79–S94. [CrossRef] [PubMed]
6. Theuretzbacher, U. Future antibiotics scenarios: Is the tide starting to turn? *Int. J. Antimicrob. Agents* **2009**, *34*, 15–20. [CrossRef] [PubMed]
7. Aslam, B.; Wang, W.; Arshad, M.I.; Khurshid, M.; Muzammil, S.; Rasool, M.H.; Nisar, M.A.; Alvi, R.F.; Aslam, M.A.; Qamar, M.U.; et al. Antibiotic resistance: A rundown of a global crisis. *Infect. Drug Resist.* **2018**, *11*, 1645–1658. [CrossRef] [PubMed]
8. Singh, S.B.; Young, K.; Silver, L.L. What is an "ideal" antibiotic? Discovery challenges and path forward. *Biochem. Pharmacol.* **2017**, *133*, 63–73. [CrossRef]
9. Nett, J.E.; Andes, D.R. Antifungal Agents: Spectrum of Activity, Pharmacology, and Clinical Indications. *Infect. Dis. Clin. N. Am.* **2016**, *30*, 51–83. [CrossRef]
10. Etubu, E.; Arikekpar, I. Antibiotics: Classification and mechanisms of action with emphasis on molecular perspectives. *Int. J. Appl. Microbiol. Biotechnol. Res.* **2016**, *4*, 90–101.
11. Kapoor, G.; Saigal, S.; Elongavan, A. Action and resistance mechanisms of antibiotics: A guide for clinicians. *J. Anaesthesiol. Clin. Pharmacol.* **2017**, *33*, 300–305. [CrossRef] [PubMed]
12. Park, Y.-K.; Kyung-Soo, H. Antimicrobial Peptides (AMPs): Peptide Structure and Mode of Action. *BMB Rep.* **2005**, *38*, 507–516. [CrossRef]
13. Ghosh, C.; Sarkar, P.; Issa, R.; Aldar, J. Alternatives to Conventional Antibiotics in the Era of Antimicrobial Resistance. *Trends Microbiol.* **2019**, *27*, 323–338. [CrossRef]
14. Singh, P.A.; Desai, S.D.; Singh, J. A Review on Plant Antimicrobials of Past Decade. *Curr. Top. Med. Chem.* **2018**, *18*, 812. [CrossRef] [PubMed]
15. Kenawy, E.R.; Worley, S.D.; Broughton, R. The chemistry and applications of antimicrobial polymers: A state-of-the-art review. *Biomacromolecules* **2007**, *8*, 1359–1384. [CrossRef] [PubMed]
16. Lemire, J.A.; Harrison, J.J.; Turner, R.J. Antimicrobial activity of metals: Mechanisms, molecular targets and applications. *Nat. Rev. Microbiol.* **2013**, *11*, 371–384. [CrossRef] [PubMed]
17. Liang, X.; Luan, S.; Yin, Z.; He, M.; He, C.; Yin, L.; Zou, Y.; Yuan, Z.; Li, L.; Song, X.; et al. Recent advances in the medical use of silver complex. *Eur. J. Med. Chem.* **2018**, *157*, 62–80. [CrossRef]
18. Cardoso, J.M.; Guerreiro, S.I.; Lourenco, A.; Alves, M.M.; Montemor, M.F.; Mira, N.P.; Leitão, J.H.; Carvalho, M.F.N. Ag(I) camphorimine complexes with antimicrobial activity towards clinically important bacteria and species of the *Candida* genus. *PLoS ONE* **2017**, *12*, e0177355. [CrossRef]
19. Carvalho, M.F.N.; Leite, S.; Costa, J.P.; Galvão, A.M.; Leitão, J.H. Ag(I) camphor complexes: Antimicrobial activity by design. *J. Inorg. Biochem.* **2019**, *199*, 110791. [CrossRef]
20. Leitão, J.H.; Sousa, S.A.; Leite, S.A.; Carvalho, M.F.N. Silver Camphor Imine Complexes: Novel Antibacterial Compounds from Old Medicines. *Antibiotics* **2018**, *7*, 65. [CrossRef]

21. Cardoso, J.M.S.; Galvão, A.M.; Guerreiro, S.I.; Leitão, J.H.; Suarez, A.C.; Carvalho, M.F.N. Antibacterial activity of silver camphorimine coordination polymers. *Dalton Trans* **2016**, *45*, 7114–7123. [CrossRef] [PubMed]
22. Cardoso, J.M.S.; Correia, I.; Galvão, A.M.; Marques, F.; Carvalho, M.F.N. Synthesis of Ag(I) camphor sulphonylimine complexes and assessment of their cytotoxic properties against cisplatin-resistant A2780cisR and A2780 cell lines. *J. Inorg. Biochem.* **2017**, *166*, 55–63. [CrossRef] [PubMed]
23. Bordwell, F.G.; Algrim, D. Nitrogen acids. 1. Carboxamides and sulfonamides. *J. Org. Chem.* **1976**, *41*, 2507–2508. [CrossRef]
24. Geary, W.J. The use of conductivity measurements in organic solvents for the characterisation of coordination compounds. *Coord. Chem. Rev.* **1971**, *7*, 81–122. [CrossRef]
25. Richau, J.A.; Leitão, J.H.; Sá-Correia, I. Enzymes leading to the nucleotide sugar precursors for exopolysaccharide synthesis in *Burkholderia cepacia*. *Biochem. Biophys. Res. Commun.* **2000**, *276*, 71–76. [CrossRef] [PubMed]
26. Doehmer, J. Predicting Drug Metabolism–dependent Toxicity for Humans with a Genetically Engineered Cell Battery. *Altern. Lab. Anim.* **2006**, *34*, 561–575. [CrossRef] [PubMed]
27. Mazu, T.K.; Bricker, B.A.; Flores-Rozas, H.; Ablordeppey, S.Y. The Mechanistic Targets of Antifungal Agents: An Overview. *Mini-Rev. Med. Chem.* **2016**, *16*, 555–578. [CrossRef] [PubMed]
28. Fernandes, T.A.; Mendes, F.; Roseiro, A.P.S.; Santos, I.; Carvalho, M.F.N. Insight into the cytotoxicity of polynuclear Cu(I) camphor complexes. *Polyhedron* **2015**, *87*, 215–219. [CrossRef]
29. Carvalho, M.F.N.; Costa, L.M.G.; Pombeiro, A.J.L.; Schier, A.; Scherer, W.; Harbi, S.K.; Verfürth, U.; Herrmann, R. Synthesis, structure, and electrochemistry of palladium complexes with camphor-derived chiral ligands. *Inorg. Chem.* **1994**, *33*, 6270–6277. [CrossRef]
30. Denmark, S.D.; Rivera, I. Asymmetric Carboalkoxyalkylidenation with a Chiral Horner-Wadsworth-Emmons Reagent. *J. Org. Chem.* **1994**, *59*, 6887–6889. [CrossRef]
31. Rice, L.B. Federal funding for the study of antimicrobial resistance in nosocomial pathogens: No ESKAPE. *J. Infect. Dis.* **2008**, *197*, 1079–1081. [CrossRef] [PubMed]
32. Sousa, S.A.; Feliciano, J.R.; Pita, T.; Guerreiro, S.I.; Leitão, J.H. *Burkholderia cepacia* Complex Regulation of Virulence Gene Expression: A Review. *Genes* **2017**, *8*, 43. [CrossRef] [PubMed]
33. Arendrup, M.C.; Cuenca-Estrella, M.; Lass-Flörl, C.; Hope, W.; EUCAST-AFST. EUCAST technical note on the EUCAST definitive document EDef 7.2: Method for the determination of broth dilution minimum inhibitory concentrations of antifungal agents for yeasts EDef 7.2 (EUCAST-AFST). *Clin. Microbiol. Infect.* **2012**, *18*, E246–E247. [CrossRef] [PubMed]
34. Van Meerloo, J.; Kaspers, G.; Cloos, J. Cell sensitivity assays: The MTT assay. *Mol. Biol.* **2011**, *731*, 237–245.
35. Carapeto, A.P.; Ferraria, A.M.; do Rego, A.M.B. Unraveling the reaction mechanism of silver ions reduction by chitosan from so far neglected spectroscopic features. *Carbohydr. Polym.* **2017**, *174*, 601–609. [CrossRef] [PubMed]

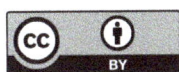

© 2019 by the authors. Licensee MDPI, Basel, Switzerland. This article is an open access article distributed under the terms and conditions of the Creative Commons Attribution (CC BY) license (http://creativecommons.org/licenses/by/4.0/).

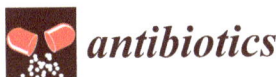

Article

Assessing National Antimicrobial Resistance Campaigns Using a Health Equity Assessment Tool (HEAT)

Graeme Hood, Lina Toleikyte and Diane Ashiru-Oredope *

Public Health England, London SE1 8UG, UK
* Correspondence: diane.ashiru-oredope@phe.gov.uk; Tel.: +44-020-7811-7240

Received: 15 June 2019; Accepted: 14 August 2019; Published: 17 August 2019

Abstract: It has been widely recognised that a significant proportion of the world's population suffer inequalities in accessing high quality healthcare and wider services. Within healthcare, antimicrobial resistance (AMR) is a global threat to public health affecting all healthcare systems and growing at an alarming pace. To ensure that national AMR campaigns developed by Public Health England are inclusive of all populations within the target audience a health equity assessment tool (HEAT) was used. The project leads for each campaign completed the HEAT independently with a follow up meeting with the study team to discuss and clarify the responses. A trend analysis was carried out with common themes being used to provide recommendations. The campaigns have demonstrated equality and diversity based on the requirements of the Equality Act 2010, particularly age, sex, and race protected characteristics. Some notable results include the translation of website materials in over 30 languages and reaching individuals in 122 countries. It was however noted that several of the protected characteristics were not applicable. The continuous development of resources with collaboration from a variety of diverse user groups would be advantageous towards aiding future campaign reach. The use of the HEAT has demonstrated the ease and cost-effective way to assess any health inequalities and would be a useful addition to antimicrobial stewardship and public health campaigns.

Keywords: antimicrobial stewardship; health inequalities; health equity assessment tool; public health

1. Introduction

Research has shown that there are inequalities in accessing high quality healthcare across the world, which affects a large proportion of people [1]. It has been estimated by the World Health Organisation (WHO) that 400 million people do not have access to one of seven essential health services, such as drugs and vaccines [2]. The variations in health inequalities have been reported both at a national and at an international level with the average life expectancy in the UK (81.2 years) lower than Japan (83.7 years) but higher than Sierra Leone (50.1 years) [1]. The health inequalities are classified as unjust differences in health and wellbeing between different groups of people which are systematic and avoidable and may be driven by (Supplementary Figure S1):

- Different experiences of the wider determinants of health or structural factors, for example the environments, income or housing.
- Differences in health behaviours or other risk factors between groups, for example smoking, diet, and physical activity levels have different social distributions. Health behaviours may be influenced by wider determinants of health, like income.
- Unequal access to or experience of health and other services between social groups.

The monitoring of health inequalities is important as it can identify progress linked to specific health policies or programmes and help to focus interventions at the most disadvantaged cohorts of the population. Through continual monitoring, the reduction or widening of health differences can be highlighted [3,4]. To aid the assessment of health interventions, policies, programmes, services and reduce health inequalities, specific assessment tools have been created such as the health equity assessment toolkit (HEAT) that was developed by the World Health Organisation (WHO) between 2014 and 2016 [5]. The WHO HEAT is a software, that contains the WHO's health equity monitor database, supporting countries to assess inequalities within the country with over 30 indicators including reproductive, maternal, new-born and child health and five dimensions of inequality (economic status, education, place of residence, subnational region and child's sex, where applicable) [5].

The reduction of health inequalities within England is a responsibility for Public Health England (PHE), an executive agency of the UK Government [6]. To help the organisation assess the impact of the public facing campaigns for health equity, PHE's Health Inequalities team designed an internal HEAT. The assessment consists of a series of questions, which are designed to support systematic assessment of health inequalities related to work programmes, initiatives, policies and identify actions that need to be taken to reduce any potential identified inequalities.

The HEAT was built on international experience from the WHO and the Ministry of Health in New Zealand [5,7]. Unlike the WHO and New Zealand HEAT, the PHE tool considers the requirements of the Equality Act 2010 and therefore the set protected characteristics (Box 1) in addition to inequalities.

Box 1. Protected characteristics (Equality Act 2010).

- age
- sex
- race
- religion or belief
- disability
- sexual orientation
- gender reassignment
- pregnancy and maternity
- marriage and civil partnership

As well as considerations about socio-economic differences, area variations by the deprivation level (IMD), service provisions, urban/rural populations or in general and excluded and underserved groups for example homeless people, people in prison, or young people leaving care were considered.

It also recommends five stages for the assessment which include prepare, assess, refine, apply and review. Each assessment is likely to be iterative and can help areas continuously improve the contribution of work streams to reducing health inequalities. There have been notable local results within New Zealand from the application of this toolkit, including health promotion and health care clinics in low decile schools; dental care for those on low incomes; free interpreter services; and mobile Māori nursing services [8]. The WHO HEAT is pre-populated with the health equity monitor database, allowing users to explore the situation in one setting of interest (e.g., a country, province, or district) to determine the latest situation of inequality and changes in inequalities over time as well as to benchmark settings/countries. The PHE and New Zealand tools can be considered quality improvement tools for assessing and developing programmes, initiatives and policies.

It is important to use the HEAT to assess that the impact of public facing campaigns. The development of an internal HEAT has helped PHE to assess such interventions and provides a pragmatic and systematic set of steps for health policy makers to assess their initiative in relation to health equity. The application of the toolkit can occur at different stages of the program or policy development including the initial planning phase, the implementation stages or in the programme review phase [7]. Within the development of proposals or policies, there can be a tendency to leave the target groups as wide as possible so that more people are included. However, this approach can potentially result in the reduction of certain cohorts of the population that would benefit most from the programme or policy. This can result in unintended and unanticipated health impacts on certain population groups [9]. The use of HEAT can potentially help to reduce this unintended outcome for which PHE has started to incorporate this toolkit within the assessment process of national campaigns. The outcome of health equity assessments can inform decisions on how to build and strengthen policies, programmes and future services that organisations provide [8]. The antimicrobial resistance team has been one of the pioneers to adopt it within its campaigns.

Antimicrobial resistance (AMR) is a global threat to public health affecting all healthcare systems and growing at an alarming pace [10,11]. The implementation of antimicrobial stewardship programmes has been used within secondary care to help reduce this burden, with a focus on the UK Government ambition to reduce inappropriate antibiotic prescribing [12]. An important element of these programmes is the use of national campaigns to increase the overall reach. There is currently a lack of research assessing the potential health inequalities within public facing antimicrobial stewardship campaigns. The primary aim of this study was to assess whether the public facing AMR initiatives are reaching a diverse population within England. The secondary aim included providing individual campaign recommendations and general trend recommendations for the overall campaigns. Following a literature review, the authors believe there is currently limited research available that specifically assesses health inequalities related to AMR national campaigns.

National Campaigns

The following four national AMR campaigns run by Public Health England were assessed:
Antibiotic Guardian

As part of the European Antibiotic Awareness Week (EAAD), this campaign was launched in September 2014. The aim was to increase commitment by healthcare professionals and members of the public to reduce AMR, change behaviour and increase knowledge. This is done through a pledge-based system where healthcare professionals and members choose a relevant pledge relating to their practice or personal situation [13].

Target audience: Broad audience

e-Bug

This campaign was developed as a European Union project and created a junior and senior school educational resource for teachers covering microbes, hygiene, antibiotics and the prevention of infection. There is both a paper based educational pack along with a web site that hosts games for young people and their families to play in the classroom or at home [14].

Target audience: School age children and teachers

TARGET (Treat Antibiotics Responsibly, Guidance, Education, Tools)

The TARGET antibiotics toolkit was developed by PHE in collaboration with the Royal College of General Practitioners (RCGP) and other professional societies. The main aim of this campaign is to improve antimicrobial prescribing in primary care through multiple channels such as guidance, interactive workshops, patient facing educational and audit materials [15].

Target audience: Prescribing clinicians

Keep Antibiotics Working

This is a consumer-led campaign to help raise awareness of antibiotic resistance to members of the public and highlight the dangers of not using antibiotics appropriately.

There are three main aims within this campaign—alert the public to the issue of AMR, reduce public expectation for antibiotics and support change amongst healthcare professionals [16].

Target audience: Women aged 20–45 and Men and women aged 50+

2. Results

The overall results assessing whether each protected characteristic as defined in the Equality Act 2010 was addressed by the campaign are summarised in Table 1.

Table 1. Campaign assessment of the protected characteristics.

Protected Characteristic	Antibiotic Guardian	e-Bug	Target	Keep Antibiotics Working
Age	All ages	Ages 9–24	All ages	Ages 20–45 and 50+
Sex	All	All	All	All
Race	Website available to all	Translated into over 30 languages	Translated into approximately 20 languages	Resources distributed throughout the UK
Religion or Belief	No specific information	No specific information	No specific information	N/A
Disability	No specific information	No specific information	Material for learning disability users	Material designed for all groups to understand (C2DE inclusive)
Sexual Orientation	N/A	N/A	N/A	N/A
Gender reassignment	N/A	N/A	N/A	N/A
Pregnancy and maternity	No specific information	N/A	Information on pregnancy within leaflets	Aimed at females responsible for family health
Marriage and civil partnership	N/A	N/A	N/A	N/A

N/A—no data available.

2.1. Antibiotic Guardian

The overall reach of this campaign was found to be extensive with 122 countries having at least one pledge [17]. This included the Antibiotic Guardian website currently being translated into 4 languages as well as English. When reviewing the population within England, it may be advantageous to offer languages in line with the latest Census (e.g., 2011 Census in England and Wales showed 7.7% of the population had another main language that was not English) [18]. The materials are open to everyone who has internet access so can be accessed by a variety of local populations and specific cultural groups. Further engagement and understanding of the culture of specific groups (e.g., Black, Asian and minority ethnic (BAME) and travelling community) or those in deprived communities would be beneficial to help promote the materials.

The Antibiotic Guardian campaign has now been embedded in the boy scouts to improve reach within younger children, an addition within the equivalent guides would help provide this key resource to more children.

The accessibility of information within the website is very good with an easy to use interface. Supportive resources, via leaflets and videos, provide a platform for those that do not have internet access. It could be beneficial to create and promote paper versions (PDF/word) of antibiotic guardian pledges that can be used by local campaign leads so that individuals without the internet can also pledge. The website supports a subtitle function on the home page video but a transcription of the video would improve accessibility. Future interface designs of the website could be done in conjunction with specific minority groups.

2.2. e-Bug

The e-Bug focuses on the education element of infections within children, young people and those hard to reach in the community. This interactive campaign has been translated into over 30 languages and has approved trainers throughout England, Wales and Northern Ireland which improves accessibility for these resources. The e-Bug trainer events should be targeted at areas with greater antibiotic use which have greater deprivation and ethnicity. It was found that all resources are freely available to download and print from the internet. The resources are developed for a range of ages and therefore abilities within the community. In the Beat the Bugs resources, each lesson plan has a range of activities to suit a range of abilities. The antibiotic Beat the Bug resources include a specific patient facing pictorial resource for the public with language or learning difficulties. There is an increased awareness within the project team of pictorial and foreign language resources, with a commitment to continue to reassess the language being used is inclusive of all, especially for disadvantaged and minority groups. There is also an increase focus in the implementation of resources in deprived areas using additional work force and targeted training to local clinical commissioning group staff.

An analytical review of the e-Bug website usage and views would help identify further development and improvement to reduce health inequalities and could be beneficial.

2.3. TARGET

The TARGET resources were found to be easily accessible to all healthcare professionals via an open access website. The distribution was extensive and resources can be accessed to permanent, training or temporary general practitioners (GPs). This was also the case for the out of hour GPs, though further publicity within this group would aid the reach. The use of community pharmacists in promoting the use of TARGET resources would help improve reach to patients. The TARGET website contains patient facing resources to share in consultations for respiratory tract infections (including a pictorial version) and urinary tract infections for patients under and over 65 years. These patient leaflets are available in the most common non-English languages spoken in the UK.

2.4. Keep Antibiotics Working

The quantitative research completed by the internal marketing team demonstrated a representative sample of the population within England, however due to the size of the sample, it was not possible or appropriate to break down the data by every protected characteristic. The choice of media via the TV ensured the campaigned reached a broad cross section of the population. During the campaign period, over 766,000 posters and leaflets were distributed to a range of partners including local authorities, health care centres and housing associations with 92% of GP practices in England engaged [19]. Prisons were also included within the distribution along with GPs who reach those from lower socioeconomic backgrounds. The advertising featured red and white pills which have no gender or racial bias. All campaign research, including campaign tracking, strategic and creative development research was carried out across all socioeconomic groups. The campaign materials were designed for all groups to understand and were C2DE—skilled working class, working class and non-working (the three lower social and economic groups in a society) inclusive. It would be recommended to conduct a review impact analysis of the campaign by age, sex and socioeconomic group, and where appropriate, change the campaign strategy based on this evidence. It was noted that more data is required to change the marketing or targeting specific populations but the use of advertising routes that are set up to engage with minority groups (e.g. radio channels focusing on certain groups, promote in religious areas, prisons) may be beneficial. It could be advantageous to translate resource leaflets into multiple languages in line with latest national Census and local population.

3. Discussion

The assessments highlight the diverse and inclusive nature of the four campaigns run by Public Health England. There have been notable successes in reaching a wider audience such as 92% of GP practices in England being engaged with the Keep Antibiotic Campaign. Interestingly, this wider reach may have contributed to a positive impact on the intended behaviour, with 78% of the public stating that they would be unlikely to ask their GP for antibiotics [19]. It is important to note that the reach of a campaign on the population can also have an influence on healthcare professionals with 93% of GPs saying they felt the materials supported them to say no to antibiotics when they were not needed [19]. As technology advances, it has been demonstrated that there is more of an emphasis being put on the use of technology within healthcare over the last few years. It is vital that campaigns use this to reach greater audiences but also remembering an ageing population who potentially do not have access to technology or would prefer not to be contacted through this means. The use of paper-based approaches are still of value and should be utilised to make sure it is inclusive of all.

The assessments were conducted by the project lead and team members which could cause bias when completing the assessment. However, through the use of an independent study team who are not actively involved within the projects, this was partially negated during the review meeting where the member of the study team provided a focus on the context of each question and did not aid or prompt the project lead around a particular response. It would be ideal to have an independent person completing the assessment without the involvement of the project lead but due to the complexities of the campaigns, specialist knowledge is required to provide meaningful results.

During the assessments, it became apparent that not all protected characteristics were appropriate for each campaign, for example, the e-Bug where the target audience is children, the marriage and civil partnership criteria for assessment was not applicable.

The way in which each campaign runs alongside each other is important with the integration and collaboration being key to improving the overall AMR message. The involvement of a senior sponsor of the proposed campaign during the review stage would aid this further integration and also make sure that organisational oversight is achieved.

The use of behavioural insight teams can also play a significant part in helping change an individual's views when it comes to antibiotic use with a greater input in all campaigns would help achieve a long-term improvement when the public use antibiotics.

One of the limitations of this study is that the analysed/numeric data from the national campaigns are not presented. However, it is important to note that whilst these are not presented within the manuscript, the data and evidence are an essential part of section A—prepare the health equities assessment tool (HEAT) (S1). This study focuses its attention on the importance of national campaigns considering and monitoring health inequalities in their development and revisions. This will ensure that interventions do not widen health inequalities and also, they can be focused at the most disadvantaged cohorts of the population.

To improve the output of future campaigns, further research on health inequalities and AMR is needed. This would provide corresponding data to help tailor campaigns to specific individuals that may not be reached. Of the limited data available, there have been significant findings, including the increase of AMR among refugees and asylum seekers in high-migrant community settings [20]. This has highlighted where future policy could be implemented, but with this data being available it can also contribute to the effectiveness of using the HEAT in other health economies. Although this study only assessed each campaign once, the use of HEAT is an iterative process which can help to continuously improve the contribution of campaigns to reduce health inequalities. To consider the impact this assessment has in reducing health inequalities, a subsequent review is advised.

4. Materials and Methods

An internal HEAT (Supplementary Figure S1) developed by PHE was used. The project leads for each campaign in England, UK were asked to complete the HEAT independently, over an eight-week period from October to November 2018, with input from their team members as required. There was a 100% (4/4) completion rate to the HEAT during the allocated period. An initial meeting was conducted with the project lead and one member of the study team to discuss the rationale of the assessment tool and explain how the tool should be used. The HEAT was sent to each project lead via email with responses also returned in the same way. A follow up meeting between the same individuals was arranged to discuss and clarify queries and to standardise the approach for each separate assessment. This was done to be able to provide trend analysis over all the assessed campaigns. All the responses were collated by one member of the study team with a summary of the responses being discussed with the remaining members of the study team. The main focus of the overall analysis was assessing whether each protected characteristic as defined in the Equality Act 2010 and is the focus of the PHE HEAT was included within the individual campaigns. A trend analysis was carried out on all four campaign assessments with common themes of the responses being used to provide recommendations for future work. A common theme was confirmed if two or more of the campaign responses identified that theme. A qualitative analysis was used to summarise each campaign against the protected characteristics. An action plan for each project was developed inclusive of common themes but also of any specific recommendations relevant to that campaign.

5. Conclusions

The use of the HEAT comes at a significant time when the threat of AMR is well publicised. Making sure any stewardship campaign is as diverse and inclusive as possible is essential to improve the reach of the target audience. The greater the reach, the more impact national campaigns have with greater flexibility to make them accessible for a diverse population. To help tailor campaigns to hard to reach groups, further research into health inequalities relating to accessing antimicrobials would be beneficial. The assessment has shown to be an easy and cost-effective way to assess any health inequalities within a campaign and could be a useful addition to local level stewardship programmes that are trying to reduce the amount of inappropriate antimicrobial use. This systematic approach helps facilitate opportunities to address any health inequalities that have been identified and can also be applied to a range of services and programmes. The communication of information within diverse populations is vital in reducing the burden of AMR and addressing health inequalities. To improve the reach of this information, the use of HEAT is also vital.

Supplementary Materials: The following are available online at http://www.mdpi.com/2079-6382/8/3/121/s1, Figure S1: The PHE Health Equity Assessment Tool. * This assessment tool is currently a working draft that the PHE's Health inequalities team is planning to revise in line with stakeholder feedback.

Author Contributions: Conceptualization, D.A.-O.; data curation, G.H.; formal analysis, G.H.; methodology, L.T. and D.A.-O.; project administration, G.H.; supervision, D.A.-O. and L.T.; writing—original draft, G.H.; writing—review and editing, G.H., L.T. and D.A.-O.

Funding: This research received no external funding and was conducted by Public Health England.

Acknowledgments: The authors would like to thank all the campaign leads that participated in the assessment process. Antibiotic Guardian: Diane Ashiru-Oredope. Keep Antibiotics Working: Eleanor Walsh, Jennie Snook. e-Bug: Cliodna McNulty, Charlotte Eley. TARGET: Cliodna McNulty, Donna Lecky.

Conflicts of Interest: The authors declare no conflicts of interest.

References

1. Global Health Inequalities. Available online: https://researchbriefings.parliament.uk/ResearchBriefing/Summary/POST-PN-0553 (accessed on 17 January 2018).
2. Tracking Universal Health Coverage: First Global Monitoring Report. Available online: https://www.who.int/healthinfo/universal_health_coverage/report/2015/en/ (accessed on 17 January 2018).
3. WHO Handbook on Health Inequality Monitoring with a Special Focus on Low and Middle Income Countries. Available online: http://www.who.int/gho/health_equity/handbook/en/ (accessed on 17 January 2018).

4. State of Inequality: Reproductive, Maternal, Newborn and Child Health. Available online: http://www.who.int/gho/health_equity/report_2015/en/ (accessed on 17 January 2018).
5. Hosseinpoor, A.R.; Nambiar, D.; Schlotheuber, A.; Reidpath, D.; Ross, Z. Health Equity Assessment Toolkit (HEAT): Software for exploring and comparing health inequalities in countries. *BMC Med. Res. Methodol.* **2016**, *16*, 141. [CrossRef] [PubMed]
6. Public Health England About Us. Available online: https://www.gov.uk/government/organisations/public-health-england/about (accessed on 17 January 2018).
7. The Health Equity Assessment Tool: A User's Guide. Available online: https://www.health.govt.nz/publication/health-equity-assessment-tool-users-guide (accessed on 17 January 2018).
8. Sheridan, N.F.; Kenealy, T.W.; Connolly, M.J.; Mahony, F.; Barber, P.A.; Bpyd, M.A.; Carswell, P.; Clinton, J.; Delvin, G.; Doughty, R.; et al. Health equity in the New Zealand health care system: A national survey. *Int. J. Equity Health* **2011**, *10*, 45. [CrossRef] [PubMed]
9. Equity Focussed Health Impact Assessment Framework. Available online: http://hiaconnect.edu.au/old/files/efhia_framework.pdf (accessed on 17 January 2018).
10. WHO Antimicrobial Resistance. Available online: http://www.who.int/mediacentre/factsheets/fs194/en/ (accessed on 17 January 2018).
11. Review on Antimicrobial Resistance. Available online: https://amr-review.org/background.html (accessed on 17 January 2018).
12. Research Reveals Levels of Inappropriate Prescriptions in England. Available online: https://www.gov.uk/government/news/research-reveals-levels-of-inappropriate-prescriptions-in-england (accessed on 17 July 2019).
13. Keston, J.M.; Bhattacharya, A.; Ashiru-Oredope, D.; Gobin, M.; Audrey, S. The Antibiotic Guardian campaign: A qualitative evaluation of an online pledge-based system focused on making better use of antibiotics. *BMC Public Health* **2017**, *18*, 5. [CrossRef] [PubMed]
14. McNulty, C.A.; Lecky, D.M.; Farrell, D.; Kostkova, P.; Adriaenssens, N.; Koprivova Herotova, T.; Holt, J.; Touboul, P.; Merakou, K.; Koncan, R.; et al. e-Bug Working Group. Overview of e-Bug: An antibiotic and hygiene educational resource for schools. *J. Antimicrob. Chemother.* **2011**, *66*, 5. [CrossRef] [PubMed]
15. Jones, L.F.; Hawking, M.K.D.; Owens, R.; Lecky, D.; Francis, N.A.; Butler, C.; Gal, M.; McNulty, C.A.M. An evaluation of the TARGET (Treat Antibiotics Responsibly; Guidance, Education, Tools) Antibiotics Toolkit to improve antimicrobial stewardship in primary care—Is it fit for purpose? *Fam. Pract.* **2017**, *35*, 4. [CrossRef] [PubMed]
16. Keep Antibiotics Working. Available online: https://campaignresources.phe.gov.uk/resources/campaigns/58-keep-antibiotics-working/Overview (accessed on 17 January 2018).
17. Newitt, S.; Oloyede, O.; Puleston, R.; Hopkins, S.; Ashiru-Oredope, D. Demographic, Knowledge and Impact Analysis of 57,627 Antibiotic Guardians Who Have Pledged to Contribute to Tackling Antimicrobial Resistance. *Antibiotics* **2019**, *8*, 21. [CrossRef] [PubMed]
18. Language in England and Wales: 2011. Available online: https://www.ons.gov.uk/peoplepopulationandcommunity/culturalidentity/language/articles/languageinenglandandwales/2013-03-04 (accessed on 17 July 2019).
19. English Surveillance Programme for Antimicrobial Utilisation and Resistance Report. Available online: https://assets.publishing.service.gov.uk/government/uploads/system/uploads/attachment_data/file/759975/ESPAUR_2018_report.pdf (accessed on 2 August 2019).
20. Nellums, L.B.; Thompson, H.; Holmes, A.; Castro-Sanchez, E.; Otter, J.A.; Norredam, M.; Friedland, J.S.; Hargreaves, S. Antimicrobial resistance among migrants in Europe: A systematic review and meta-analysis. *Lancet Infect. Dis.* **2018**, *18*, 796–811. [CrossRef]

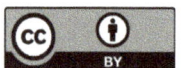

© 2019 by the authors. Licensee MDPI, Basel, Switzerland. This article is an open access article distributed under the terms and conditions of the Creative Commons Attribution (CC BY) license (http://creativecommons.org/licenses/by/4.0/).

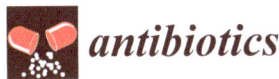

Article

General Practitioners' Attitudes toward Municipal Initiatives to Improve Antibiotic Prescribing—A Mixed-Methods Study

Marthe Sunde [1,†], **Marthe Marie Nygaard** [1,†] **and Sigurd Høye** [2,*]

1 Faculty of Medicine, University of Oslo, 0318 Oslo, Norway
2 Antibiotic Centre for Primary Care, Department of General Practice, Institute of Health and Society, University of Oslo, 0318 Oslo, Norway
* Correspondence: sigurd.hoye@medisin.uio.no
† These authors contributed equally to this work, and share first authorship.

Received: 12 July 2019; Accepted: 15 August 2019; Published: 17 August 2019

Abstract: Antimicrobial stewardship (AMS) interventions directed at general practitioners (GPs) contribute to an improved antibiotic prescribing. However, it is challenging to implement and maintain such interventions at a national level. Involving the municipalities' Chief Medical Officer (MCMO) in quality improvement activities may simplify the implementation and maintenance, but may also be perceived challenging for the GPs. In the ENORM (Educational intervention in NORwegian Municipalities for antibiotic treatment in line with guidelines) study, MCMOs acted as facilitators of an AMS intervention for GPs. We explored GPs' views on their own antibiotic prescribing, and their views on MCMO involvement in improving antibiotic prescribing in general practice. This is a mixed-methods study combining quantitative and qualitative data from two data sources: e-mail interviews with 15 GPs prior to the ENORM intervention, and online-form answers to closed and open-ended questions from 132 GPs participating in the ENORM intervention. The interviews and open-ended responses were analyzed using systematic text condensation. Many GPs admitted to occasionally prescribing antibiotics without medical indication, mainly due to pressure from patients. Too liberal treatment guidelines were also seen as a reason for overtreatment. The MCMO was considered a suitable and acceptable facilitator of quality improvement activities in general practice, and their involvement was regarded as unproblematic (scale 0 (very problematic) to 10 (not problematic at all): mean 8.2, median 10). GPs acknowledge the need and possibility to improve their own antibiotic prescribing, and in doing so, they welcome engagement from the municipality. MCMOs should be involved in quality improvement and AMS in general practice.

Keywords: quality improvement; general practitioners; primary care; antibiotics; guideline

1. Introduction

The presence of antibiotic resistance is closely connected to the consumption of antibiotics, both at a societal and an individual level, and most antibiotics consumed by humans are prescribed in primary care [1]. Compared to other European countries, the use of antibiotics in Norwegian primary care is relatively low, but there is still room for improvement [2]. Accordingly, in 2016 the Norwegian Ministry of Health and Care Services published an action plan with the aim of an overall 30% reduction in the use of antibiotics by 2020 [3].

As general practitioners (GPs) have a key role in regulating the amount of consumed antibiotics in primary care, numerous antimicrobial stewardship interventions directed at GPs have been tried out. In the Norwegian *Rx*-PAD (Prescription Peer Academic Detailing) study [4], effective strategies such as educational outreach visits [5] and audit and feedback [6] were combined, resulting in a relative reduction in antibiotic prescribing of 9%, and an increased proportion of narrow spectrum antibiotic of 24%.

The participating GPs found the intervention acceptable [7], and especially valued that the intervention was implemented by a peer GP and not by an external authority.

In Norway, GPs are mainly self-employed and have no clinical superiors. Professional autonomy is highly valued [8]. The municipality, with which the GP has a contract to deliver primary care services, has a legal responsibility to ensure quality improvement and patient safety measures for the GPs [9]. However, how this responsibility should be interpreted and implemented is very unclear [10].

The *Rx-PAD* intervention was resource intensive, as it included training, travel expenses, and payment for the GPs who acted as peer academic detailers. Hence, the intervention has not been implemented as a freely available course for Norwegian GPs. The same is the case for many antimicrobial stewardship interventions both in primary and secondary care. To overcome these challenges, we developed the ENORM (Educational intervention in NORwegian Municipalities for antibiotic treatment in line with guidelines) study [11], which aims at testing an antimicrobial stewardship intervention that, if effective and acceptable, can be easily implemented throughout primary care. The intervention; a 15-hour course consisting of 3 e-learning sessions and 3 Continuing Medical Education (CME) group meetings where the GPs are to discuss their personal prescription reports, is rolled out by a representative of the municipality, the Municipal Chief Medical Officer (MCMO). In small municipalities, the MCMO post usually is a part-time position for a GP, while full-time MCMO position is the norm in large municipalities. The ENORM intervention was tested in 30 randomly selected, medium-size (5.000–25.000 inhabitants), high-antibiotic-consumption Norwegian municipalities between February 2017 and September 2018. The effect of the intervention will be reported in a separate publication.

The aim of this study is to explore the GPs' judgment of their own antibiotic prescribing, and their views and attitudes toward MCMOs' involvement in antimicrobial stewardship efforts toward GPs.

2. Results

2.1. Part 1—E-Mail Interviews

During our analysis, we defined three main themes: antibiotic prescribing, reduction, and quality improvement.

2.1.1. Antibiotic Prescribing

The GPs were divided in their views of own antibiotic prescribing without medical indication. Many stated that this was rarely or never the case. An equally common statement was that the GP admitted to doing this on some occasions. A view was held that the correct prescription practice is not easily defined:

"I don't prescribe antibiotics without a medical indication, but here I mean there are grey areas of right/wrong use, and not a black/white picture on indication." (GP, board member)

Perceived pressure from patients was the most common explanation as to why the GPs prescribed antibiotics without medical indication. While some GPs had recently experienced patients to be more knowledgeable in their views on antibiotic use, the majority still experienced pressure from patients to prescribe antibiotics. They expressed that this demand could be challenging to withstand. Fear of under-treating, the patient's strong opinion of the need for antibiotic treatment, and lack of time to explain and convince the patient that the treatment is unnecessary, were pointed out as reasons for not withstanding the pressure. Some pointed out patients' lack of understanding the difference between bacterial and viral infections, and a perception of antibiotics as an easy quick-fix.

Treatment guidelines were mentioned within the topic of reasons for antibiotic overuse. Some GPs claimed that the actual guidelines on antibiotic use are an obstacle for reducing antibiotic prescribing, and pointed to several areas where they found that this was the case. Otitis, respiratory tract infections, uncomplicated cystitis, and acne were some of the indications suggested for revision.

"I think (...) the indications are too spacious. We are over-treating when we follow guidelines." (GP with board membership)

2.1.2. Reduction

The GPs held that antimicrobial resistance is a serious threat, and they strongly agreed that antibiotic use had to be greatly reduced. The GPs that reflected on their own ability to contribute to reducing prescription rates were concerned about the goal being set too high. The majority stated that they were unsure of their ability to cut their own prescription rates to match the 30% reduction goal set by the Government. One GP stated that their prescription rate was at a level where 30% reduction would not be a justifiable correction.

The GPs had several ideas on how to reduce antibiotic prescribing. Guideline revision, information to the patients and public on antibiotic resistance, and the use of delayed prescribing were suggested. Although most examples of ways to reduce antibiotic prescriptions were very specific, one GP had thoughts on a more long-term measure:

"Make the GPs proud of their professional mandate, including their ability to single out the few seriously ill patients who actually need antibiotics." (GP with board membership)

This view was opposed by another GP who pointed out how their professional freedom is rightfully challenged when matters of serious public concern are debated:

"As all my colleagues, I value my independence as a general practitioner, but certain cases (like the problem of bacterial resistance) are too important not to manage centrally." (GP without board membership)

2.1.3. Quality Improvement

The GPs welcomed the MCMO as a facilitator of quality improvement activities in primary care. It was described as a praiseworthy and reasonable use of the MCMO's time, and an interesting quality improvement approach. Some informants explicitly missed the municipalities' engagement in quality improvement.

"(If the municipality initiated quality improvement measures) I would probably faint by the surprise of it. My municipality does nothing to improve the content of the primary care service." (GP with board membership)

A view was held that the MCMO would be in an appropriate professional position to initiate quality improvement initiatives toward GPs.

"Professional independence is a sensitive topic for general practitioners. An arrangement like this by the pharmacy, for an example, would end up wrong. A municipality doctor or infection doctor would possibly be acceptable." (GP without board membership)

2.2. Part 2—Online-Form Answers

2.2.1. Own Potential for Improvement

We received 132 answers to the question "What do you consider to be your potential for improvement?" All respondents presented one or several specific goals for their antibiotic prescribing. They pointed out specific diagnoses and age groups where they could reduce their use of antibiotics, and considered tools to help them achieving their goals, such as enhanced consultation techniques. Some of the respondents also set a time limit for when they should have reached their goals. Even though the specificity and comprehensiveness of the answers varied, no respondents argued that they saw small, or no, room for improvement.

2.2.2. The Municipal Chief Medical Officer's Role

About 85% (112) of the 132 participants responded to the rating scale question "What is your opinion on the Municipal Chief Medical Officer's role in this course?" On the 11 points scale (0: very problematic to 10: not problematic at all), the mean value was 8.2 (95% CI: 7.6–8.7), and the median value was 10.

Twenty five percent (33) of the 132 participants responded to the open-ended question "Provide comments on the Municipal Chief Medical Officer's role." Four respondents commented that their MCMO did not have any role in the implementation of the ENORM course in their CME group, and five respondents commented that they themselves were MCMOs, in addition to being GPs. The remaining 24 respondents all gave positive comments on the MCMOs role. Two main explanations were identified: First, the participants appreciated having a designated course facilitator. They experienced that the MCMO coordinated and structured the meeting, gave useful information and reminders, and initiated valuable group discussions with relevant and relatable cases. Second, it was appreciated that the MCMO engaged in the issue of antibiotic prescribing and set an example by recommending national guidelines.

Some of the respondents commented that the MCMO also participated in the course as a GP, or that they knew them as a GP, and that they considered the MCMO to be more a peer than a manager.

3. Discussion

3.1. Main Findings

The general practitioners in this study stated that there is an overuse of antibiotics in general practice, and that the use should be reduced. Perceived pressure from patients, lack of time, fear of under-treatment, and too liberal guidelines were pointed out as drivers of unnecessary antibiotic prescribing. Both arguments that GPs themselves could bring about the needed reduction and that external efforts were justified for GPs to reduce prescribing existed among the GPs. The Municipal Chief Medical Officer (MCMO) was seen as a suitable and acceptable facilitator of quality improvement activities in general practice. This view was supported by GPs taking part in the ENORM intervention, facilitated by their MCMO.

3.2. Strengths and Limitations

This study has some limitations. The response rate on the open-ended questions was relatively low in both part 1 (15% of invited GPs without board position) and part 2 (25% of participating GPs) of the study. GPs with strong views on antimicrobial stewardship and GP's autonomy, work frames, and quality improvement may have been more inclined to participate, as suggested by the fact that 62% of GPs with board positions responded. However, the aim in qualitative studies is not to recruit a representative sample of informants within the given population, but to explore existing views among a variety of informants [12]. We find that the selection of GPs was diverse, including both opinion leaders and GPs without any board membership, and we achieved variety with respect to geography, gender, municipality's size, and municipality's antibiotic consumption.

Our selection of informants is quite small. In a paper on sample sizes in qualitative studies [13], Malterud presents "information power" as a concept. Malterud suggests that the more relevant information a sample holds for a study, the lower number of participants is needed. Our informants may be considered to provide information of high value, as they included both potential participants of a planned intervention and participants of the actual intervention.

The respondents gave relatively short answers to the open-ended questions, ranging from 1 to 180 words. As held by Meho [14], e-mail interviewing can be a viable alternative to face-to-face interviews in qualitative research. The opportunity of easy outreach to informants over a large geographic area was a great benefit in our study. The challenge of using this method, however, is the less opportunity for continuous correspondence, and the information gathered is less in-depth than what could be expected in a face-to-face interview. We also experienced that some GPs agreed to participate but did not respond when the e-mail with the actual interview was sent, suggesting that e-mail interviews may be perceived as less binding than a face-to-face interview.

Due to the wording of the question "What do you consider to be your potential for improvement?" respondents may have felt obliged to suggest such a potential, even if they found that there was no need for improvement. Also, the respondents in part 2 had agreed to participate in a course facilitated by the MCMO. GPs with negative views on such cooperation may have rejected the MCMOs invitation, thus introducing a selection bias in this part of the study. However, no negative remarks regarding the MCMOs' involvement were expressed in part 1 of the study.

3.3. Results and Discussion

Many of the informants admitted to occasionally prescribing antibiotics without clinical indication. Their reasons for doing so were to a large extent coherent with previous findings on "non-pharmacological" antibiotic prescribing [15]: the lack of opportunity for continued care, pressure from patients, and the GP's uncertainty. However, the view that antibiotic overtreatment may be due to adherence to guidelines is to our knowledge a new finding. GPs experience that obligations to adhere to several single-disease guidelines may lead to polypharmacy and overtreatment in multimorbid patients [16]. Especially, guidelines on prevention of cardiovascular disease are held to be inadequate and cause overtreatment in primary care [17]. The existence of this view among GPs when it comes to guidelines for antibiotic use may indicate that the guidelines could be stricter, but at the same time it also indicates that there is a risk of under-treatment of infections in primary care.

The MCMO's role as facilitator and organizer of quality improvement activities in general practice was approved, both as a general idea among GPs not exposed to such activities, and based on the experience of GPs taking part in the ENORM intervention. Previous research has demonstrated the importance for GPs that quality improvement tutors are "one of them," and independent of health authorities [7]. The MCMO is indeed a representative of the health authorities, but to a large extent, the participants regarded the MCMO as a peer, since many of them worked as both GP and MCMO. Also, the MCMOs in the ENORM intervention seem to have acted as facilitators, organizers, and initiators rather than experts or superiors.

There is an ongoing frustration among GPs, both in Norway and internationally, that GPs are imposed an increasing number of tasks and obligations without corresponding financial and organizational support [18,19]. The participants in our study valued the engagement from the municipality, possibly indicating that quality improvement and antimicrobial stewardship are perceived as necessary and wanted activities within general practice and not as obligations imposed by external authorities.

Preliminary results from part 1 of this study have been utilized to develop and tailor the content and implementation of the ENORM intervention.

4. Materials and Methods

This is a mixed-methods study combining quantitative and qualitative data from two data sources:
Part 1: E-mail interviews with a sample of GPs prior to the ENORM intervention.
Part 2: Online-form answers to closed and open-ended questions from GPs participating in the ENORM intervention.

4.1. Part 1—E-Mail Interviews

4.1.1. Interview Guide

We developed a list of open-ended questions covering the themes—unnecessary antibiotic prescribing, own potential for reducing antibiotic prescribing, and the MCMO's potential role in quality improvement in primary care. The questions were piloted among three GPs and modified according to the GPs' comments (Supplementary File 1).

4.1.2. Selection and Recruitment

Two groups of informants were recruited:

(1) GPs who were considered to be opinion leaders among their peers, especially concerning clinical practice and quality improvement; board members of the General Practitioners' Association (Allmennlegeforeningen), the Norwegian College of General Practitioners (Norsk forening for allmennmedisin) and the General Practice committee for Quality and Patient Safety (Allmennmedisinsk utvalg for kvalitet og pasientsikkerhet), a subcommittee of the Norwegian College of General Practitioners.

(2) GPs in high-antibiotic-consuming, medium-size (5.000–25.000 inhabitants) municipalities, aiming at variety with respect to geography, gender, municipality size, and municipality antibiotic consumption.

Invitations were sent out by either mail or e-mail. GPs that consented to participate were sent the questions by e-mail, and asked to reply to the e-mail. We aimed at about equal numbers of informants in group (1) and (2), and continued to recruit GPs to group (2) until this was achieved. In group (1), 8 out of 13 GPs consented to participate, and in group (2), 7 out of 47 GPs consented to participate, resulting in a total of 15 respondents. The interviews were performed between June 2016 and June 2017. None of the informants were exposed to the ENORM intervention.

4.1.3. Analysis

The e-mail answers were anonymized and then analyzed using systematic text condensation [20]. MS and SH read all the text thoroughly, and agreed upon a list of initial themes, resulting in a coding frame. MS coded the text. The analysis followed four steps: (1) reading the complete material to obtain an overall impression; (2) identifying units of meaning representing different aspects of antibiotic use and antimicrobial stewardship efforts, and coding for these units; (3) condensing and summarizing the contents of each of the coded groups; and (4) generalizing descriptions and concepts. MS and SH read the condensates and agreed to the analysis. Illustrative quotes were translated into English. The software tool NVIVO was used in the analysis.

4.2. Part 2—Online-Form Answers

4.2.1. Online Form

We developed an online form to be filled out by the participating GPs in the ENORM intervention directly after the first group meeting. The form had three purposes—to register completion of each participant's group meeting, to aid as a quality improvement tool as part of a Plan-Do-Study-Act (PDSA) cycle [21], and to register the participants views on the Municipal Chief Medical Officers' role in the intervention. Three of the online-form questions are used in this study:

- What do you consider to be your potential for improvement?
- What is your opinion on the Municipal Chief Medical Officer's role in this course? (11-points rating scale, from 0 (very problematic) to 10 (not problematic at all))
- Provide comments on the Municipal Chief Medical Officer's role.

The first question was mandatory in order to register completion of the group meeting, while the two other questions were optional. Hence, all GPs participating in the ENORM intervention were asked to fill the online form.

4.2.2. Selection, Recruitment, and Analysis

MCMOs in the 30 ENORM intervention municipalities were informed that they belonged to a high-antibiotic-consuming municipality, and invited to recruit their local GPs to participate in a 15-hour antibiotic-prescribing improvement course. MCMOs who were also GPs could participate alongside the other GPs in their municipality. Participating GPs gave written consent to analysis of their online-form answers. By the end of the ENORM intervention in September 2018, 132 GPs had completed the first group meeting, resulting in 132 online-form answers.

The material was analyzed in the same manner as described in Part 1. MMN and SH read through all the responses, and MMN coded the text. The rating scale answers were analyzed using Microsoft Excel 2016.

4.3. Ethics (Part 1 and 2)

All participants gave informed consent to the study. The ENORM project was presented for the Regional Ethics Committee South/East (2016/1491/REK sør-øst C), which concluded that ethical approval was not mandatory. Data protection was approved by NSD—Norwegian Centre for Research Data (48136/3 and 50740/3).

5. Conclusions

GPs acknowledge the need and possibility to improve their own antibiotic prescribing. In doing so, they welcome engagement from the municipality, and they find that the MCMO is a suitable and acceptable quality improvement facilitator. MCMOs should be involved in quality improvement and antimicrobial stewardship efforts in general practice.

Supplementary Materials: The following are available online at http://www.mdpi.com/2079-6382/8/3/120/s1, File 1: E-mail with questions sent to general practitioners who consented to take part in the interview study.

Author Contributions: Idea, S.H.; Data Collection, M.S. and S.H.; Validation, M.S., M.M.N., and S.H.; Formal Analysis M.S. (Part 1), M.M.N (Part 2), and S.H.; writing—original draft preparation, M.S. and M.M.N.; writing—review and editing, M.S., M.M.N., and S.H.; supervision, S.H.; project administration, S.H.; funding acquisition, S.H.

Funding: This research was funded through a postdoctoral scholarship to S.H. from The Research Council of Norway, grant 228971/H10.

Acknowledgments: We thank the participating GPs. The online form was developed in collaboration with SKIL (Senter for kvalitet i legekontor; The Norwegian Quality Centre for Outpatient Clinics).

Conflicts of Interest: The authors declare no conflict of interest.

References

1. NORM/NORM-VET. Usage of Antimicrobial Agents and Occurrence of Antimicrobial Resistance in Norway; Tromsø/Oslo 2017. 2016. Available online: https://unn.no/Documents/Kompetansetjenester,%20-sentre%20og%20fagr%C3%A5d/NORM%20-%20Norsk%20overv%C3%A5kingssystem%20for%20antibiotikaresistens%20hos%20mikrober/Rapporter/NORM_NORM-VET_2017.pdf (accessed on 16 August 2019).
2. Gjelstad, S.; Straand, J.; Dalen, I.; Fetveit, A.; Strom, H.; Lindbaek, M. Do general practitioners' consultation rates influence their prescribing patterns of antibiotics for acute respiratory tract infections? *J. Antimicrob. Chemother.* **2011**, *66*, 2425–2433. [CrossRef] [PubMed]
3. National strategy against antibiotic resistance 2015–2020. Available online: https://www.regjeringen.no/contentassets/5eaf66ac392143b3b2054aed90b85210/antibiotic-resistance-engelsk-lavopploslig-versjon-for-nett-10-09-15.pdf (accessed on 16 August 2019).
4. Gjelstad, S.; Høye, S.; Straand, J.; Brekke, M.; Dalen, I.; Lindbæk, M. Improving antibiotic prescribing in acute respiratory tract infections: Cluster randomised trial from Norwegian general practice (prescription peer academic detailing (Rx-PAD) study). *B.M.J.* **2013**, *347*, f4403. [CrossRef] [PubMed]
5. Thomson O'Brien, M.A.; Oxman, A.D.; Davis, D.A.; Haynes, R.B.; Freemantle, N.; Harvey, E.L. Educational outreach visits: effects on professional practice and health care outcomes. *Cochrane Database Syst. Rev.* **2000**, *2*. [CrossRef]
6. Ivers, N.; Jamtvedt, G.; Flottorp, S.; Young, J.M.; Odgaard-Jensen, J.; French, S.D.; O'Brien, M.A.; Johansen, M.; Grimshaw, J.; Oxman, A.D. Audit and feedback: effects on professional practice and healthcare outcomes. *Cochrane Database Syst. Rev.* **2012**, *6*. [CrossRef]

7. Frich, J.C.; Høye, S.; Lindbæk, M.; Straand, J. General practitioners and tutors' experiences with peer group academic detailing: A qualitative study. *BMC. Fam. Pract.* **2010**, *11*, 12. [CrossRef] [PubMed]
8. Spehar, I.; Sjovik, H.; Karevold, K.I.; Rosvold, E.O.; Frich, J.C. General practitioners' views on leadership roles and challenges in primary health care: A qualitative study. *Scand. J. Prim. Health Care* **2017**, *35*, 105–110. [CrossRef] [PubMed]
9. Regulations on the general practitioner scheme in the municipalities. Ministry of Health and Care Services: 2012. Available online: https://lovdata.no/dokument/SF/forskrift/2012-08-29-842 (accessed on 16 August 2019).
10. Gaski, M.; Abelsen, B. Reinforced medical service in the municipalities. Effects on the municipalities of a new regular general practitioner regulation. Available online: https://norut.no/sites/default/files/norut_alta_rapport_2013_8_legetjeneste.pdf (accessed on 16 August 2019).
11. The ENORM study. Available online: https://www.riktigantibiotika.no/the-enorm-study/ (accessed on 08 September 2019).
12. Malterud, K. Qualitative research: Standards, challenges, and guidelines. *Lancet* **2001**, *358*, 483–488. [CrossRef]
13. Malterud, K.; Siersma, V.D.; Guassora, A.D. Sample Size in Qualitative Interview Studies: Guided by Information Power. *Qual. Health Res.* **2016**, *13*, 1753–1760. [CrossRef] [PubMed]
14. Meho, L.I. E-mail interviewing in qualitative research: A methodological discussion. *J. Am. Soc. Inf. Sci. Tec.* **2006**, *57*, 1284–1295. [CrossRef]
15. Petursson, P. GPs' Reasons for "non-pharmacological" prescribing of antibiotics. A phenomenological study. *Scand. J. Prim. Health Care* **2005**, *23*, 120–125. [CrossRef] [PubMed]
16. Austad, B.; Hetlevik, I.; Mjolstad, B.P.; Helvik, A.S. Applying clinical guidelines in general practice: A qualitative study of potential complications. *BMC. Fam. Pract.* **2016**, *17*, 92. [CrossRef] [PubMed]
17. Getz, L.; Sigurdsson, J.A.; Hetlevik, I.; Kirkengen, A.L.; Romundstad, S.; Holmen, J. Estimating the high risk group for cardiovascular disease in the Norwegian HUNT 2 population according to the 2003 European guidelines: modelling study. *BMJ.* **2005**, *331*, 551. [CrossRef] [PubMed]
18. Croxson, C.H.; Ashdown, H.F.; Hobbs, F.R. GPs' perceptions of workload in England: A qualitative interview study. *Br. J. Gen. Pract.* **2017**, *67*, e138–e147. [CrossRef] [PubMed]
19. Theie, M.G.; Lind, L.H.; Haugland, L.M.; Skogli, E. The regular general practitioner scheme in crisis—what do the numbers say? Menon Economics: Oslo, 2018. Available online: https://beta.legeforeningen.no/contentassets/1f3039425ea744adab5e11ac5706b85a/fastlegeordningen-i-krise-hva-sier-tallene-endelig-rapport.pdf (accessed on 16 August 2019).
20. Malterud, K. *Qualitative Research Methods for Medicine and Health Sciences [Kvalitative Forskningsmetoder for Medisin og Helsefag]*, 3rd ed.; Universitetsforlaget: Oslo, Norway, 2017.
21. Plan-Do-Study-Act (PDSA) Worksheet. Available online: http://www.ihi.org/resources/Pages/Tools/PlanDoStudyActWorksheet.aspx (accessed on 24 June 2019).

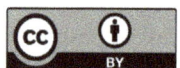

© 2019 by the authors. Licensee MDPI, Basel, Switzerland. This article is an open access article distributed under the terms and conditions of the Creative Commons Attribution (CC BY) license (http://creativecommons.org/licenses/by/4.0/).

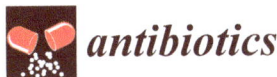

Article

Qualitative Analysis of Primary Care Provider Prescribing Decisions for Urinary Tract Infections

Larissa Grigoryan [1,*], Susan Nash [1], Roger Zoorob [1], George J. Germanos [1], Matthew S. Horsfield [1], Fareed M. Khan [1], Lindsey Martin [2,3] and Barbara W. Trautner [2,3]

1. Department of Family and Community Medicine, Baylor College of Medicine, Houston, TX 77098, USA; sgnash@bcm.edu (S.N.); Roger.Zoorob@bcm.edu (R.Z.); George.Germanos@bcm.edu (G.J.G.); Matthew.Horsfield@bcm.edu (M.S.H.); fkhan@bcm.edu (F.M.K.)
2. Center for Innovations in Quality, Effectiveness and Safety (IQuESt), Michael E. DeBakey Veterans Affairs Medical Center, Houston, TX 77030, USA; Lindsey.Martin@bcm.edu (L.M.); trautner@bcm.edu (B.W.T.)
3. Section of Health Services Research, Department of Medicine, Baylor College of Medicine, Houston, TX 77030, USA
* Correspondence: grigorya@bcm.edu; Tel.: +1-713-798-9181; Fax: +1-832-787-1307

Received: 14 May 2019; Accepted: 14 June 2019; Published: 19 June 2019

Abstract: Inappropriate choices and durations of therapy for urinary tract infections (UTI) are a common and widespread problem. In this qualitative study, we sought to understand why primary care providers (PCPs) choose certain antibiotics or durations of treatment and the sources of information they rely upon to guide antibiotic-prescribing decisions. We conducted semi-structured interviews with 18 PCPs in two family medicine clinics focused on antibiotic-prescribing decisions for UTIs. Our interview guide focused on awareness and familiarity with guidelines (knowledge), acceptance and outcome expectancy (attitudes), and external barriers. We followed a six-phase approach to thematic analysis, finding that many PCPs believe that fluoroquinolones achieve more a rapid and effective control of UTI symptoms than trimethoprim-sulfamethoxazole or nitrofurantoin. Most providers were unfamiliar with fosfomycin as a possible first-line agent for the treatment of acute cystitis. PCPs may be misled by advanced patient age, diabetes, and recurrent UTIs to make inappropriate choices for the treatment of acute cystitis. For support in clinical decision making, few providers relied on guidelines, preferring instead to have decision support embedded in the electronic medical record. Knowing the PCPs' knowledge gaps and preferred sources of information will guide the development of a primary care-specific antibiotic stewardship intervention for acute cystitis.

Keywords: antibiotic stewardship; antibiotics; fluoroquinolones; guidelines; urinary tract infections

1. Introduction

Antimicrobial resistance is increasingly being recognized as one of the major threats to human health globally [1]. The 2015 United States (U.S.) National Action Plan for Combatting Antibiotic Resistant Bacteria set a goal to reduce inappropriate antibiotic use by 50% in outpatient settings [2]. Primary care providers (PCPs) constitute the largest proportion of antibiotic prescribers in the U.S.; therefore, engaging these practitioners is essential to improving outpatient antibiotic stewardship [3]. In 2011, outpatient healthcare providers in the U.S. prescribed 262.5 million courses of antibiotics, with the largest proportion (24%) being prescribed by family medicine physicians [3].

Most studies in outpatient settings have addressed implementing antibiotic stewardship for upper respiratory infections, typically viral infections in which antibiotics are not indicated [4,5]. Few studies have addressed inappropriately prescribing for urinary tract infections (UTI) [6], one of the top three diagnoses for which antibiotics are prescribed in outpatient settings [7]. The first-line agents recommended by the updated 2010 Infectious Diseases Society of America (IDSA) guidelines to treat uncomplicated cystitis are nitrofurantoin, trimethoprim-sulfamethoxazole, and fosfomycin [8]. However, inappropriate choices and durations of antibiotic therapy for UTI are a common problem in primary care [9–11]. Providers often choose fluoroquinolones as a first-line agent for uncomplicated cystitis and prescribe antibiotics for longer than the guidelines' recommended treatment duration [9,10]. Fluoroquinolone use is one of the factors that has led to the emergence and spread of multidrug-resistant *Escherichia coli (E.coli)* strain sequence type 131 [12]. In addition, the U.S. Food and Drug Administration (FDA) issued black box warnings for fluoroquinolones in 2016 [13] and 2018 [14,15] that fluoroquinolones should not be used for uncomplicated UTIs in patients who have other treatment options. These FDA warnings are based on studies indicating an association between fluoroquinolone use and tendonitis and tendon rupture [16,17], QT-prolongation [18], dysglycemia [19,20], neuropathy [21–23], and potentially aortic rupture [15].

Unfortunately, the 2010 IDSA guidelines had little impact on national outpatient national antibiotic prescribing practices for UTI [24], with fluoroquinolones as the most commonly prescribed antibiotic class in young women both before and after the release of the guidelines [24]. In order to design an effective antibiotic stewardship intervention for outpatient UTI management, we first need to understand why primary care providers are choosing certain antibiotics or certain durations of treatment and what sources of information they rely on to guide their antibiotic-prescribing behavior. To acquire these insights, we used qualitative semi-structured interviews to explore primary care provider prescribing decisions for UTI.

2. Results

We interviewed 18 primary care providers working in two private academically affiliated family medicine clinics. We reached data saturation after 13 interviews with our homogeneous sample [25,26].

Our thematic analysis identified seven themes related to providers' prescribing decisions for acute cystitis (Figure 1). The themes were mapped to the Cabana framework for understanding the barriers to physician adherence to clinical practice guidelines [27]. Four of these themes reflected factors influencing antibiotic prescribing decisions for acute cystitis, two themes described the sources of information they rely upon to guide antibiotic-prescribing decisions, and one theme explored the perceptions of antibiotic resistance in providers' practices.

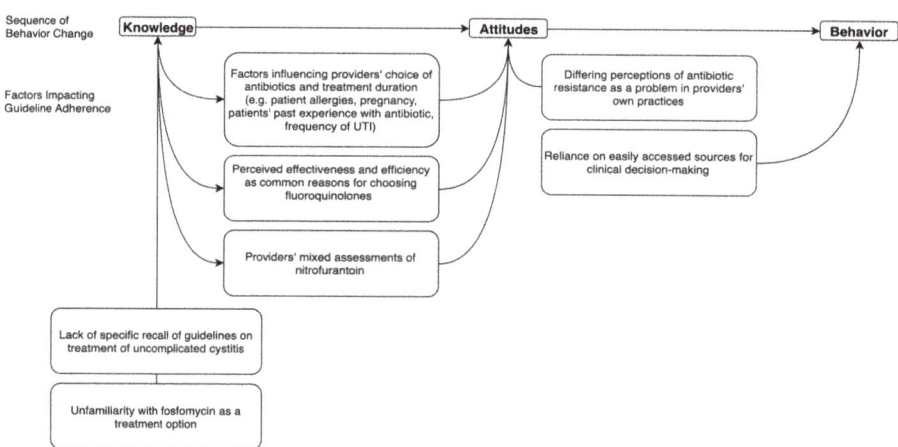

Figure 1. Mapping of the identified themes to the Cabana framework.

2.1. Theme 1: Perceived Effectiveness and Efficiency were Common Reasons for Choosing Fluoroquinolones

Most providers reported that they would prescribe trimethoprim-sulfamethoxazole (TMP-SMX) or nitrofurantoin in the case scenario; however, the treatment duration suggested was sometimes longer than recommended by the guideline. Specifically, the preferred treatment duration of nitrofurantoin was 7 days instead of the guideline recommendation of 5 days among approximately half of the providers who selected this medication as their first choice for treatment. The suggested duration of TMP-SMX was 5 days instead of the guideline recommendation of 3 days among a few providers who selected this medication as a first choice, though most providers correctly chose a guideline concordant with the 3-day duration. Relatively few providers chose fluoroquinolones in the case scenario, though a third listed fluoroquinolones second among their top three choices of antibiotics most frequently prescribed for uncomplicated cystitis in response to a different question. In all quotations below, alias initials of providers were included to indicate that the quotations presented come from a variety of participants.

Common reasons given for why providers might choose fluoroquinolones included prescribing familiarity, "I think a lot of it has to do with familiarity and comfort." (DS); perceived effectiveness, "No matter what kind of bacteria it is, it would be responsive to Cipro." (WC); short course of treatment, "In most instances, I just choose Cipro, and it's easy; it's for three days." (WC); broad-spectrum coverage, "Ciprofloxacin is a very strong antibiotic, and it is broad-spectrum." (JG); and previous patient experience, "If the patient had reported that Cipro had worked well before for them in the past, that might be a consideration." (SL). Providers also expressed confidence in the ability of ciprofloxacin to kill a wide range of bacteria, reporting, for example, "Physicians don't want the patient to have a treatment failure and come back in for a second antibiotic." (AA).

2.2. Theme 2: Factors Influencing Providers' Choice of Antibiotics and Treatment Duration

Providers described multiple considerations when choosing the best antibiotic for acute cystitis. These considerations included allergies, patient sex, pregnancy, patients' past experience with the antibiotic, familiarity with the antibiotic, previous antibiotic susceptibilities, older age, shorter treatment duration and better compliance, frequency of UTI, presence of diabetes, and cost of antibiotics. A few providers mentioned the potential effect of fluoroquinolones on tendons. For example, one provider noted, "There is concern about the fluoroquinolones and their effect on tendons, but I don't know whether it's a media sort of blown up case of concern or whether it's real." (MB). Another provider described various factors affecting their choice of antibiotic for particular patients, "Age, whether or not they have frequent UTI, maybe information from their previous urine cultures which shows sensitivities." (AA).

When the interviewer asked probing questions about the treatment of older patients, some providers mentioned that they would be more likely to choose ciprofloxacin and a longer duration of treatment, while others mentioned that the management of UTI would not change. Similarly, when questioned about recurrent UTIs and the management of diabetic patients with UTI, some providers reported that they would go with "a stronger, broad-spectrum antibiotic such as ciprofloxacin" (BC) and a longer treatment duration. When questioned about male UTIs, providers emphasized the need to rule out a sexually transmitted infection and recommended a treatment duration of up to 14 days.

2.3. Theme 3: Providers' Mixed Assessments of Nitrofurantoin

Few side effects, low cost, and good tolerance were mentioned by the majority of providers as the benefits of nitrofurantoin, with providers giving such responses as, "Nitrofurantoin, it is one of my "go to". It is a good medication for uncomplicated cystitis." (JQ). However, many providers also mentioned that nitrofurantoin is not as "strong" and not as "quick" as fluoroquinolones. One provider explained, "We have a patient population that wants their symptoms to be resolved immediately. Therefore, nitrofurantoin is not a good choice as it is bacteriostatic, and I want to make sure the patient is satisfied and just want to give them something that will resolve symptoms faster." (BC).

A few providers were concerned about birth defects based on published case-control studies [28,29], while others thought nitrofurantoin is much safer than TMP-SMX or fluoroquinolones for pregnant women with UTIs, reporting, for example, "It's one of the ones I use the most, especially in women of childbearing age." (AV). Provider-reported drawbacks included concerns about lung problems with prolonged use, "When I was on the pulmonary rotation, they were talking about the risk of nitrofurantoin causing pulmonary fibrosis, and I've never forgotten that." (JS), as well as contraindication in patients with low creatinine clearance or in older patients in general, "It's on the Beers list." (AA).

2.4. Theme 4: Unfamiliarity with Fosfomycin as a Treatment Option

Most providers were unfamiliar with fosfomycin as a possible treatment option for cystitis, although it is a first-line agent per guidelines [8]. Providers gave such responses as, "I don't use fosfomycin. I've read about it maybe once or twice." (AV) and "I don't think one can use it in the United States. I've never seen anyone try it, and I've never looked into it." (WC). One provider reported having had a patient who had been prescribed fosfomycin by an infectious disease specialist.

2.5. Theme 5: Reliance on Easily Accessed Sources for Clinical Decision-making

In terms of sources of support for clinical decision-making, few providers directly relied on guidelines. Instead, many reported that they use clinical decision support resources, such as UpToDate, accessed through the institution's electronic health record, "I use UpToDate. That's simple. I can click from Epic, so it's right there on my chart. [I'm] talking to the patient, and I just click and pop it up." (AZ) or through a mobile phone app for staying informed about new information on antibiotics, "I use UpToDate. I have the app on my phone, so I am always searching." (BC). A few providers mentioned publications such as *Prescriber's Letter* and resources available from the American Academy of Family Physicians.

2.6. Theme 6: Lack of Specific Recall of Guidelines on Treatment of Uncomplicated Cystitis

Only two providers mentioned the IDSA guidelines, though most respondents reported varying degrees of familiarity with unspecified guidelines, saying, for example, "I think I am reasonably up-to-date." (SC), "I guess I would be fairly familiar." (JQ), and "It's been about 10 years since I reviewed the guidelines." (AV). A few providers acknowledged limited recall of the details of any guidelines regarding the treatment of uncomplicated cystitis, as indicated in the following statements: "Not very. There's very little reason in something as simple as acute cystitis for me to go searching out the guidelines." (MB), "Try to stay away from Cipro first line. That's about all I remember." (DT), and "I have to admit I'm not particularly conversant. I will usually look at UpToDate and just refresh my memory." (JS).

2.7. Theme 7: Differing Perceptions of Antibiotic Resistance as a Problem in Providers' Own Practices

When discussing the extent to which antibiotic resistance is a problem in their own practices, providers had widely differing opinions, ranging from little or no resistance, "I have never noticed resistance within my practice." (GS), to clear, affirmative responses, "Yes, based on cultures, I have had patients who have had organisms identified that have a pretty concerning resistance profile." (DS). Some providers expressed uncertainty regarding the extent of antibiotic resistance, for example, "It is so hard for me to predict what's going to be resistant." (EJ), while others indicated a need for an antibiogram. One provider stated, "I don't know if there's actually resistance in this area or not. It would be nice to get, like, a report to say that." (AA).

3. Discussion

In our study PCPs' antibiotic choices and durations in the case scenario of acute uncomplicated cystitis were generally in line with the guidelines' recommended first-line therapy. Most providers correctly chose TMP-SMX or nitrofurantoin for the treatment of uncomplicated cystitis in the case scenario. However, ciprofloxacin was often the second antibiotic mentioned when providers responded to the question about the top three most frequently prescribed antibiotics for uncomplicated cystitis.

A number of providers chose treatment durations longer than the guideline recommendations. In particular, many were unaware that the current recommended duration of therapy for nitrofurantoin has been reduced to 5 days [8] compared with the 7-day duration in the previous 1999 IDSA guideline [30].

We found that many PCPs believe that fluoroquinolones are more likely to achieve rapid and effective control of UTI symptoms than TMP-SMX or nitrofurantoin. This finding is in line with a previous qualitative study on the effects of knowledge, attitudes, and practices of PCPs on antibiotic selection [31]. Belief that broad-spectrum antibiotics may be more likely to cure an infection was the main reason for a lack of adherence to the guidelines [31]. However, clinical trials have shown that fluoroquinolones are comparable with first-line recommended agents in both clinical and microbiological efficacy in UTIs [32]. Although fluoroquinolones are highly efficacious for uncomplicated cystitis if the uropathogens are susceptible, increasing resistance rates may hamper the effectiveness of fluoroquinolones for empirical antibiotic use. Fluroquinolone resistance increased dramatically in recent years, with >10–30% of community-associated Enterobacteriaceae being quinolone resistant in many parts of the United States and with even higher rates (>50%) in other parts of the world [33]. Furthermore, fluoroquinolones have been moved to the last class of agents (after β-lactams) and should be used only when no other oral options are available because of three warnings from the U.S. FDA that the risk for serious harms outweighs the benefits for patients with uncomplicated UTIs [13–15]. Of note, the initial warning preceded our interviews by approximately a year.

In our study, PCPs' prescribing decisions took into account multiple factors in determining the best course of treatment for patients with acute cystitis such as pregnancy, patients' past experience with a specific antibiotic, previous antibiotic susceptibilities, frequency of UTI, older age, and presence of diabetes. Some PCPs chose a longer duration of treatment when the patient was older or had diabetes. These results are consistent with our previous observational database study, performed in the same setting, showing that older age and the presence of diabetes were independent, significant predictors of a longer treatment duration for UTIs [10]. Older women were also more likely to receive fluoroquinolones for uncomplicated UTIs in a study on national antibiotic prescribing trends in outpatient settings in the U.S. [9]. Advanced age, diabetes, and recurrent UTIs may be cognitive biases that drive inappropriate antibiotic use for uncomplicated UTI. Treatment recommendations for otherwise healthy older women, with or without diabetes, are similar to those for younger women [34–36]. Similarly, antibiotic choice and duration for sporadic and recurrent UTIs are not different. Broadening the antibiotic spectrum or lengthening the treatment course have not been proven efficacious and elicit concern for potential harm to the individual and the community [37].

Another condition that triggered uncertainty for choosing the right antibiotic among the PCPs was UTI in pregnancy. Some were concerned about the association between the use of nitrofurantoin and birth defects reported in case-control studies [28,29]. However, no relationship between nitrofurantoin use and birth defects was observed in a recent large cohort study [38]. An alternative first-line antibiotic that can be used in pregnancy is fosfomycin. However, PCPs in our study were not familiar with fosfomycin as a possible treatment option for cystitis, although it is a first-line agent per IDSA guidelines.

The fact that our providers did not seem to be aware of fosfomycin as a first-line recommended antibiotic for uncomplicated UTI was not surprising. Fosfomycin was not prescribed in any visits for UTIs in our previous database study [10], and it was prescribed in less than 0.1% of all visits in a recent study of national antibiotic prescribing practices for UTIs in the U.S. [24]. Some of the reasons may be that susceptibility to fosfomycin is not included in the reports received by the providers from the lab, as well as insurance barriers and higher cost of fosfomycin compared with other UTI-relevant antibiotics.

Primary care physicians increasingly have multiple and sometimes conflicting guidelines [39] for patient care and are challenged to maintain the knowledge base represented by the array of guidelines for common problems. In a nationally representative sample of family physicians, Wolff and colleagues [40] found that time constraints, concern for patient well-being, and consideration of particular circumstances were all potential obstacles to guideline adherence; such concerns (e.g., compliance concerns, patient preferences, and previously reported side effects) were noted by the physicians interviewed for the current study. Likewise, nearly half of our study sample thought it would be useful to have guidelines as a component of an electronic medical record, implying that speed and ease of access are important to them. Most providers interviewed were unable to quote from guidelines presented in monograph form but reported routinely accessing various electronic media (e.g., UpToDate or Family Practice Notebook) for prescribing support.

Although most of the primary care providers were concerned about antibiotic resistance in their practice, some did not consider antibiotic resistance to be a problem in their own practice, citing greater resistance problems in inpatient settings or in non-UTI conditions. Likewise, in a Swedish qualitative study, providers were aware of antibiotic resistance but thought of it as a national problem that does not concern their own practice [41]. Some of our interviewed providers indicated a need for an antibiogram specific to their setting to guide their empiric choices and a tool that can help predict the risk of resistance in a specific patient. Unfortunately, an outpatient-specific antibiogram is not available for the participating clinics, and we suspect that few settings have an outpatient-specific antibiogram [42,43].

The main limitation of our study is the relatively small sample size. However, we performed this qualitative study in a preparatory phase of a stewardship intervention and included all PCPs working in two clinics. As with any qualitative study, the results are not meant to be generalizable. In particular, our findings may not be generalizable to public clinics or clinics that are not academically affiliated. Our findings represent an in-depth exploration of the attitudes and beliefs of the study sample. However, findings are transferable as the issues we identified have been seen in other settings [9,31,41]. We are using these findings to develop provider-focused materials for a subsequent clinic-based intervention designed to support providers in their efforts to reduce the risks of drug resistance, to minimize serious side effects, and to enhance overall patient care.

Our findings highlight the necessity of providing point-of-care information for primary care providers from a trusted and easy to access source. This information will help providers to choose the right antibiotic with the right duration, a fundamental aspect of antimicrobial stewardship for UTI.

4. Materials and Methods

4.1. Ethics

The study was conducted in accordance with the Declaration of Helsinki, and the protocol was approved by the Ethics Committee of Baylor College of Medicine on 7 February 2019 (H-38265).

4.2. Setting and Participants

We selected individual interviews as the data collection strategy most appropriate for our research objectives of exploring individual prescribing decisions. Individual interviews allow for in-depth data collection and minimize the potential influence of group interaction or seniority and supervisory relationships that could have been introduced with focus groups. In addition, individual interviews allowed a much greater flexibility with scheduling, making it more feasible to reach and engage participants. We conducted brief (30 minutes or less), individual, semi-structured interviews with 18 primary care providers (15 family medicine physicians and three physician assistants) in two private, academically affiliated family medicine clinics in a large urban area between late July 2017 and early November 2017. Both clinics utilize Epic Electronic Health Records. The characteristics of our study sample are described in Table 1.

Table 1. The characteristics of the primary care providers.

Characteristic	n (%)
Female	9 (50)
Provider type	
Physician	15 (83)
Physician assistant	3 (17)
Years in practice	
Fewer than ten years	9 (50)
10–20 years	3
Over 21 years	6
Board certified in Family Medicine	14
Board certified in other specialty	1 [a]
Race/ethnicity	
White	6
Hispanic/Latino	3
Black	1
Asian	8

[a] One physician was board certified in Internal Medicine.

On average, 19,777 patients attend 3248 appointments at these clinics each month. Patients in both clinics are predominantly female (58%) and white (54%). Fluoroquinolones were the most common antibiotic class prescribed (51.6%) for uncomplicated UTI, and 75% of all prescriptions were longer than the recommended duration in these clinics in our previous study in the period of 2011–2014 [10].

4.3. Interview Guide Development

The concepts included in our interview guide were based on the Cabana framework for understanding barriers to physician adherence to clinical practice guidelines [27]. According to this framework, three factors affect physician compliance with evidence-based guidelines: knowledge, attitudes, and external factors. Our interview guide (Figure 2) focused on the following issues: awareness and familiarity with the guidelines (knowledge), acceptance and outcome expectancy (attitudes), and external barriers. To assess awareness and familiarity, we included the following questions: "How familiar are you with any guidelines on the treatment of uncomplicated cystitis?", "What do you recall about these guidelines?", and "Do these guidelines apply to your practice?". To assess the acceptance and outcome expectancy, we asked probing questions about the treatment of recurrent UTIs and situations in which the patients were older, diabetic, or male. To help elucidate external factors that might be driving treatment decisions, we included a clinical vignette about a patient who had a diagnosis of acute uncomplicated cystitis and asked the participants to explain their rationale for antibiotic choice and treatment duration and some reasons other primary care providers might prescribe a fluoroquinolone for this condition.

> **Case Scenario:** A 44-year-old female patient comes to see you. Yesterday she began to experience urgency leading to frequent urination and dysuria. She has had urinary tract infections in the past, but not in the last two years. Her urinalysis is positive for leukocyte esterase and reveals 20-40 white blood cells. She has no medication allergies and is otherwise healthy. You diagnose her with acute uncomplicated cystitis.
>
> 1. What antibiotic would you prescribe and for how long?
> 2. Data show that many of your peers choose broad-spectrum antibiotics like ciprofloxacin for this condition. Can you tell me some reasons ciprofloxacin is frequently prescribed for this condition?
> 3. What do you think makes a fluoroquinolone a frequent choice?
> 4. What factors influence your choice of antibiotics?
>   - Can you describe some specific examples?
> 5. What are the top 3 antibiotics that you use most frequently for acute cystitis?
> 6. Can you tell me about your experiences with these antibiotics?
> 7. Can you tell me about any experiences you've had with fosfomycin?
>   - What are some of the benefits and drawbacks of this antibiotic?
> 8. How do you keep up-to-date on new information about antibiotics?
> 9. How familiar are you with any guidelines on treatment of uncomplicated cystitis?
>   - What do you recall about these guidelines? (specific examples)
> 10. Do you think antibiotic resistance is a problem in your practice?
>   - Can you tell me more about this?

Figure 2. Sample interview questions.

The interview guide also included questions about clinical and nonclinical factors influencing antibiotic choice and treatment duration, such as patient comorbidities or expected patient compliance. We asked open-ended questions about providers' experience with the specific antibiotics and their preferred sources of support for clinical decision making. We also asked whether they perceived antibiotic resistance to be a problem in their practices. Before starting the study, we pilot-tested our interview guide with two primary care providers at another institution and adapted the guide as per their suggestions.

4.4. Interview Procedures

Primary care providers were recruited by the research team during a weekly clinic meeting and provided an overview of the study. After these meetings, individual follow-up recruitment emails were sent by the research interviewer, a doctoral level social psychologist with substantial experience in conducting qualitative interviews (SN). If providers were interested in participating, the interviewer negotiated a convenient time for the session before or after regularly scheduled patient care responsibilities. At the meeting, the interviewer responded to any additional questions or concerns and obtained consent to participate. All invited providers agreed to participate and received a U.S. $20 gift card for their participation. Each individual participated only once.

4.5. Data Collection and Analysis

To protect participant confidentiality, the interviewer asked each participant to select an alias, which we designated by initials during the interview and in the resulting transcripts. The interviews were digitally recorded and transcribed verbatim by professional medical transcriptionists. The interviewer listened to all recordings to verify the accuracy of the transcripts before entering them into NVivo 10 software, a qualitative analysis package (QSR International, 2014) that facilitates the management of qualitative data. Based on a preliminary review of the transcripts and the aims of the study, we determined that the interview questions and subsequent probes provided an appropriate outline for the initial identification of key themes [44,45].

Two authors (LG and SN) met regularly to read, code, and discuss the transcribed interviews, maintaining a shared consensus on the coding process. We elected to focus on the explicit content of providers' reported experiences and perspectives [46]. Overall, we followed the six-phase approach to thematic analysis described by Braun and Clark [47], a sequential but flexible set of guidelines that encompasses familiarization with the data; initial coding; searching, reviewing, and defining themes; and finally, integrating the analytic narrative and data extracts by incorporating illustrative quotes from providers into the description of the final themes [44,47]. Although our sample size was limited to the total number of providers in the clinic setting, we judged that the last 5 to 6 interviews coded were redundant to those previously coded, in repetition without an expansion of the themes, and were confident that data saturation for this sample had been reached [25].

5. Conclusions

Our qualitative analysis found that many PCPs believe that fluoroquinolones achieve more rapid and effective control of UTI symptoms than trimethoprim-sulfamethoxazole or nitrofurantoin. The majority of the providers were unfamiliar with fosfomycin as a possible treatment option for cystitis, although it is a first-line agent per guidelines. For recurrent UTI, older patients, or those with diabetes, some providers reported that they would go with "a stronger, broad-spectrum antibiotic such as ciprofloxacin" and longer treatment duration. For support in clinical decision making, few providers relied on guidelines, preferring instead to have decision support embedded in the electronic medical record. Understanding primary care providers' clinical challenges and knowing their preferred sources of information will enable us to develop a primary care-specific antibiotic stewardship intervention for acute cystitis.

Author Contributions: L.G., B.W.T., S.N. and R.Z. conceived and designed the study; S.N. and L.G. analyzed the data; L.G., S.N., M.S.H., F.M.K., L.M., G.J.G. and B.W.T. provided input on the study concept and design and the interpretation of the data; L.G. wrote the paper.

Funding: This research was funded by Zambon Pharmaceuticals, grant number 47271-I.

Acknowledgments: This investigator-initiated research study was funded by Zambon Pharmaceuticals. Trautner's work is supported in part by the Houston Veterans Affairs Health Services Research & Development Center for Innovations in Quality, Effectiveness, and Safety (CIN 13-413) and by Veterans Affairs funding (HSR&D 16-025).

Conflicts of Interest: Grigoryan and Trautner report grants from the National Institutes of Health and the U.S. Department of Veterans Affairs Health Services Research & Development Service.

References

1. Centers for Disease Control and Prevention. Antibiotic/Antimicrobial Resistance. Biggest Threats. Available online: https://www.cdc.gov/drugresistance/biggest_threats.html (accessed on 17 June 2019).
2. National Action Plan for Combating Antibiotic-Resistant Bacteria. Available online: https://aspe.hhs.gov/system/files/pdf/258516/ProgressYears1and2CARBNationalActionPlan.pdf (accessed on 17 June 2019).
3. The Pew Charitable Trusts. Antibiotic Use in Outpatient Settings. Available online: http://www.pewtrusts.org/~/media/assets/2016/05/antibioticuseinoutpatientsettings.pdf (accessed on 17 June 2019).
4. Meeker, D.; Linder, J.A.; Fox, C.R.; Friedberg, M.W.; Persell, S.D.; Goldstein, N.J.; Knight, T.K.; Hay, J.W.; Doctor, J.N. Effect of Behavioral Interventions on Inappropriate Antibiotic Prescribing Among Primary Care Practices: A Randomized Clinical Trial. *JAMA* **2016**, *315*, 562–570. [CrossRef] [PubMed]
5. Drekonja, D.M.; Filice, G.A.; Greer, N.; Olson, A.; MacDonald, R.; Rutks, I.; Wilt, T.J. Antimicrobial stewardship in outpatient settings: A systematic review. *Infect. Control Hosp. Epidemiol.* **2015**, *36*, 142–152. [CrossRef] [PubMed]

6. Hecker, M.T.; Fox, C.J.; Son, A.H.; Cydulka, R.K.; Siff, J.E.; Emerman, C.L.; Sethi, A.K.; Muganda, C.P.; Donskey, C.J. Effect of a stewardship intervention on adherence to uncomplicated cystitis and pyelonephritis guidelines in an emergency department setting. *PLoS ONE* **2014**, *9*, e87899. [CrossRef] [PubMed]
7. Fleming-Dutra, K.E.; Hersh, A.L.; Shapiro, D.J.; Bartoces, M.; Enns, E.A.; File, T.M.; Finkelstein, J.A., Jr.; Gerber, J.S.; Hyun, D.Y.; Linder, J.A.; et al. Prevalence of Inappropriate Antibiotic Prescriptions Among US Ambulatory Care Visits, 2010–2011. *JAMA* **2016**, *315*, 1864–1873. [CrossRef] [PubMed]
8. Gupta, K.; Hooton, T.M.; Naber, K.G.; Wullt, B.; Colgan, R.; Miller, L.G.; Moran, G.J.; Nicolle, L.E.; Raz, R.; Schaeffer, A.J.; et al. International clinical practice guidelines for the treatment of acute uncomplicated cystitis and pyelonephritis in women: A 2010 update by the Infectious Diseases Society of America and the European Society for Microbiology and Infectious Diseases. *Clin. Infect. Dis.* **2011**, *52*, e103–e120. [CrossRef]
9. Kobayashi, M.; Shapiro, D.J.; Hersh, A.L.; Sanchez, G.V.; Hicks, L.A. Outpatient Antibiotic Prescribing Practices for Uncomplicated Urinary Tract Infection in Women in the United States, 2002–2011. *Open Forum Infect. Dis.* **2016**, *3*, ofw159. [CrossRef] [PubMed]
10. Grigoryan, L.; Zoorob, R.; Wang, H.; Trautner, B.W. Low Concordance With Guidelines for Treatment of Acute Cystitis in Primary Care. *Open Forum Infect. Dis.* **2015**, *2*, ofv159. [CrossRef]
11. Shively, N.R.; Buehrle, D.J.; Clancy, C.J.; Decker, B.K. Prevalence of Inappropriate Antibiotic Prescribing in Primary Care Clinics within a Veterans Affairs Health Care System. *Antimicrob. Agents Chemother.* **2018**, *62*. [CrossRef]
12. Petty, N.K.; Ben Zakour, N.L.; Stanton-Cook, M.; Skippington, E.; Totsika, M.; Forde, B.M.; Phan, M.D.; Gomes Moriel, D.; Peters, K.M.; Davies, M.; et al. Global dissemination of a multidrug resistant Escherichia coli clone. *Proc. Natl. Acad. Sci. USA* **2014**, *111*, 5694–5699. [CrossRef] [PubMed]
13. U.S Food and Drug Administration. FDA Advises Restricting Fluoroquinolone Antibiotic Use for Certain Uncomplicated Infections; Warns about Disabling Side Effects that Can Occur Together. 2016. Available online: https://www.fda.gov/downloads/Drugs/DrugSafety/UCM500591.pdf (accessed on 17 June 2019).
14. U.S Food and Drug Administration. FDA Updates Warnings for Fluoroquinolone Antibiotics on Risks of Mental Health and Low Blood Sugar Adverse Reactions. Available online: https://www.fda.gov/newsevents/newsroom/pressannouncements/ucm612995.htm (accessed on 17 June 2019).
15. U.S. Food and Drug Administration. FDA Warns about Increased Risk of Ruptures or Tears in the Aorta Blood Vessel with Fluoroquinolone Antibiotics in Certain Patients. 2018. Available online: https://www.fda.gov/Drugs/DrugSafety/ucm628753.htm (accessed on 17 June 2019).
16. Stephenson, A.L.; Wu, W.; Cortes, D.; Rochon, P.A. Tendon Injury and Fluoroquinolone Use: A Systematic Review. *Drug Saf.* **2013**, *36*, 709–721. [CrossRef]
17. Wise, B.L.; Peloquin, C.; Choi, H.; Lane, N.E.; Zhang, Y. Impact of age, sex, obesity, and steroid use on quinolone-associated tendon disorders. *Am. J. Med.* **2012**, *125*, e1223–e1228. [CrossRef] [PubMed]
18. Briasoulis, A.; Agarwal, V.; Pierce, W.J. QT prolongation and torsade de pointes induced by fluoroquinolones: Infrequent side effects from commonly used medications. *Cardiology* **2011**, *120*, 103–110. [CrossRef] [PubMed]
19. Aspinall, S.L.; Good, C.B.; Jiang, R.; McCarren, M.; Dong, D.; Cunningham, F.E. Severe dysglycemia with the fluoroquinolones: A class effect? *Clin. Infect. Dis.* **2009**, *49*, 402–408. [CrossRef] [PubMed]
20. Chou, H.W.; Wang, J.L.; Chang, C.H.; Lee, J.J.; Shau, W.Y.; Lai, M.S. Risk of severe dysglycemia among diabetic patients receiving levofloxacin, ciprofloxacin, or moxifloxacin in Taiwan. *Clin. Infect. Dis.* **2013**, *57*, 971–980. [CrossRef] [PubMed]
21. Ali, A.K. Peripheral neuropathy and Guillain-Barre syndrome risks associated with exposure to systemic fluoroquinolones: A pharmacovigilance analysis. *Ann. Epidemiol.* **2014**, *24*, 279–285. [CrossRef] [PubMed]
22. Aoun, M.; Jacquy, C.; Debusscher, L.; Bron, D.; Lehert, M.; Noel, P.; van der Auwera, P. Peripheral neuropathy associated with fluoroquinolones. *Lancet* **1992**, *340*, 127. [CrossRef]
23. Etminan, M.; Brophy, J.M.; Samii, A. Oral fluoroquinolone use and risk of peripheral neuropathy: A pharmacoepidemiologic study. *Neurology* **2014**, *83*, 1261–1263. [CrossRef]
24. Durkin, M.J.; Keller, M.; Butler, A.M.; Kwon, J.H.; Dubberke, E.R.; Miller, A.C.; Polgreen, P.M.; Olsen, M.A. An Assessment of Inappropriate Antibiotic Use and Guideline Adherence for Uncomplicated Urinary Tract Infections. *Open Forum Infect. Dis.* **2018**, *5*, ofy198. [CrossRef]
25. Saunders, B.; Sim, J.; Kingstone, T.; Baker, S.; Waterfield, J.; Bartlam, B.; Burroughs, H.; Jinks, C. Saturation in qualitative research: Exploring its conceptualization and operationalization. *Qual. Quant.* **2018**, *52*, 1893–1907. [CrossRef]

26. Guest, G.; Bunce, A.; Johnson, L. How Many Interviews Are Enough? *Field Methods* **2006**, *18*, 59–82. [CrossRef]
27. Cabana, M.D.; Rand, C.S.; Powe, N.R.; Wu, A.W.; Wilson, M.H.; Abboud, P.A.; Rubin, H.R. Why don't physicians follow clinical practice guidelines? A framework for improvement. *JAMA* **1999**, *282*, 1458–1465. [CrossRef] [PubMed]
28. Ailes, E.C.; Gilboa, S.M.; Gill, S.K.; Broussard, C.S.; Crider, K.S.; Berry, R.J.; Carter, T.C.; Hobbs, C.A.; Interrante, J.D.; Reefhuis, J.; et al. Association between antibiotic use among pregnant women with urinary tract infections in the first trimester and birth defects, National Birth Defects Prevention Study 1997 to 2011. *Birth Defects Res. A Clin. Mol. Teratol.* **2016**, *106*, 940–949. [CrossRef] [PubMed]
29. Crider, K.S.; Cleves, M.A.; Reefhuis, J.; Berry, R.J.; Hobbs, C.A.; Hu, D.J. Antibacterial medication use during pregnancy and risk of birth defects: National Birth Defects Prevention Study. *Arch. Pediatr. Adolesc. Med.* **2009**, *163*, 978–985. [CrossRef] [PubMed]
30. Warren, J.W.; Abrutyn, E.; Hebel, J.R.; Johnson, J.R.; Schaeffer, A.J.; Stamm, W.E. Guidelines for antimicrobial treatment of uncomplicated acute bacterial cystitis and acute pyelonephritis in women. Infectious Diseases Society of America (IDSA). *Clin. Infect. Dis.* **1999**, *29*, 745–758. [CrossRef] [PubMed]
31. Sanchez, G.V.; Roberts, R.M.; Albert, A.P.; Johnson, D.D.; Hicks, L.A. Effects of knowledge, attitudes, and practices of primary care providers on antibiotic selection, United States. *Emerg. Infect. Dis.* **2014**, *20*, 2041–2047. [CrossRef] [PubMed]
32. Grigoryan, L.; Trautner, B.W.; Gupta, K. Diagnosis and management of urinary tract infections in the outpatient setting: A review. *JAMA* **2014**, *312*, 1677–1684. [CrossRef]
33. Spellberg, B.; Doi, Y. The Rise of Fluoroquinolone-Resistant Escherichia coli in the Community: Scarier Than We Thought. *J. Infect. Dis.* **2015**, *212*, 1853–1855. [CrossRef]
34. Mody, L.; Juthani-Mehta, M. Urinary tract infections in older women: A clinical review. *JAMA* **2014**, *311*, 844–854. [CrossRef]
35. Grigoryan, L.; Zoorob, R.; Wang, H.; Horsfield, M.; Gupta, K.; Trautner, B.W. Less workup, longer treatment, but no clinical benefit observed in women with diabetes and acute cystitis. *Diabetes Res. Clin. Pract.* **2017**, *129*, 197–202. [CrossRef]
36. Schneeberger, C.; Stolk, R.P.; Devries, J.H.; Schneeberger, P.M.; Herings, R.M.; Geerlings, S.E. Differences in the pattern of antibiotic prescription profile and recurrence rate for possible urinary tract infections in women with and without diabetes. *Diabetes Care* **2008**, *31*, 1380–1385. [CrossRef]
37. Smith, A.L.; Brown, J.; Wyman, J.F.; Berry, A.; Newman, D.K.; Stapleton, A.E. Treatment and Prevention of Recurrent Lower Urinary Tract Infections in Women: A Rapid Review with Practice Recommendations. *J. Urol.* **2018**, *200*, 1174–1191. [CrossRef] [PubMed]
38. Muanda, F.T.; Sheehy, O.; Berard, A. Use of antibiotics during pregnancy and the risk of major congenital malformations: A population based cohort study. *Br. J. Clin. Pharmacol.* **2017**, *83*, 2557–2571. [CrossRef] [PubMed]
39. Markowitz, M.A.; Wood, L.N.; Raz, S.; Miller, L.G.; Haake, D.A.; Kim, J.H. Lack of uniformity among United States recommendations for diagnosis and management of acute, uncomplicated cystitis. *Int. Urogynecol. J.* **2018**. [CrossRef] [PubMed]
40. Wolff, M.; Bower, D.J.; Marbella, A.M.; Casanova, J.E. US family physicians' experiences with practice guidelines. *Fam. Med. Kans. City* **1998**, *30*, 117–121.
41. Bjorkman, I.; Berg, J.; Viberg, N.; Stalsby Lundborg, C. Awareness of antibiotic resistance and antibiotic prescribing in UTI treatment: A qualitative study among primary care physicians in Sweden. *Scand. J. Prim. Health Care* **2013**, *31*, 50–55. [CrossRef] [PubMed]
42. Rank, E.L.; Lodise, T.; Avery, L.; Bankert, E.; Dobson, E.; Dumyati, G.; Hassett, S.; Keller, M.; Pearsall, M.; Lubowski, T.; et al. Antimicrobial Susceptibility Trends Observed in Urinary Pathogens Obtained From New York State. *Open Forum Infect. Dis.* **2018**, *5*, ofy297. [CrossRef]
43. Delisle, G.; Quach, C.; Domingo, M.C.; Boudreault, A.A.; Gourdeau, M.; Bernatchez, H.; Lavallee, C. Escherichia coli antimicrobial susceptibility profile and cumulative antibiogram to guide empirical treatment of uncomplicated urinary tract infections in women in the province of Quebec, 2010–2015. *J. Antimicrob. Chemother.* **2016**, *71*, 3562–3567. [CrossRef]
44. King, N. Using templates in the thematic analysis of text. In *Essential Guide to Qualitative Methods in Organizational Research*; Cassell, C., Symon, G., Eds.; Sage Publications Ltd.: Thousand Oaks, CA, USA, 2004; pp. 257–270.

45. Rowley, J. Conducting research interviews. *Manag. Res. Rev.* **2012**, *35*, 260–271. [CrossRef]
46. Riessman, C.K. *Narrative Methods for the Human Sciences*; Sage Publications Inc.: Thousand Oaks, CA, USA, 2008.
47. Braun, V.; Clarke, V. Using thematic analysis in psychology. *Qual. Res. Psychol.* **2006**, *3*, 77–101. [CrossRef]

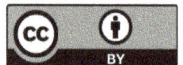

© 2019 by the authors. Licensee MDPI, Basel, Switzerland. This article is an open access article distributed under the terms and conditions of the Creative Commons Attribution (CC BY) license (http://creativecommons.org/licenses/by/4.0/).

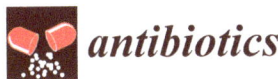

Article

Antibiotic Prescribing Quality in Out-of-Hours Primary Care and Critical Appraisal of Disease-Specific Quality Indicators

Annelies Colliers [1,*,†], Niels Adriaenssens [1,†], Sibyl Anthierens [1], Stephaan Bartholomeeusen [1], Hilde Philips [1], Roy Remmen [1] and Samuel Coenen [1,2,3]

1. Department of Primary and Interdisciplinary Care (ELIZA)—Centre for General Practice, Faculty of Medicine and Health Sciences, University of Antwerp, Doornstraat 331, B-2610 Antwerp, Belgium; niels.adriaenssens@uantwerpen.be (N.A.); sibyl.anthierens@uantwerpen.be (S.A.); stephaan.bartholomeeusen@uantwerpen.be (S.B.); hilde.philips@uantwerpen.be (H.P.); roy.remmen@uantwerpen.be (R.R.); samuel.coenen@uantwerpen.be (S.C.)
2. Department of Epidemiology and Social Medicine (ESOC), Faculty of Medicine and Health Sciences, University of Antwerp, Universiteitsplein 1, B-2610 Antwerp, Belgium
3. Vaccine & Infectious Disease Institute (VAXINFECTIO), Faculty of Medicine and Health Sciences, University of Antwerp, Universiteitsplein 1, B-2610 Antwerp, Belgium
* Correspondence: annelies.colliers@uantwerpen.be; Tel.: +32-3-265-18-32
† The first two authors made equal contributions.

Received: 15 May 2019; Accepted: 7 June 2019; Published: 12 June 2019

Abstract: Outpatient antibiotic use in Belgium is among the highest in Europe. The most common reason for an encounter in out-of-hours (OOH) primary care is an infection. In this study, we assessed all consultations from July 2016 to June 2018 at five OOH services. We described antibiotic prescribing by diagnosis, calculated disease-specific antibiotic prescribing quality indicators' (APQI) values and critically appraised these APQI. We determined that 111,600 encounters resulted in 26,436 (23.7%) antibiotic prescriptions. The APQI diagnoses (i.e., bronchitis, upper respiratory infection, cystitis, tonsillitis, sinusitis, otitis media, and pneumonia) covered 14,927 (56.7%) antibiotic prescriptions. Erysipelas (1344 (5.1%)) and teeth/gum disease (982 (3.7%)) covered more prescriptions than sinusitis or pneumonia. Over 75% of patients with tonsillitis and over 50% with bronchitis, sinusitis, and otitis media were prescribed an antibiotic. Only for otitis media the choice of antibiotic was near the acceptable range. Over 10% of patients with bronchitis or pneumonia and over 25% of female patients with an acute cystitis received quinolones. The APQI cover the diagnoses for only 57% of all antibiotic prescriptions. As 5.1% and 3.7% of antibiotic prescriptions are made for erysipelas and teeth/gum disease, respectively, we propose to add these indications when assessing antibiotic prescribing quality in OOH primary care.

Keywords: antibiotics; out-of-hours care; primary care; quality of care; quality indicators; practitioners cooperative

1. Introduction

Antibiotic use in Belgium is among the highest in Europe, especially in ambulatory care, and thus the risk for antimicrobial resistance is high [1]. The European Surveillance of Antimicrobial Consumption (ESAC) [2] project has developed a set of 21 disease-specific antibiotic prescribing quality indicators (APQI) to assess the quality of antibiotic prescribing in primary care [3]. These APQI have been adopted in several evaluations of antibiotic prescribing in Europe [4–6].

Out-of-hours (OOH) care covers a large part of hours during a week. In Belgium, but also in the rest of Europe, the on-going establishment of large-scale general practitioner cooperatives

(GPCs) represents one of the most important developments for primary OOH health care. The most common reason for an encounter in Flemish (Northern part of Belgium) OOH primary care is an infection [7]. Many infections are self-limiting and no antimicrobial treatment is necessary. However, in our qualitative work general practitioners (GPs) describe the difficulties they encounter in OOH care not to prescribe antibiotics relating to contextual factors such as a larger uncertainty due to an unknown patient, type of patients (e.g., children, elderly, Non-Native Speakers, ...), workload, and the lack of diagnostic tools or follow-up. They have a feeling that their professional identity is different compared to in-hours care [8,9]. However, previous research in Belgium showed similar APQI values for in- and out-of-hours care, using the data of a singular general practitioner cooperative (GPC) from 2004–2009 [4], which is similar to findings in Norway and Sweden [10,11]. In the Netherlands, research showed higher prescribing rates in OOH care but with equal or even better quality compared to in-hours care [12]. In the United Kingdom, researchers found an increase in antibiotic prescribing in OOH primary care in contrast to in-hours care, however, this study did not explore the quality of the prescriptions [13,14]. Moreover, in Danish OOH care, antibiotics are the most prescribed drugs, but there was no evaluation on the quality of prescribing [15].

Therefore, the objective of this study is to assess the quality of antibiotic prescribing in OOH primary care to inform the implementation of future interventions to improve the antibiotic prescribing quality in this specific setting [16]. More specifically, we aim to describe antibiotic prescribing in Belgian OOH primary care by indication, assess its quality by updating values for ESAC's disease-specific APQI [3] and critically appraise these APQI [4].

2. Methods

2.1. Database and GPCs

Data were extracted from the Improving Care and Research Electronic Data Trust Antwerp (iCAREdata) database, a research database of linked data on OOH primary care [17,18]. On a weekly basis, routine clinical data and patient characteristics are automatically collected from GPCs, emergency departments (EDs) and pharmacists' electronic records completed during OOH-care. For this study we only used data from GPCs.

iCAREdata currently covers nine GPCs, that cover a population of 1,127,153. Only data from five GPCs were withheld for this study, because of the level of completeness of their data and availability at the start of the study. Together, they cover a population of around 811,000 inhabitants (11% of the Flemish population; i.e., the Northern Dutch speaking part of Belgium). The characteristics of these five GPCs are presented in Table 1. Because of a lack of registration of home visits in OOH care, only data from consultations at the GPC itself were used.

Table 1. Characteristics of the five general practitioner cooperatives (GPCs) providing data for this study.

GPC	Population	Number of GPs	Rural/Urban
Antwerp-East	148,366	112	Urban
Antwerp-North	141,110	119	Urban/rural
Antwerp-Centre	185,358	171	Urban
Tienen	84,430	80	Rural
Zuiderkempen	251,833	270	Rural
Total	811,097	752	

2.2. Study Setting

Since the beginning of the year 2000, Belgian OOH care is increasingly being organized in GPCs in regions that typically cover 80–180 GPs. All practicing GPs in such an area are obliged to participate in this service following a rotation-based system of being 'on call' during the weekends in their own region and they work in shifts of on average 12 h. GPCs are mostly organized in a fee-for-service system. There are 80–180 GPs per GPC. Belgian GPs do not have a gatekeeper function. There is free access to primary, secondary, and tertiary care. They use an electronic medical health record to register every patient contact. The software can differ depending on the GPC, but diagnoses are always selected using Thesaurus terms in the Belgian Bilingual Biclassified Thesaurus (3BT). By selecting a diagnosis in 3BT, an International Classification of Primary Care (ICPC-2-R) code is automatically linked [19]. Prescriptions are registered using the database of the Belgian Centre for Pharmacotherapeutic Information [20], which is linked to the Anatomical Therapeutic Chemical (ATC) classification system [21,22].

2.3. Data Analysis

Data extraction was done using Microsoft SQL server 2012. We performed descriptive analyses using Microsoft Excel 2016. Data from 1 July 2016 until 30 June 2018 were included.

2.3.1. Antibiotic Prescribing by Indication

To describe antibiotic prescribing by indication, first we only analyzed all antibiotic prescriptions (ATC code J01: antibacterials for systemic use) delivered during the consultations in five GPCs during a two-year timeframe and linked them with the diagnosis that was registered in the electronic medical health record.

2.3.2. Quality of Antibiotic Prescribing: Disease-Specific APQI

Second, we used information on all encounters to assess the quality of antibiotic prescribing using the disease-specific APQI introduced by ESAC (European Surveillance of Antimicrobial Consumption project) in 2007 [3]. The seven most common indications for antibiotic prescribing are in descending order: acute bronchitis (ICPC code R78), acute upper respiratory tract infection (RTI) (R74), cystitis/other urinary infection (UTI; U71), acute tonsillitis (R76), acute/chronic sinusitis (R75), and acute otitis media (H71). For pneumonia (R81), values of three valid APQI were calculated:

a = the percentage of patients with age and/or gender limitation (see legend Table 3) prescribed an antibiotic;
b = a and receiving the guideline recommended antibiotic;
c = a and receiving quinolones.

We compared them with the findings of an earlier study with data from 2004–2009 from one GPC [4].

2.3.3. Critical Appraisal

We evaluated if APQI is a sufficient method when describing the quality of antibiotic prescribing in OOH care. We used and adapted the concept of drug utilization 90% (DU90%) [23], which analyzes the number of drugs accounting for 90% of drug use. We used it to see if using APQI-diagnoses covers 90% of all antibiotic prescriptions.

2.4. Ethics

The study was approved by the Ethics Committee of the Antwerp University Hospital/University of Antwerp (reference number 17/08/089), and registered at clinicaltrials.gov (NCT03082521). The study was approved by the scientific advisory board of ICAREdata and the different GPCs.

3. Results

From 1/7/2016 until 30/6/2018, 26,436 antibiotic prescriptions were registered in 111,600 visits (excluding home visits) covering a population of 811,097 persons.

For 93.65% of the prescriptions, a diagnosis was registered in the same consultation. A diagnosis was missing for 1612 (6.35%) antibiotic prescriptions.

3.1. Antibiotic Prescribing by Indication

Table 2 shows the number of prescriptions linked to the ICPC chapters. Of them, 44% of the prescriptions are linked to diagnoses related to respiratory infections, 13% to urinary tract infections, 12% skin infections, 11% ear infections, and 6% digestive infections. Other diagnoses represent less than 5% of the prescriptions and are grouped in other diagnoses.

Table 2. Number of antibiotic prescriptions in a two-year time frame linked to diagnostic group (total patient contacts (excluding home visits) = 111,600).

ICPC-Code	Number of Antibiotic Prescriptions	Percentage
R	11,526	44%
U	3448	13%
S	3125	12%
H	2839	11%
D	1707	6%
missing	1612	6%
Other diagnoses (A, Y, L, X, B, F, W, K, P, N, T)	2179	8%
TOTAL	26,436	100%

ICPC: International Classification of Primary Care; R: respiratory; U: urinary; S: skin; H: ear; D: digestive; A: general and unspecified; Y: Male genital system; L: Musculoskeletal; X: female genital system and breast; B: blood forming organs, lymphatics, spleen; F: eye; W: pregnancy, childbirth, family planning; K: circulatory; P: Psychological; N: neurological; T: endocrine, metabolic and nutritional.

3.2. The Quality of Antibiotic Prescribing

Table 3 shows the results of the quality appraisal using APQI. We complemented this table with similar indicators for erysipelas and dental abscess, because they both cover respectively 5% and 4% of antibiotic prescriptions. There are not yet quality indicators for these two indications [24], but we chose to use following age limitations: older than one year for erysipelas and older than 18 year for dental abscess. Overall, for all conditions the percentage of antibiotics prescribed for common conditions exceed the upper limit (i.e., 20% for otitis media, upper RTI, sinusitis and tonsillitis, and 30% for bronchitis). Despite the fact that the highest amount of prescribed antibiotics are linked to upper RTI (Table 3), indicator 2A shows that 30% of patients diagnosed with upper RTI receive a prescription. Of the patients diagnosed with tonsillitis, 77% received an antibiotic prescription. For the latter two conditions, the use of the recommended antibiotics is less than 10% (3% for upper RTI and 6% for tonsillitis). For most other conditions, the use of recommended antibiotics ranges from 40–46% (40% for sinusitis, 42% for bronchitis, 42% for teeth/gum disease, erysipelas, and 46% for pneumonia). For cystitis and otitis media, the use of recommended antibiotics is higher, 69% and 74% respectively. No conditions reached the goal of 80–100%. Comparing these results with the APQI OOH study from 2004–2009, there is an improvement in choosing the recommended antibiotic. (otitis media: 42% → 74%; acute sinusitis: 23% → 40%; cystitis 40% → 69%; bronchitis 34% → 42%). Other values are in the same range as in 2004–2009 (Table S1 in the online Supplementary Materials).

For four conditions, the 5% upper limit of quinolone use was exceeded, i.e., in ascending order sinusitis (7%), bronchitis (11%), pneumonia (15%), and cystitis (25%).

GPs can choose to enter a symptom diagnosis. (such as fever, cough, etc.), but only 3.8% of all antibiotic prescriptions are linked to this type of diagnosis (Table S2 in the online Supplementary Materials).

Table 3. Quality appraisal using disease-specific antibiotic prescribing quality indicators (APQI) complemented with self-generated indicators for erysipelas and dental abscess.

ICPC-Code	Label	% of Patients Prescribed AB	% of Patients Receiving the Guideline Recommended AB	% of Patients Receiving Quinolones
		(<20%)	(>80%)	(<5%)
H71	Acute otitis media	64 [52–71]	74 [72–81]	1 [0–1]
R74	Acute upper respiratory tract infection	30 [15–41]	3 [2–7]	2 [0–2]
R75	Acute sinusitis	51 [39–57]	40 [35–51]	7 [2–9]
R76	Acute tonsillitis	77 [65–87]	6 [3–15]	1 [0–1]
		(<30%)	(>80%)	(<5%)
R78	Acute bronchitis	69 [58–75]	42 [37–54]	11 [5–15]
		(>80%)	(>80%)	(<5%)
R81	Pneumonia	80 [70–85]	46 [42–62]	15 [2–20]
U71	Acute cystitis	91 [77–95]	69 [64–77]	25 [18–32]
		(? > 80%?)	(>80%)	(<5%)
S76	Erysipelas	80 [64–83]	44 [36–59]	1 [0–2]
		(? < 30%?)	(>80%)	(<5%)
D82	Teeth/gum disease	67 [53–72]	42 [38–52]	1 [0–2]

ICPC: International Classification of Primary Care; AB: antibiotics; (): the acceptable range []: variation between the individual GPCs; R78: patients aged between 18 and 75 years with acute bronchitis/bronchiolitis; R74: patients older than one year with acute upper respiratory infection; U71: female patients older than 18 years with cystitis/other urinary infection; R76: patients older than one year with for acute tonsillitis; R75: patients older than 18 years with acute/chronic sinusitis; H71: patients older than two years with acute otitis media/myringitis; R81: patients aged between 18 and 65 years with pneumonia; S76: patients older than one year with erysipelas; D82: patients older than 18 years with teeth/gum disease.

3.3. Critical Appraisal of APQI to Describe Antibiotic Prescribing Quality in OOH Care

In 31,596/111,600 consultations, a diagnosis covered by APQI or erysipelas or dental abscess was made in OOH. Detailed diagnoses linked to antibiotic prescription are shown in Table 4. Most prescriptions are linked to upper respiratory tract infections (13%), followed by prescriptions for acute cystitis (12%), acute tonsillitis (9%) acute bronchitis (8%), and acute otitis media (8%). Most antibiotic prescriptions for skin infections are made for erysipelas (5%). Sinusitis, teeth/gum disease and pneumonia represent 4%, 4%, and 3% of the total of antibiotic prescriptions, respectively. When only using APQI diagnoses, 57% of antibiotic prescriptions are covered. When including erysipelas and teeth/gum disease, these nine diagnoses represent 66% of all antibiotic prescription. DU90% normally describes the number of drugs. When applying this concept on the coverage of indications, we do not reach 90% of all antibiotic prescriptions. The 220 other diagnoses represent in total 28% of the prescriptions but represent less than 3% each.

Table 4. Total antibiotic prescriptions and percentage linked to the diagnosis in a two-year time frame. (total patient contacts (excluding home visits) = 111,600).

ICPC-Code	Label	Total Prescriptions	Percentage
R74 [†]	Acute upper respiratory tract infection	3564	13%
U71 [†]	Acute cystitis	3068	12%
R76 [†]	Acute tonsillitis	2294	9%
R78 [†]	Acute bronchitis	2223	8%
H71 [†]	Acute otitis media	2129	8%
missing	Diagnosis missing	1612	6%
S76	Erysipelas	1344	5%
D82	Teeth/gum disease	982	4%
R75 [†]	Acute sinusitis	965	4%
R81 [†]	Pneumonia	684	3%
Other diagnoses	Group of diagnoses representing less than 3% each	7571	29%
Total		26,436	100%

[†] Diagnosis used in antibiotic prescribing quality indicators (APQI).

4. Discussion

4.1. Main Findings

Although most respiratory tract infections are self-limiting and usually caused by viral pathogens, at least half of the patients diagnosed with acute otitis media, sinusitis, tonsillitis, and bronchitis receive a prescription for an antibiotic at the GPC. Patients diagnosed with acute tonsillitis receive in 77% of the cases an antibiotic. Only for patients diagnosed with acute upper respiratory tract infection is the proportion of antibiotic prescriptions lower, but still higher than acceptable (30% while the acceptable range is between 0–20%). For nearly all indications the recommended type of antibiotics, according to the guidelines, are not prescribed apart from for otitis media, which is almost within the accepted range. Quinolone use is outside the acceptable range for following respiratory infections: sinusitis (7%), bronchitis (11%), and pneumonia (15%), which is in line with previous studies. The highest proportion of quinolones are still found among antibiotics prescribed for female patients with acute cystitis (25%). Looking at the total amount of antibiotic prescribing, we noticed a high number of prescriptions for erysipelas and dental problems, again with a high prescribing rate of non-guideline recommended antibiotics. There is not yet an acceptable range of prescribing determined for these two conditions. We suggest an acceptable range for the recommended antibiotic of more than 80% and respectively >80% and <30% of total antibiotic prescribing for erysipelas and teeth/gum disease.

For acute tonsillitis and acute upper respiratory tract infection, the very low percentage of recommended antibiotics (6% and 3%, respectively, acceptable range 80–100%) can be explained by the frequent unavailability of small spectrum penicillin in the Belgian pharmacies, therefore GPs most often choose to prescribe amoxicillin as an alternative (63% and 66% of all antibiotic prescriptions for upper RTI and tonsillitis respectively are for amoxicillin, see Tables S2 and S3) [4]. It is likely that conditions with recommended use around 40–44% (40% for sinusitis, 42% for bronchitis, 43% for teeth/gum disease, and 44% for erysipelas and 46% for pneumonia) are of more interest to policy makers, as for these conditions the GP decides to deviate from the guidelines mostly in favor of a broader spectrum antibiotic e.g., amoxicillin with clavulanic acid instead of amoxicillin alone). More detailed research is needed to identify appropriate use of broader spectrum antibiotic (e.g., treatment failure of initiated small spectrum antibiotic) versus inappropriate use driven by other factors such as lack of knowledge of the guideline, disagreement with the guideline, etc. [8]. These factors have been suggested as drivers for the use of quinolones for respiratory tract infections [25].

In Belgium, since 1 May 2018, the conditions for the reimbursement of quinolones and fluoroquinolones have been changed. These antibiotics are no longer reimbursed for the treatment of respiratory tract infections or uncomplicated urinary tract infections. Immediately after 1 May 2018, this measure seemed to have had an effect on quinolone prescribing [26]. However, whether or not this effect is causal and whether this trend will continue will be further monitored and analyzed using iCAREdata [17,18].

We have used the disease-specific APQI to describe the quality of antibiotic prescribing during OOH care. In our study, all seven diagnoses included in these APQI represent a considerable proportion of the total antibiotic use. In addition, we noticed that a substantial number of antibiotic prescriptions was also linked to two other diagnoses, i.e., erysipelas, dental problems (erysipelas (ICPC S76), and teeth/gum disease (ICPC D82), the latter most often representing a dental abscess based on notes review in a sample of the data. Therefore, we propose to add these two diagnoses (ICPC codes) when assessing the quality of antibiotic prescribing in OOH care. Further validation and more studies are necessary to confirm their relevance. However, when using these nine indications, only 66% of antibiotic prescriptions are covered and it could be argued that this is not enough to describe antibiotic quality. In accordance with the DU90% [23] concept, it would be more relevant to use indicators to be able to describe 90% of prescriptions. Dolk et al. found that the majority of antibiotic prescriptions in English primary care were for infections of the respiratory and urinary tracts, followed by skin infections and only a small number for dental problems [27].

According to the Belgian antibiotic guidelines, the primary treatment of acute dental problems is dental care by a dentist [28]. However, patients with acute tooth ache often visit the GPC to seek help during weekends and receive antibiotics. This has also been shown in previous studies in the UK [29]. GPs feel that general practice is not the best setting for managing dental problems [30] and one could argue whether or not the care for dental problems falls within the remit of GPs. Access to dental care during the weekends is limited, but patients should be redirected to these services.

APQI's were calculated for 1 GPC from data from 2004 to 2009. In the current study, with five GPCs (including the one GPC that was used in the 2004–2009 APQI OOH study) we noticed similar results in the percentage of patients who received an antibiotic, but an improvement in choice of antibiotics.

4.2. Strengths and Limitations

We have used electronic data that were routinely registered by GPs in their electronic health record for each patient contact. We used these observational routinely collected data retrospectively and GPs had no knowledge of an ongoing study. We included five GPCs (rural as well as urban GPCs) covering a large population that reflects the general population in Flanders (Belgium). Only GPCs with complete datasets were included. All GPs of the region are obliged to participate in the OOH care. Therefore, maximal coverage of GPs is guaranteed. In this way, we were able to achieve high validity and completeness of the data.

The use of electronic primary care databases such as iCAREdata can produce valid APQI values [4]. These values were originally developed for primary care, but not specifically for OOH care. Previous research showed minimal differences in antibiotic prescribing between in and out of hours care [4]. The quality of the data depends on the quality of the registrations by the GPs. We suspect that these APQI values give an incomplete picture of antibiotic prescribing. Antibiotics prescriptions linked to a symptom diagnosis, i.e., coding the diagnosis with a code for reasons for encounter such as fever, ear ache, cough, sore throat, etc., were not included in calculating APQI values. However, Flemish GPs not often register symptom diagnoses [7]. Indeed, when looking at the total number of antibiotic prescriptions, only a small percentage was made for symptom diagnosis. Handwritten prescriptions are still possible at the GPC, but are discouraged. Diagnosis shifting is possible as well, i.e., registering an incorrect diagnosis to justify a prescription [8]. Every prescription made by a GP is registered, and no difference is made between an immediate or a delayed prescription in the data. Although delayed prescriptions will add to the quantity of antibiotic prescribing, we know that around 40–60% of patients will collect their antibiotic anyway [31–34]. We register antibiotic prescribing and not antibiotic consuming or adherence to the prescribed course [31].

4.3. Implications for Practice and Future Research

Feedback of APQI values could serve as benchmarks of (in)appropriate prescribing. Each GPC could compare their antibiotic prescribing quality with the range of acceptable use to help quantify the magnitude of inappropriate prescribing in OOH primary care. It gives the opportunity to focus on the specific challenges in every organization and to work on prescribing more accurately.

These data could inform future tailored interventions to improve the quality of antibiotic prescribing in OOH primary care, such as we plan to do in the BAbAR project [16], and may also be used to monitor effects of other interventions to improve quality of care at the level of GPCs [35]. However, these indications do not cover all antibiotic prescribing.

5. Conclusions

Flemish GPs too often prescribe antibiotics for self-limiting infections in OOH primary care and do not choose the guideline recommended antibiotics. When using disease-specific APQI to define the quality of antibiotic prescribing in OOH care, we suggest to calculate indicator values for two additional disease entities, since a substantial amount of antibiotics are also prescribed for dental abscess and erysipelas.

Supplementary Materials: The following are available online at http://www.mdpi.com/2079-6382/8/2/79/s1: Table S1: Average value (%) for the disease-specific antibiotic prescribing quality indicators over a six-year period from 1 January 2004 to 31 December 2009 during out-of-hours vs. value (%) for the disease-specific antibiotic prescribing quality indicators over a two-year period from 1 July 2016 to 30 June 2018, Table S2: Number of antibiotic prescriptions in a 2 year time frame linked to symptom diagnosis * (total antibiotic prescriptions = 26,436), Table S3: Number of antibiotic prescriptions in a 2 year time frame linked to ICPC code R74, Table S4: Number of antibiotic prescriptions in a 2 year time frame linked to ICPC code R76.

Author Contributions: Conceptualization: A.C., N.A., S.A., H.P., S.B., R.R., and S.C.; methodology, A.C., N.A., and S.C.; data management: S.B. and H.P.; formal analysis: A.C. and N.A.; writing—original draft preparation: A.C. and N.A.; writing—review and editing: A.C., N.A., S.A., H.P., S.B., R.R., and S.C.

Funding: The study is part of the BAbAR study and has been granted a Ph.D. fellowship by the Faculty of Medicine and Health Sciences of the University of Antwerp. The iCAREdata database is funded by the Research Foundation Flanders.

Acknowledgments: We would like to thank the GPCs who gratefully provided consent to use the data from their organisation: Antwerp-East, Antwerp-North, Antwerp-Centre, Tienen, and Zuiderkempen.

Conflicts of Interest: The authors declare no conflict of interest.

References

1. European Centre for Disease Prevention and Control: Summary of the Latest Data on Antibiotic Consumption in the European Union: 2017. Available online: https://ecdc.europa.eu/en/publications-data/summary-latest-data-antibiotic-consumption-eu-2017 (accessed on 10 May 2019).
2. European Surveillance of Antimicrobial Consumption Network (ESAC-Net). Available online: https://ecdc.europa.eu/en/about-us/partnerships-and-networks/disease-and-laboratory-networks/esac-net (accessed on 10 May 2019).
3. Adriaenssens, N.; Coenen, S.; Tonkin-Crine, S.; Verheij, T.J.M.; Little, P.; Goossens, H.; Grp, E.P. European Surveillance of Antimicrobial Consumption (ESAC): Disease-specific quality indicators for outpatient antibiotic prescribing. *BMJ Qual. Saf.* **2011**, *20*, 764–772. [CrossRef] [PubMed]
4. Adriaenssens, N.; Bartholomeeusen, S.; Ryckebosch, P.; Coenen, S. Quality of antibiotic prescription during office hours and out-of-hours in Flemish primary care, using European quality indicators. *Eur. J. Gen. Pract.* **2014**, *20*, 114–120. [CrossRef]
5. Glinz, D.; Reyes, S.L.; Saccilotto, R.; Widmer, A.F.; Zeller, A.; Bucher, H.C.; Hemkens, L.G. Quality of antibiotic prescribing of Swiss primary care physicians with high prescription rates: A nationwide survey. *J. Antimicrob. Chemother.* **2017**, *72*, 3205–3212. [CrossRef] [PubMed]
6. Tyrstrup, M.; Van der Velden, A.; Engstrom, S.; Goderis, G.; Molstad, S.; Verheij, T.; Coenen, S.; Adriaenssens, N. Antibiotic prescribing in relation to diagnoses and consultation rates in Belgium, the Netherlands and Sweden: Use of European quality indicators. *Scand. J. Prim. Health Care* **2017**, *35*, 10–18. [CrossRef]
7. Smits, M.; Colliers, A.; Jansen, T.; Remmen, R.; Bartholomeeusen, S.; Verheij, R. Examining differences in out-of-hours primary care use in Belgium and the Netherlands: A cross-sectional study. *Eur. J. Public Health* **2019**. [CrossRef] [PubMed]
8. Colliers, A.; Coenen, S.; Remmen, R.; Philips, H.; Anthierens, S. How do general practitioners and pharmacists experience antibiotic use in out-of-hours primary care? An exploratory qualitative interview study to inform a participatory action research project. *BMJ Open* **2018**, *8*, e023154. [CrossRef] [PubMed]
9. Williams, S.J.; Halls, A.V.; Tonkin-Crine, S.; Moore, M.V.; Latter, S.E.; Little, P.; Eyles, C.; Postle, K.; Leydon, G.M. General practitioner and nurse prescriber experiences of prescribing antibiotics for respiratory tract infections in UK primary care out-of-hours services (the UNITE study). *J. Antimicrob. Chemother.* **2018**, *73*, 795–803. [CrossRef]
10. Lindberg, B.H.; Gjelstad, S.; Foshaug, M.; Høye, S. Antibiotic prescribing for acute respiratory tract infections in Norwegian primary care out-of-hours service. *Scand. J. Prim. Health Care* **2017**, *35*, 178–185. [CrossRef]
11. Cronberg, O. Infections and antibiotic prescribing in Swedish primary care. In *Abstracts of the GRIN Meeting*; Oral Presentation; UMC Utrecht: Zeist, The Netherlands, 2018; p. 26.
12. Debets, V.E.; Verheij, T.J.; van der Velden, A.W. SWAB's Working Group on Surveillance of Antimicrobial Use. Antibiotic prescribing during office hours and out-of-hours: A comparison of quality and quantity in primary care in The Netherlands. *Br. J. Gen. Pract.* **2017**, *67*, e178–e186. [CrossRef]

13. Edelstein, M.; Agbebiyi, A.; Ashiru-Oredope, D.; Hopkins, S. Trends and patterns in antibiotic prescribing among out-of-hours primary care providers in England, 2010–14. *J. Antimicrob. Chemother.* **2017**, *72*, 3490–3495. [CrossRef]
14. Hayward, G.N.; Fisher, R.F.; Spence, G.T.; Lasserson, D.S. Increase in antibiotic prescriptions in out-of-hours primary care in contrast to in-hours primary care prescriptions: Service evaluation in a population of 600,000 patients. *J. Antimicrob. Chemother.* **2016**, *71*, 2612–2619. [CrossRef] [PubMed]
15. Christensen, M.B.; Noroxe, K.B.; Moth, G.; Vedsted, P.; Huibers, L. Drug prescriptions in Danish out-of-hours primary care: A 1-yearpopulation-based study. *Scand. J. Prim. Health Care* **2016**, *34*, 453–458. [CrossRef] [PubMed]
16. Colliers, A.; Coenen, S.; Philips, H.; Remmen, R.; Anthierens, S. Optimising the quality of antibiotic prescribing in out-of-hours primary care in Belgium: A study protocol for an action research project. *BMJ Open* **2017**, *7*, e017522. [CrossRef]
17. Bartholomeeusen, S.; Philips, H.; Van Royen, P.; Remmen, R.; Coenen, S. iCAREdata: Improving Care And Research Electronic Data Trust Antwerp. *Zenodo* **2017**. [CrossRef]
18. Colliers, A.; Bartholomeeusen, S.; Remmen, R.; Coenen, S.; Michiels, B.; Bastiaens, H.; Van Royen, P.; Verhoeven, V.; Holmgren, P.; De Ruyck, B.; et al. Improving Care And Research Electronic Data Trust Antwerp (iCAREdata): A research database of linked data on out-of-hours primary care. *BMC Res. Notes* **2016**, *9*, 259. [CrossRef] [PubMed]
19. Verbeke, M.; Schrans, D.; Deroose, S.; De Maeseneer, J. The International Classification of Primary Care (ICPC-2): An essential tool in the EPR of the GP. *Stud. Health Technol. Inform.* **2006**, *124*, 809–814. [PubMed]
20. The Belgian Centre for Pharmacotherapeutic Information. Available online: http://www.bcfi.be (accessed on 10 May 2019).
21. WHO Collaborating Centre for Drug Statistics Methodology. *Anatomical Therapeutic Chemical (ATC) Classification System: Guidelines for ATC Classification and DDD Assignment 2011*; Norwegian Institute of Public Health: Oslo, Norway, 2011; Available online: http://www.whocc.no/filearchive/publications/2011guidelines.pdf (accessed on 10 May 2019).
22. Lamberts, H.; Wood, M. *International Classification of Primary Care*; Oxford University Press: Oxford, UK, 1987.
23. Bergman, U.; Popa, C.; Tomson, Y.; Wettermark, B.; Einarson, T.R.; Aberg, H.; Sjoqvist, F. Drug utilization 90%—A simple method for assessing the quality of drug prescribing. *Eur. J. Clin. Pharmacol.* **1998**, *54*, 113–118. [CrossRef] [PubMed]
24. Saust, L.T.; Monrad, R.N.; Hansen, M.P.; Arpi, M.; Bjerrum, L. Quality assessment of diagnosis and antibiotic treatment of infectious diseases in primary care: A systematic review of quality indicators. *Scand. J. Prim. Health Care* **2016**, *34*, 258–266. [CrossRef] [PubMed]
25. Coosemans, N.; Anthierens, S.; Adriaenssens, N. Waarom schrijven huisartsen chinolonen voor bij luchtweginfecties? *Huisarts Nu* **2016**, *45*, 186–189. [CrossRef]
26. GPs More Cautious When Prescribing Antibiotics. Available online: https://www.uantwerpen.be/popup/nieuwsonderdeel.aspx?newsitem_id=3391&c=HOMEEN&n=101352 (accessed on 10 May 2019).
27. Dolk, F.C.K.; Pouwels, K.B.; Smith, D.R.M.; Robotham, J.V.; Smieszek, T. Antibiotics in primary care in England: Which antibiotics are prescribed and for which conditions? *J. Antimicrob. Chemother.* **2018**, *73*, 2–10. [CrossRef]
28. Belgian Antibiotic Policy Coordination Committee (BAPCOC). Available online: https://consultativebodies.health.belgium.be/en/advisory-and-consultative-bodies/commissions/BAPCOC (accessed on 10 May 2019).
29. Cope, A.L.; Chestnutt, I.G.; Wood, F.; Francis, N.A. Dental consultations in UK general practice and antibiotic prescribing rates: A retrospective cohort study. *Br. J. Gen. Pract.* **2016**, *66*, e329–e336. [CrossRef] [PubMed]
30. Cope, A.L.; Wood, F.; Francis, N.A.; Chestnutt, I.G. General practitioners' attitudes towards the management of dental conditions and use of antibiotics in these consultations: A qualitative study. *BMJ Open* **2015**, *5*, e008551. [CrossRef] [PubMed]
31. Francis, N.A.; Gillespie, D.; Nuttall, J.; Hood, K.; Little, P.; Verheij, T.; Goossens, H.; Coenen, S.; Butler, C.C. Delayed antibiotic prescribing and associated antibiotic consumption in adults with acute cough. *Br. J. Gen. Pract.* **2012**, *62*, e639–e646. [CrossRef] [PubMed]
32. Hoye, S.; Gjelstad, S.; Lindbk, M. Effects on antibiotic dispensing rates of interventions to promote delayed prescribing for respiratory tract infections in primary care. *Br. J. Gen. Pract.* **2013**, *63*, e777–e786. [CrossRef]

33. Little, P.; Moore, M.; Kelly, J.; Williamson, I.; Leydon, G.; McDermott, L.; Mullee, M.; Stuart, B.; Investigators, P. Delayed antibiotic prescribing strategies for respiratory tract infections in primary care: Pragmatic, factorial, randomised controlled trial. *BMJ-Br. Med. J.* **2014**, *348*, g1606. [CrossRef]
34. Francis, N.A.; Gillespie, D.; Nuttall, J.; Hood, K.; Little, P.; Verheij, T.; Coenen, S.; Cals, J.W.; Goossens, H.; Butler, C.C.; et al. Antibiotics for acute cough: An international observational study of patient adherence in primary care. *Br. J. Gen. Pract.* **2012**, *62*, e429–e437. [CrossRef] [PubMed]
35. Willems, L.; Denckens, P.; Philips, H.; Henriquez, R.; Remmen, R. Can we improve adherence to guidelines for the treatment of lower urinary tract infection? A simple, multifaceted intervention in out-of-hours services. *J. Antimicrob. Chemother.* **2012**, *67*, 2997–3000. [CrossRef]

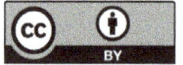

© 2019 by the authors. Licensee MDPI, Basel, Switzerland. This article is an open access article distributed under the terms and conditions of the Creative Commons Attribution (CC BY) license (http://creativecommons.org/licenses/by/4.0/).

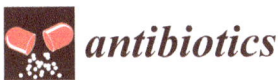

Article

Determination of Florfenicol, Thiamfenicol and Chloramfenicol at Trace Levels in Animal Feed by HPLC–MS/MS

Rosa Elvira Gavilán [1], Carolina Nebot [1,*], Ewelina Patyra [2], Beatriz Vazquez [1], Jose Manuel Miranda [1] and Alberto Cepeda [1]

[1] Department of Analytical Chemistry, Nutrition and Bromatology, Faculty of Veterinary Medicine, University of Santiago de Compostela, 27002 Lugo, Spain; rosaelviraclg@yahoo.es (R.E.G.); beatriz.vazquez@usc.es (B.V.); josemanuel.miranda@usc.es (J.M.M.); alberto.cepeda@usc.es (A.C.)
[2] Department of Hygiene of Animal Feedingstuffs, National Veterinary Research Institute, 24–100 Pulawy, Poland; ewelinapatyra@gmail.com
* Correspondence: carolina.nebot@usc.es

Received: 20 March 2019; Accepted: 30 April 2019; Published: 7 May 2019

Abstract: Administration of florfenicol and thiamfenicol through medicated feed is permitted within the European Union, always following veterinary prescription and respecting the withdrawal periods. However, the presence of low levels of florfenicol, thiamfenicol, and chloramfenicol in non-target feed is prohibited. Since cross-contamination can occur during the production of medicated feed and according to Annex II of the European Regulation 2019/4/EC, the control of residue levels of florfenicol and thiamfenicol in non-target feed should be monitored and avoided. Based on all the above, a sensitive and reliable method using liquid chromatography tandem mass spectrometry was developed for the simultaneous detection of chloramfenicol, florfenicol, and thiamfenicol at trace levels in animal feed. Analytes were extracted from minced feed with ethyl acetate. Then, the ethyl acetate was evaporated, the residue was resuspended in Milli-Q water and the extract filtered. The method was in-house validated at carryover levels, with concentration ranging from 100 to 1000 µg/kg. The validation was conducted following the European Commission Decision 2002/657/EC and all performance characteristics were successfully satisfied. The capability of the method to detect amfenicols at lower levels than any prior perspective regulation literature guarantees its applicability in official control activities. The developed method has been applied to non-compliant feed samples with satisfactory results.

Keywords: non-target feed; florfenicol; thiamfenicol; chloramfenicol; HPLC–MS/MS; validation; swine

1. Introduction

Globalization permits food produced in one country to be sold in other countries, sometimes on an intercontinental level. However, globalization also contributes to competition between production companies. The final goal of any type of business is to have low production cost and high benefits. Low production cost is very important in food of animal origin, for which farmers fight with animal disease. The use of certain veterinary medicine is permitted to control, prevent, and treat illness. The most employed medicines, in this case, include antibiotics and antiparasitic agents. Antimicrobial medicines are sold as premixes, oral powders, oral solutions, injections, intramammary preparations pastes, oral pastes, boluses and intrauterine preparations [1]. Fenicols (chloramfenicol, thiamfenicol, and florfenicol) belong to this group of antibiotics; however, even if chloramfenicol is very effective on a broad spectrum, it is prohibited in food-producing animals within the European Union [2]. On the other hand, thiamfenicol and florfenicol can be administrated through feed, but always respecting the withdrawal periods. Regulation 2019/4/EC [3] includes these two antibiotics as an active substance for medicated feed and also in Annex II of the Regulation, indicating that cross-contamination level should be investigated during the production of medicated feed.

Techniques such as phase sorptive extraction [4], indirect competitive enzyme-linked immunosorbent assays [5], molecularly imprinted solid-phase extraction [6], high performance liquid chromatography (HPLC) with ultraviolet (UV) detection [7], capillary electrophoresis [8], and QuEChERS [9] were employed for amfenicol analysis.

The European Decision Commission 2002/657/EC states that positive samples need to be confirmed with confirmatory methods, and that HPLC–MS/MS is a good technique for confirmatory methods [10]. The use of HPLC–MS/MS has been reported for amfenicol analysis in food matrices. However, when compared with other antibiotics, such as tetracyclines, sulfonamides or penicillin, there are few methods available for amfenicols. According to the ESVAC 2015 report, these three groups of antibiotics (tetracyclines, sulfonamides, and penicillin) accounted for approximately 70% of the total sales of antibiotics in the European Union. The reported HPLC–MS/MS methods include one described by Van de Riet et al. (2013) [11] for chloramfenicol, thiamfenicol, and florfenicol in fish muscle, one developed by Barreto et al. (2016) [12] to detect the same amfenicols in poultry, swine, bovine, and fish muscle, another published by Anderson et al. (2016) [13] for florfenicol and thiamfenicol in white-tailed deer, one described for detection in milk and honey [9], and the most recent one reported for detection in egg [14].

Regarding feed samples, Pietroń et al. (2014) [15] reported an HPLC–UV method for the quantification of florfenicol and thiamfenicol in medicated feed. Later, in 2017, a similar method was reported, but the feed extract was purified by thigh layer chromatography (TLC) (Yang et al., 2017) [16]. For residue levels of amfenicols in feed, the technique most frequently employed is HPLC combined with different types of mass spectrometry. Between 30 and 300 active compounds (veterinary drugs, pesticides, and others) can be identified with low limits of detection (20 μg/kg). However, some of these methods are for screening [17–21] while others purify the extract with primary secondary amine (PSA) [22] or solid-phase extraction (SPE) [23].

To the best of the authors' knowledge, no method has been found in the scientific literature that is capable of analyzing all three amfenicols (chloramfenicol, thiamfenicol, and florfenicol) at the residual levels that fulfill the requirements of the European Commission Decision 2002/657/EC. Therefore, the aim of this research article is to report a simple extraction protocol followed by HPLC–MS/MS detection of amfenicols in feed samples from different animal species.

2. Results

The objective of this article is to describe a simple extraction protocol and an HPLC–MS/MS method to confirm the presence of amfenicols in feed samples at trace levels.

Figures 1 and 2 show multiple reaction monitoring (MRM) transitions of the different analytes in blank feed samples and in the same blank feed samples spiked with amfenicols to a final concentration of 100 μg/kg.

2.1. HPLC–MS/MS Conditions

Standard solutions of 1 μg/mL of florfenicol, thiamfenicol, chloramfenicol, and chloramfenicol-d_5 were employed to optimize their detection by the MS. The objective was to achieve a high signal intensity of representative ions through modifications in parameters such as curtain gas, ion spray voltage, source temperature, and curtain gas flow. Once precursor ions were selected for each amfenicol and optimized by manual tuning, automatic optimization was conducted (Table 1). This process permitted the evaluation of parameters such as entrance potential, collision cell potential, collision energy, and collision cell exit potential for four representative production ions. From these four ions, two were selected to conduct MRM analysis. Amfenicols were ionized by employing negative electrospray, due to the chemistry of the molecule; this ionization mode has been previously employed by other researchers in this field [14,17–24]. Acetonitrile was the first tested organic solvent as it is preferential to methanol. Acetonitrile was combined with water and buffers (ammonium acetate, ammonium formate, and ammonium hydroxide), resulting in a good intensity signal. The best resolution between peaks and signal intensity was obtained with the combination of acetonitrile and water with ammonium formate and 0.1% of formic acid.

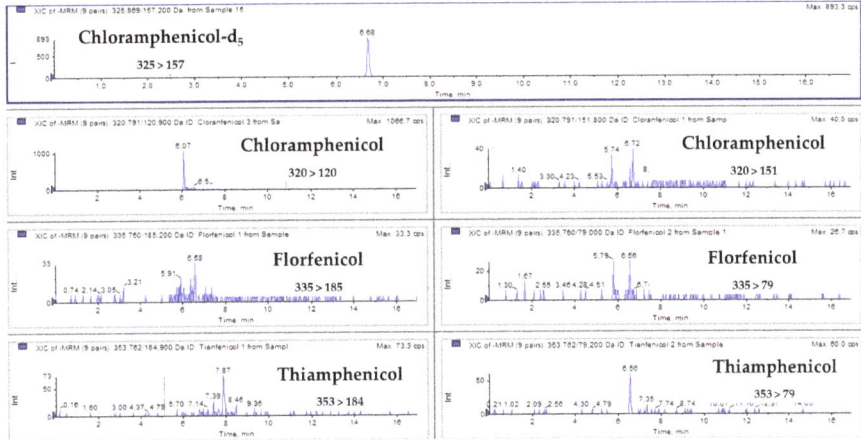

Figure 1. The total ion chromatogram (TIC) of a blank feed sample.

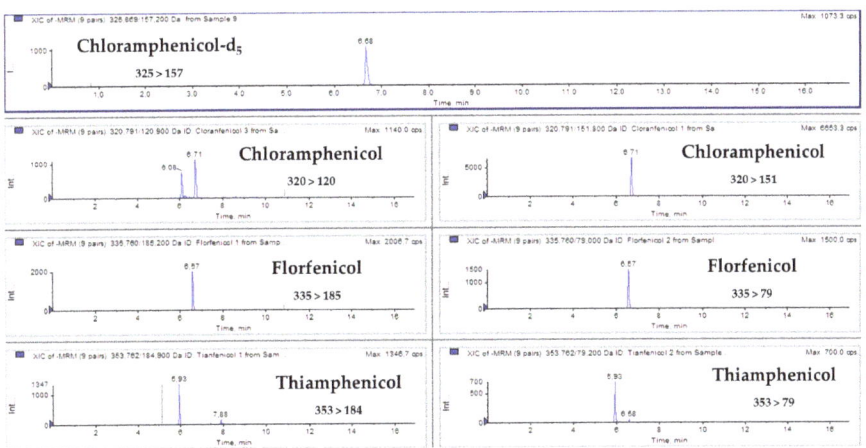

Figure 2. MRM chromatograms of feed samples spiked with amfenicols at the validation level of 200 µg/kg.

Table 1. Retention time (Rt), cone voltage (CV), collision energy, and precursor and product ions employed for ion identification.

Tetracycline	Rt (min)	m/z Transition	CV	Collision Energy
Chloramfenicol	6.71	320 > 151	46	26
Chloramfenicol		320 > 120	46	32
Thiamfenicol	5.93	353 > 184	56	20
Thiamfenicol		353 > 79	56	27
Florfenicol	6.57	335 > 185	61	23
Florfenicol		335 > 79	61	23
Chloramfenicol-d5	6.69	325 > 157	41	32

Following the requirement of the Decision 2002/657/EC, four identification points were achieved with the use of two MRM transitions for each amfenicol and the internal standard (IS). While both MRM transitions gave identification information, quantification was implemented from the MRM that gave the higher signal to noise ratio (S/N). The ions selected for chloramfenicol and florfenicol were also employed by Cronly et al. (2010) [25] and by Shinoda et al. (2011) [26] for detection in feed matrices. Similar results occurred between the selected ion for florfenicol and the work described by Shinoda et al. (2011) and Cronly et al. (2010), though the latter reference does not include florfenicol in its method. The same ions have also employed in other type of matrices, such as wastewater [27], manure [27], poultry tissues [28], pork, porcine liver, porcine kidney, beef, bovine liver, fish, chicken [29], milk, and honey [9]. The chromatography separation was performed with various C18 columns, including LiChrospher, Symmetry Shield RP18, ZORBAX Eclipse Plus, XTerra C18, and Hypersil C18-BD. For the present work, Sunfire C18 columns were selected.

2.2. Extraction

Independently of the matrix, most methods described in the scientific literature employ ethyl acetate to extract amfenicols [12,24,28,30]. Xiao et al. (2015) also employed ethyl acetate for poultry tissue but with a pressurized liquid extraction system [28]. Acetone and dichloromethane were selected by Van de Riet et al. (2013) to extract the drugs from fish muscle [11]. Acetonitrile with formic acid was employed by Boix et al. (2014) in feed samples and water combined with buffered acetonitrile by Leon et al. (2016) also for feed samples [21]. More sophisticated extraction techniques, such as QuEChERS, were employed by Liu et al. (2016) for milk and honey [9]. An immunoaffinity column was used by Luo et al. (2010) [31] for swine muscle and imprinted polymer by Ge et al. (2010) for animal tissue [6]. For the extraction of trace-level amfenicols from feed samples, 2 mL of water and 5 mL of ethyl acetate were employed with satisfactory results. However, after shaking for 20 minutes and centrifugation for the separation of the different phases, only 2 mL of the organic layer was evaporated. The evaporation of greater volumes (3, 3.5, and 4 mL) was investigated to increase the limit of detection (LOD), however, a higher matrix effect was observed, and the idea discarded.

2.3. Method Validation

The research group has developed, validated, and published various methods for the analysis of trace levels of veterinary drugs (coccidiostats, sulfonamides, and other antibiotics) in animal food and feed samples [32–35]. Validation for this type of sample and the matrix has typically been conducted following the European guideline (Decision 2002/657/EC) [10], which permits method implementation and comparisons in EU reference laboratories.

The Decision 2002/657/EC indicates that when no certificate reference material is available, trueness of measurements is assessed through recovery of additions of knowns amount of the analytes to a blank matrix. For amfenicols, recoveries were between −20% and +10% for the three investigated analytes (Table 2).

As with recovery, the precision under conditions of repeatability and reproducibility were evaluated using a standard addition method. Precision values were within the range provided by the European Decision; they ranged from 12% to 21% for chloramfenicol, 6.5% to 22% for thiamfenicol, and 12% to 19% for florfenicol. Currently, the presence of residue of amfenicols in non-target feed is prohibited; therefore, CCα and CCβ were calculated through employing formula for non-permitted substances. After peak identification, the area was plotted against the added concentration. CCα was the corresponding concentration at the y-intercept plus 2.33 times the standard deviation of the within-laboratory reproducibility. Similarly, for CCβ calculation, the peak area was plotted against the added concentration, and the CCα plus 1.64 times the standard deviation of the within-laboratory reproducibility of the mean measured content at the CCα equals the CCβ (2002/657/EC). While CCα values were 108, 140, and 110 µg/kg for chloramfenicol, thiamfenicol, and florfenicol, respectively, CCβ values were 116, 180, and 122 µg/kg for chloramfenicol, thiamfenicol, and florfenicol, respectively.

For the selected analytes, the S/N at the CCα was around 100; values for LOD and limit of quantification (LOQ) were calculated with the feed samples spiked with amfenicols. Results indicated that the LOD and LOQ values could reach 50 µg/kg. However, to further validate the method, validation was conducted at 200 µg/kg to confirm satisfactory S/N at the CCα level of each compound and to fulfill the EU requirements.

The technique itself is very selective/specific as it uses an MRM detection mode; the use of two MRM transitions reduces the detection of other interfering peaks. Selective/specific proxies were investigated with 20 blank feed samples for different animal species. The same 20 samples were spiked at 100 µg/kg with amfenicols and other antibiotics (sulfadiazine, trimethoprim, tetracycline, and ciprofloxacin). Both the absence of interfering peaks at the Rt of the amfenicols in the two MRM transitions of each analyte and the correct identification of the analytes demonstrate the selectivity/specificity of the developed method.

Table 2. Recovery (%), repeatability (CV%), reproducibility (CV%), CCα (µg/kg), CCβ (µg/kg), LOD (µg/kg) and LOQ (µg/kg) of Chloramfenicol, Tiamfenicol and Florfenicol.

	Fortification Level (µg/kg)	Recovery (n = 18)	Repeatability (n = 6)	Reproducibility (n = 18)	CCα	CCβ	LOD	LOQ
Chloramfenicol	100	81	21	16	108	116	25	40
	200	88	12	16				
	300	89	15	19				
	Mean	86	16	17				
Tiamfenicol	100	81.41	6.5	22.35	140	180	75	100
	200	97.69	12.58	21.61				
	300	103.83	18.97	21.98				
	Mean	94.31	12.69	21.98				
Florfenicol	100	96.61	14.64	18.77	110	122	50	75
	200	94.680	12.97	12.32				
	300	90.342	13.22	15.22				
	Mean	93.88	13.61	15.44				

2.4. Real Sample Collection and Analysis

Interlaboratory studies gave satisfactory results indicating the reliability and applicability of the developed method. Furthermore, the presence of the three amfenicols was investigated in 30 feed samples from feed mills. Florfenicol was the only amfenicol detected, and it was detected in one individual sample at a concentration of 0.36 mg/kg. This sample belonged to a group of four samples used to monitor florfenicol carryover after the production of a bath of medicated feed with 80 mg/kg of florfenicol. These results indicated that florfenicol carryover may occur during the manufacture of medicated feed and should be investigated in more detail. None of the samples collected from pig farms gave positive results.

3. Materials and Methods

3.1. Chemicals, Reagents, and Stock Solutions

Florfenicol, thiamfenicol, chloramfenicol, and chloramfenicol-d_5 (purity > 98%) were purchased from Sigma-Aldrich (St. Louis, MO, USA). Chloramfenicol-d_5 was employed as internal standard (IS). Ethyl acetate and acetonitrile was obtained from Scharlau Chemie (Barcelona, Spain), and formic acid and ammonium acetate (purity >99% for analysis) were obtained from Acros Organics (Geel, Belgium). Purified water was prepared in-house with a Milli-Q water system from Millipore (Bedford, MA, USA).

Nitrogen gas was generated using an in-house nitrogen generator from Peak Scientific Instruments, Ltd (Chicago, IL, USA).

In 20 mL volumetric flasks, 20 ± 0.01 mg of each analyte (florfenicol, thiamfenicol, chloramfenicol, and chloramfenicol-d_5) were precisely weighed to prepare stock solutions of individual compounds in acetonitrile (to yield a final concentration of 1 mg/mL; the purity was considered when calculating specific concentrations). To prepare the intermediate stock solution (10 µg/mL), the individual solutions were mixed and diluted with acetonitrile. Each day, a working stock solution (1 µg/mL) was freshly prepared by diluting the intermediate stock solution with acetonitrile. All standards solutions were stored in the dark at −18 °C for no longer than three months.

3.2. Conditions for HPLC–MS/MS Analysis

The HPLC–MS/MS analyses were performed using a 1100 HPLC from Agilent Technologies (Waldbronn, Germany) attached to a QTRAP 2000™ MS from Applied Biosystems/MDS-Sciex (Toronto, Canada). The software Analyst 1.4.1 from Applied Biosystems (Toronto, Canada) was employed to control the system.

The analysis of the extracts with amfenicols was achieved with a Sunfire C18 (3.5 µm 2.1 × 150 mm) HPLC column from Waters (Milford, PA, USA), water with formic acid (185 µL), and 370 µL of ammonium formate (6.3% in water; mobile phase A), and acetonitrile (mobile phase B). Mobile phase components A and B were freshly prepared with each batch of sample. The solvents were mixed at a constant flow rate of 250 µL/min, the column temperature was maintained at 50 °C, and the injection volume was 40 µL. The gradient program was as follows: 0 min, 90% A; 1 min, 50% A; 5 min, 20% A; 7 min, 90% A; 17 min, 90% A.

The MS analysis was performed using negative electrospray ionization mode (ESI). The dwell time was 150 ms between transitions. The system uses nitrogen as nebulized gas set up at 50 psi for ion source gases 1 and 2. The source temperature was 475 °C, the ion spray voltage was −4500 V, and the curtain gas flow was 25 psi. Analytes were identified by retention time (Rt) and two multiple reaction monitoring (MRM) transitions. Table 1. compiles the MS parameters employed for the identification of each analyte.

3.3. Sample Extraction

To confirm the absence of chloramfenicol, feed samples were sent to an accredited laboratory. Once the results were obtained, these samples were employed as blank feed samples to prepare matrix-matched calibration.

Quantification of the analytes was performed with matrix-matched samples spiked with the analytes at concentrations of 100, 200, 300, 400, and 1000 µg/kg. Samples were ground on a Minimoka GR-020 grinder (Lleida, Spain), and 1 g was transferred to a 15 mL Falcon conical-bottom tube. Then, 2 mL of Milli-Q water and 5 mL of ethyl acetate were added to the tube. The mixture was mixed with an IKA Minishaker MS2 (Staufen, Germany) for 20 s, shaken for 30 min at 200 rpm on a New Brunswick Scientific G25 orbital shaker (NJ, USA), and centrifuged at 7000 rpm for 10 minutes on a Kokusan H-103N centrifuge (Tokyo, Japan). Then, a volume of 2 mL was transferred to a conical glass tube and evaporated to dryness with a stream of nitrogen on a TurboVap® II evaporator from Zymark (MA, USA). The dry residue was dissolved in 500 µL of Milli-Q water, filtered with a GHP Acrodisc syringe filter (0.2 µm; Waters Corporation, MA, USA), and transferred to an HPLC amber vial with an insert. The extract was stored at −20 °C until analysis, which was conducted within a day. Figure 1 shows the total ion chromatogram (TIC) of a blank feed sample, and Figure 2 shows MRM chromatograms of feed samples spiked with amfenicols at the validation level of 200 µg/kg.

3.4. Method Validation

Linearity range, recovery, precision (repeatability and reproducibility), selectivity/specificity, limit of detection (LOD), limit of quantification (LOQ), decision limit (CCα), and detection capability

(CCβ) of the developed method were obtained, along with validation of the method. The validation was conducted following the criteria included in the Commission Decision 657/2002/EC. Blank feed samples were spiked with the amfenicols at 100, 200, 300, 400, and 1000 µg/kg for linearity verification. Calibration curves were prepared over four different days; for each day, peak area was correlated against analyte concentrations for linear regression analysis. The accuracy of the method could not be determined as certified reference materials were no available. Therefore, trueness and precision were obtained with blank feed samples spiked at 100, 200, and 300 µg/kg. Six replicates of each concentration were extracted and analyzed on the same day to obtain intra-day precision (repeatability). The same procedure was repeated over three different days for inter-day precision (reproducibility).

The selectivity/specificity was evaluated with blank feed samples spiked and non-spiked with amfenicols at the validation level (100 µg/kg). The different feed samples were provided by the manufacturers. Selectivity/specificity was evaluated with feed samples for different animal species (swine, poultry, and cattle).

3.5. Sample Collection and Analysis

Feed producers provided non-targeted feed samples ($n = 30$) to the laboratory. Four of these samples belonged to a feed mill and were collected after being manufactured in the same production line of medicated feed and after the cleaning batches to evaluate carryover contamination. The other feed samples were collected in pig farms and were feed employed for pig crowing. Once in the laboratory, all samples were ground and keep in plastic bottles in the dark until analysis. Interlaboratory samples from 2018 RIKILT proficiency tests were also conducted.

4. Conclusions

The article describes a simple a rapid confirmatory method based on HPLC–MS/MS for the simultaneous identification and quantification of residue of chloramfenicol, thiamfenicol and florfenicol in non-target feed. Since the method was validated following the EU guidelines and fulfilled the requirements of the Decision, the method can be applied by different laboratories, including reference laboratories.

Author Contributions: Investigation, R.E.G. and C.N.; Methodology, R.E.G. and E.P.; Supervision, J.M.M. and A.C.; Validation, C.N.; Writing—original draft, C.N. and B.V.

Funding: This research was funded by FEADER (The European Agricultural Fund for Rural Development (EAFRD)), grant number 2018/001B and ED431C 2018/05.

Conflicts of Interest: The authors do not have any conflict of interest.

References

1. ESVAC (2015) Fifth ESVAC Report—Sales of Veterinary Antimicrobial Agents in 26 EU/EEA Countries in 2013. Available online: www.ema.europa.eu/docs/en_GB/document_library/Report/2015/10/WC500195687.pdf (accessed on 29 January 2017).
2. Europe Comission. Regulation 37/2010. Commission Regulation (EU) No 37/2010 of 22 December 2009 on pharmacologically active substances and their classification regarding maximum residue limits in foodstuffs of animal origin. *Off. J. Eur. Union* **2010**, *15*, 1–72.
3. Europe Comission. Regulation 2019/4. Commission Regulation (EU) 2019/4 of the European Parliament and of the Council of 11 December 2018 on the manufacture, placing on the market and use of medicated feed, amending Regulation (EC) No 183/2005 of the European Parliament and of the Council and repealing Council Directive 90/167/EEC (Text with EEA relevance). *Off. J. Eur. Union* **2019**, *4*, 1–23.
4. Samanidou, V.; Kaltzi, I.; Kabir, A.; Furton, K.G. Simplifying sample preparation using fabric phase sorptive extraction technique for the determination of benzodiazepines in blood serum by high performance liquid chromatography. *Biomed. Chromatogr.* **2016**, *30*, 829–836. [CrossRef] [PubMed]

5. An, L.; Wang, Y.; Pan, Y.; Tao, Y.; Chen, D.; Liu, Z.; Yuan, Z. Development and validation of a sensitive indirect competitive enzyme-linked immunosorbent assay for the screening of florfenicol and Tiamfenicol in edible animal tissue and feed. *Food Anal. Method* **2016**, *9*, 2434–2443. [CrossRef]
6. Ge, S.; Yan, M.; Cheng, X.; Zhang, C.; Yu, J.; Zhao, P.; Gao, W. On-line molecular imprinted solid-phase extraction flow-injection fluorescence sensor for determination of florfenicol in animal tissues. *J. Pharm. Biomed.* **2010**, *52*, 615–619. [CrossRef] [PubMed]
7. Hayes, J. Determination of florfenicol in fish feeds at high inclusion rates by HPLC-UV. *J. AOAC Int.* **2013**, *96*, 7–11. [CrossRef] [PubMed]
8. Kowalski, P.; Konieczna, L.; Chmielewska, A.; Olędzka, I.; Plenis, A.; Bieniecki, M.; Lamparczyk, H. Comparative evaluation between capillary electrophoresis and high-performance liquid chromatography for the analysis of florfenicol in plasma. *J. Pharm. Biomed.* **2005**, *39*, 983–989. [CrossRef]
9. Liu, H.Y.; Lin, S.L.; Fuh, M.R. Determination of chloramfenicol, Tiamfenicol and florfenicol in milk and honey using modified QuEChERS extraction coupled with polymeric monolith-based capillary liquid chromatography tandem mass spectrometry. *Talanta* **2016**, *150*, 233–239. [CrossRef] [PubMed]
10. Europe Comission. Comission Decission 2002/657/EC. Commission Decision of 12 August 2002 implementing Council Directive 96/23/EC concerning the performance of analytical methods and the interpretation of results. *Off. J. Eur. Union* **2002**, *221*, 8–36.
11. Van de Riet, J.M.; Potter, R.A.; Christie-Fougere, M.; Burns, B.G. Simultaneous determination of residues of chloramfenicol, tiamfenicol, florfenicol, and florfenicol amine in farmed aquatic species by liquid chromatography/mass spectrometry. *J. AOAC Int.* **2003**, *86*, 510–514. [PubMed]
12. Barreto, F.; Ribeiro, C.; Hoff, R.B.; Dalla Costa, T. Determination of chloramfenicol, Tiamfenicol, florfenicol and florfenicol amine in poultry, swine, bovine and fish by liquid chromatography-tandem mass spectrometry. *J. Chromatogr. A* **2016**, *1449*, 48–53. [CrossRef]
13. Anderson, S.C.; Subbiah, S.; Gentles, A.; Austin, G.; Stonum, P.; Brooks, T.A.; Smith, E.E. Qualitative and quantitative drug residue analyses: Florfenicol in white-tailed deer (Odocoileus virginianus) and supermarket meat by liquid chromatography tandem-mass spectrometry. *J. Chromatogr. B* **2016**, *1033*, 73–79. [CrossRef] [PubMed]
14. Xie, X.; Wang, B.; Pang, M.; Zhao, X.; Xie, K.; Zhang, Y.; Dai, G. Quantitative analysis of chloramfenicol, tiamfenicol, florfenicol and florfenicol amine in eggs via liquid chromatography-electrospray ionization tandem mass spectrometry. *Food Chem.* **2018**, *269*, 542–548. [CrossRef]
15. Pietro, W.J.; Woźniak, A.; Pasik, K.; Cybulski, W.; Krasucka, D. Amfenicols stability in medicated feed–development and validation of liquid chromatography method. *Bull. Vet. Inst. Pulawy* **2014**, *58*, 621–629. [CrossRef]
16. Yang, J.; Sun, G.; Qian, M.; Huang, L.; Ke, X.; Yang, B. Development of a high-performance liquid chromatography method for the determination of florfenicol in animal feedstuffs. *J. Chromatogr. B* **2017**, *1068*, 9–14. [CrossRef] [PubMed]
17. Boix, C.; Ibáñez, M.; Sancho, J.V.; León, N.; Yusá, V.; Hernández, F. Qualitative screening of 116 veterinary drugs in feed by liquid chromatography–high resolution mass spectrometry: Potential application to quantitative analysis. *Food Chem.* **2014**, *160*, 313–320. [CrossRef]
18. Robert, C.; Gillard, N.; Brasseur, P.Y.; Ralet, N.; Dubois, M.; Delahaut, P. Rapid multiresidue and multi-class screening for antibiotics and benzimidazoles in feed by ultra-high performance liquid chromatography coupled to tandem mass spectrometry. *Food Control* **2015**, *50*, 509–515. [CrossRef]
19. Aguilera-Luiz, M.M.; Romero-González, R.; Plaza-Bolaños, P.; Vidal, J.L.M.; Frenich, A.G. Wide-scope analysis of veterinary drug and pesticide residues in animal feed by liquid chromatography coupled to quadrupole-time-of-flight mass spectrometry. *Anal. Bioanal. Chem.* **2013**, *405*, 6543–6553. [CrossRef] [PubMed]
20. Gómez-Pérez, M.L.; Romero-González, R.; Martínez Vidal, J.L.; Garrido Frenich, A. Analysis of veterinary drug and pesticide residues in animal feed by high-resolution mass spectrometry: Comparison between time-of-flight and Orbitrap. *Food Addit. Contam. A* **2015**, *32*, 1637–1646. [CrossRef]
21. León, N.; Pastor, A.; Yusà, V. Target analysis and retrospective screening of veterinary drugs, ergot alkaloids, plant toxins and other undesirable substances in feed using liquid chromatography–high resolution mass spectrometry. *Talanta* **2016**, *149*, 43–52. [CrossRef]

22. Boscher, A.; Guignard, C.; Pellet, T.; Hoffmann, L.; Bohn, T. Development of a multi-class method for the quantification of veterinary drug residues in feedingstuffs by liquid chromatography-tandem mass spectrometry. *J. Chromatogr. A* **2010**, *1217*, 6394–6404. [CrossRef]
23. Piatkowska, M.; Jedziniak, P.; Zmudzki, J. Multiresidue method for the simultaneous determination of veterinary medicinal products, feed additives and illegal dyes in eggs using liquid chromatography–tandem mass spectrometry. *Food Chem.* **2016**, *197*, 571–580. [CrossRef]
24. Zhang, S.; Liu, Z.; Guo, X.; Cheng, L.; Wang, Z.; Shen, J. Simultaneous determination and confirmation of chloramfenicol, tiamfenicol, florfenicol and florfenicol amine in chicken muscle by liquid chromatography–tandem mass spectrometry. *J. Chromatogr. B* **2008**, *875*, 399–404. [CrossRef]
25. Cronly, M.; Behan, P.; Foley, B.; Malone, E.; Martin, S.; Doyle, M.; Regan, L. Rapid multi-class multi-residue method for the confirmation of chloramfenicol and eleven nitroimidazoles in milk and honey by liquid chromatography-tandem mass spectrometry (LC-MS). *Food Addit. Contam.* **2010**, *27*, 1233–1246. [CrossRef] [PubMed]
26. Shinoda, N.; Kojima, F.; Sugiura, K. Simultaneous determination of residues of chloramfenicol and florfenicol in animal feed by liquid chromatography tandem mass spectrometry. *J. Resid. Sci. Technol.* **2011**, *8*, 125–129.
27. Wei, R.; Ge, F.; Chen, M.; Wang, R. Occurrence of ciprofloxacin, enrofloxacin, and florfenicol in animal wastewater and water resources. *J. Environ. Qual.* **2012**, *41*, 1481–1486. [CrossRef]
28. Xiao, Z.; Song, R.; Rao, Z.; Wei, S.; Jia, Z.; Suo, D.; Fan, X. Development of a subcritical water extraction approach for trace analysis of chloramfenicol, tiamfenicol, florfenicol, and florfenicol amine in poultry tissues. *J. Chromatogr. A* **2015**, *1418*, 29–35. [CrossRef]
29. Chou, K.Y.; Cheng, T.Y.; Chen, C.M.; Hung, P.L.; Tang, Y.Y.; Chung-Wang, Y.J.; Shih, Y.C. Simultaneous determination of residual tiamfenicol and florfenicol in foods of animal origin by HPLC/electrospray ionization-MS/MS. *J. AOAC Int.* **2009**, *92*, 1225–1232. [PubMed]
30. Peng, L.I.; Yueming, Q.I.U.; Huixia, C.A.I.; Ying, K.O.N.G.; Yingzhang, T.A.N.G.; Daning, W.A.N.G.; Mengxia, X.I.E. Simultaneous determination of chloramfenicol, tiamfenicol, and florfenicol residues in animal tissues by gas chromatography/mass spectrometry. *Chin. J. Chromatogr.* **2006**, *24*, 14–18.
31. Luo, P.; Chen, X.; Liang, C.; Kuang, H.; Lu, L.; Jiang, Z.; Shen, J. Simultaneous determination of thiamfenicol, florfenicol and florfenicol amine in swine muscle by liquid chromatography–tandem mass spectrometry with immunoaffinity chromatography clean-up. *J. Chromatogr. B* **2010**, *878*, 207–212. [CrossRef] [PubMed]
32. Nebot, C.; Iglesias, A.; Regal, P.; Miranda, J.; Cepeda, A.; Fente, C. Development of a multi-class method for the identification and quantification of residues of antibiotics, coccidiostats and corticosteroids in milk by liquid chromatography–tandem mass spectrometry. *Int. Dairy J.* **2012**, *22*, 78–85. [CrossRef]
33. Nebot, C.; Guarddon, M.; Seco, F.; Iglesias, A.; Miranda, J.M.; Franco, C.M.; Cepeda, A. Monitoring the presence of residues of tetracyclines in baby food samples by HPLC-MS/MS. *Food Control* **2014**, *46*, 495–501. [CrossRef]
34. Gavilán, R.; Nebot, C.; Miranda, J.; Martín-Gómez, Y.; Vázquez-Belda, B.; Franco, C.; Cepeda, A. Analysis of tetracyclines in medicated feed for food animal production by HPLC-MS/MS. *Antibiotics* **2016**, *5*, 1. [CrossRef] [PubMed]
35. Gavilán, R.E.; Nebot, C.; Patyra, E.; Miranda, J.M.; Franco, C.M.; Cepeda, A. Simultaneous analysis of coccidiostats and sulphonamides in non-target feed by HPLC-MS/MS and validation following the Commission Decision 2002/657/EC. *Food Addit. Contam. A* **2018**, *35*, 1093–1106. [CrossRef] [PubMed]

© 2019 by the authors. Licensee MDPI, Basel, Switzerland. This article is an open access article distributed under the terms and conditions of the Creative Commons Attribution (CC BY) license (http://creativecommons.org/licenses/by/4.0/).

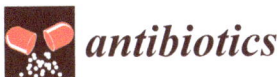

Article

Antimicrobial and Synergistic Effects of Commercial Piperine and Piperlongumine in Combination with Conventional Antimicrobials

Eunice Ego Mgbeahuruike [1,*], Milla Stålnacke [2], Heikki Vuorela [1] and Yvonne Holm [1]

[1] Division of Pharmaceutical Biosciences, Faculty of Pharmacy, University of Helsinki, P.O. Box 56, FI-00014 Helsinki, Finland; Heikki.vuorela@helsinki.fi (H.V.); Yvonne.holm@helsinki.fi (Y.H.)
[2] Department of Pharmacology, Institute of Neuroscience and Physiology, The Sahlgrenska Academy, University of Gothenburg, Box 431, SE-40530 Gothenburg, Sweden; gusstami@student.gu.se
* Correspondence: eunice.mgbeahuruike@helsinki.fi or euny_ego2007@yahoo.com; Tel.: +358442399653

Received: 15 April 2019; Accepted: 2 May 2019; Published: 4 May 2019

Abstract: Microbial resistance to currently available antibiotics is a public health problem in the fight against infectious diseases. Most antibiotics are characterized by numerous side effects that may be harmful to normal body cells. To improve the efficacy of these antibiotics and to find an alternative way to minimize the adverse effects associated with most conventional antibiotics, piperine and piperlongumine were screened in combination with conventional rifampicin, tetracycline, and itraconazole to evaluate their synergistic, additive, or antagonistic interactions against *Staphylococcus aureus*, *Pseudomonas aeruginosa*, and *Candida albicans*. The fractional inhibitory concentration index was used to estimate the synergistic effects of various combination ratios of the piperamides and antibiotics against the bacterial and fungal strains. Both piperine and piperlongumine showed synergistic effects against *S. aureus* when combined at various ratios with rifampicin. Synergistic interaction was also observed with piperine in combination with tetracycline against *S. aureus*, while antagonistic interaction was recorded for piperlongumine and tetracycline against *S. aureus*. All the piperamide/antibacterial combinations tested against *P. aeruginosa* showed antagonistic effects, with the exception of piperine and rifampicin, which recorded synergistic interaction at a ratio of 9:1 rifampicin/piperine. No synergistic interaction was observed when the commercial compounds were combined with itraconazole and tested against *C. albicans*. The results showed that piperine and piperlongumine are capable of improving the effectiveness of rifampicin and tetracycline. Dosage combinations of these bioactive compounds with the antibiotics used may be a better option for the treatment of bacterial infections that aims to minimize the adverse effects associated with the use of these conventional antibacterial drugs.

Keywords: piperine; piperlongumine; antibacterial; antifungal; synergy

1. Introduction

Infectious diseases caused by bacteria and fungi are one of the leading causes of death worldwide [1–3]. The emergence of multidrug resistance in microbes and the nonavailability of antibiotics to combat and treat microbial infections have led to a constant search for new antimicrobial agents from natural sources. Previous research has shown that about 13 million deaths are recorded throughout the world each year as a result of bacterial and fungal diseases that are often caused by multidrug-resistant pathogens [4,5]. Natural products of plant origin include novel therapeutic and highly effective antimicrobial agents [6,7]. In clinical practice, one of the leading new advances in the fight against microbial resistance is antimicrobial combination therapy [8–10]. Alternatively, bioactive compounds from natural sources could also be screened for leads to the discovery of new antibiotics to combat microbial resistance [5,11,12]. The mode of activity of antimicrobial combination therapy in antimicrobial treatments differs from that of the same individual antibiotics when administered as single drugs [8,13]. Bioactive compounds and extracts from plants can also potentiate the effect of antimicrobial drugs, thereby acting as antibiotic adjuvants [5,11]. Another strategic approach to the fight against multidrug-resistant bacteria in clinical practice is to deactivate the resistance mechanism of the bacteria to the existing antibiotics. In addition, pharmacological studies have shown that synergistic interaction is necessary and could greatly enhance the activity of antimicrobial compounds with moderate or weak activity. Thus, these bioactive plant compounds can serve as inhibitors against multidrug-resistant pathogens [5,14].

Piperine (1) and piperlongumine (2) are novel alkaloids found in most *Piper* species. Piperlongumine (2), also known as piplartin, is a piperamide compound found in Indian long pepper *Piper longum* L. [15]. It is a bioactive compound of clinical importance that is active against multidrug-resistant pathogens such as *Pseudomonas aeruginosa* (Schroeter) Mogul and *Staphylococcus aureus* Rosenbach [16]. Piperine (1) is a piperamide compound found in *Piper guineense* Schumach. & Thonn., black pepper *Piper nigrum* L., and other *Piper* species [17–19]. The chemical structures of piperine and piperlongumine are shown in Figure 1. Previous research has shown that piperine is a potent antibacterial agent acting as an inhibitor of the efflux pump of *S. aureus* [20,21]. Recent pharmacological research on piperine and piperlongumine [22–25] led us to hypothesize that these piperamide compounds may potentiate the antibiotic effect of some conventional antimicrobials, thereby acting as antibiotic adjuvants.

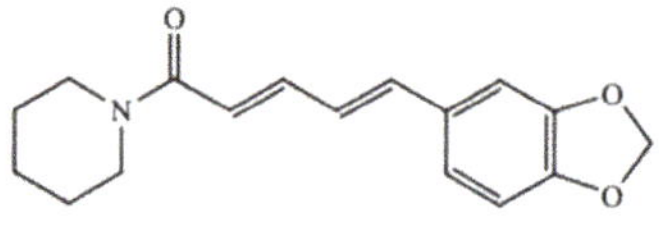

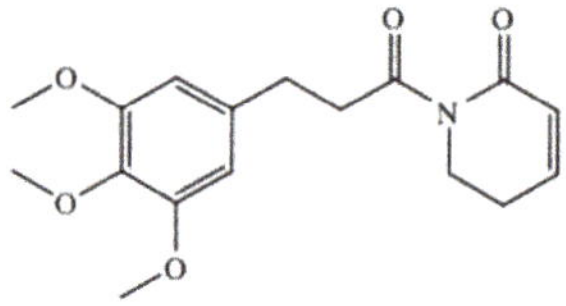

Figure 1. Chemical structures of piperine and piperlongumine.

The aim of this study was to investigate the in vitro antimicrobial effects of piperine and piperlongumine when used in combination at various ratios with some conventional antimicrobials (tetracycline, rifampicin, and itraconazole) against *P. aeruginosa*, *S. aureus*, and *Candida albicans*. It was aimed at evaluating whether piperine and piperlongumine interact synergistically when combined with tetracycline, rifampicin, or itraconazole at various ratios. This is the first report on the synergistic activity of piperlongumine in combination with conventional antimicrobials. The study of the synergistic interaction of these piperamide compounds with conventional antibiotics may aid in addressing the problem of microbial resistance and provide new strategies for improving the use of antibiotics in the treatment of infectious diseases. Piperine and piperlongumine as antibiotic adjuvants may help to reduce the adverse effects associated with these conventional antibiotics.

2. Results

To evaluate an alternative way to fight multidrug-resistant pathogens and to minimize the adverse effects associated with most conventional antibiotics, piperine and piperlongumine were screened singly and in combination with conventional antimicrobials to determine their synergistic, additive, or antagonistic interactions against *S. aureus*, *P. aeruginosa*, and *C. albicans* (Table 1, Figures 2 and 3). The aim was to investigate the synergistic effects of piperine and piperlongumine when used singly and in combination with conventional antimicrobials against *S. aureus*, *P. aeruginosa*, and *C. albicans*. *S. aureus*, *P. aeruginosa*, and *C. albicans* are pathogens that are capable of causing systemic infections in humans. As such, 90–95% of *S. aureus* strains are resistant to most conventional antibiotics [8,26]. The fractional inhibitory concentration (FIC) index was used to determine the synergistic interaction between the commercial piperamides and the antimicrobials. The FIC index method is one of the most accurate means for determining synergistic interactions when two inhibitors are studied in various combinations [27,28]. A synergistic effect was observed when the FIC index value of the compound of interest was ≤ 0.5 [26]. Previous research has also shown that the ratio of combination of two inhibitors could influence the degree of their interaction, such that the interactions could vary depending on the ratio by which the two inhibitors are combined [28].

Table 1. Inhibition zone diameters (mm) of the antibacterial and antifungal effects of piperine, piperlongumine (P. longumine), rifampicin, tetracycline, itraconazole, and 70% ethanol tested individually against *Staphylococcus aureus*, *Pseudomonas aeruginosa*, and *Candida albicans*, using the agar diffusion method.

Bacteria/Fungi	Piperine	P. longumine	Tetracycline	Rifampicin	70% Ethanol	Itraconazole
S. aureus	15.2 ± 0.31	12.4 ± 0.31	49.1 ± 0.32	47.2 ± 0.17	NA	NP *
P. aeruginosa	14.4 ± 0.33	11.5 ± 0.33	34.6 ± 0.33	30.3 ± 0.33	NA	NP *
C. albicans	16.5 ± 0.31	18.2 ± 0.31	NP *	NP *	NA	15.2 ± 0.33

NA, not active; *, not performed. The inhibition zone diameters (mm) represent the means of three replicates ($n = 3$) ± the SEM (standard error of the mean).

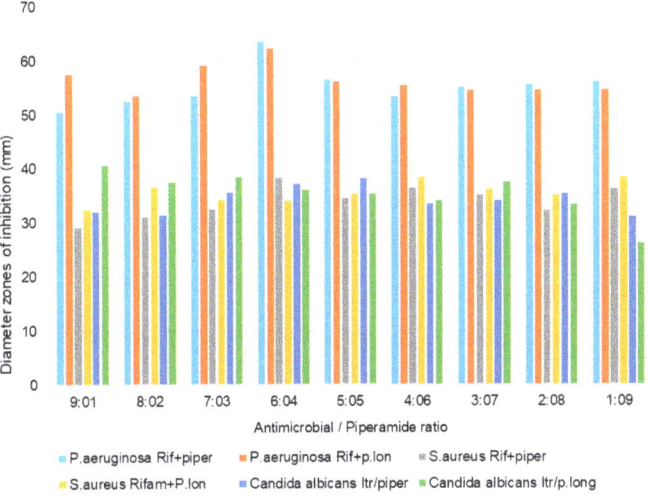

Figure 2. Inhibition zone diameters (mm) of the antibacterial and antifungal effects of piperine and piperlongumine combined at various ratios with rifampicin/itraconazole against *S. aureus*, *P. aeruginosa*, and *C. albicans*, using the agar diffusion method. Rif, rifampicin; Itr, itraconazole; piper, piperine; p.long, piperlongumine; 200 μL of the piperamide/antimicrobial combinations were applied in the wells.

The results of the first preliminary agar diffusion method performed singly on the piperamide compounds and antibacterials against *S. aureus* showed that the inhibition zone diameters of tetracycline, rifampicin, piperine, and piperlongumine were 49.1 mm, 47.2 mm, 15.2 mm, and 12.4 mm, respectively (Table 1). Preliminary agar diffusion screening was also performed on the various piperamide/antimicrobial combinations to ascertain the five best combinations to screen for the minimum inhibitory concentrations (MICs) and FIC index calculations for synergistic or antagonistic evaluations (Figures 2 and 3).

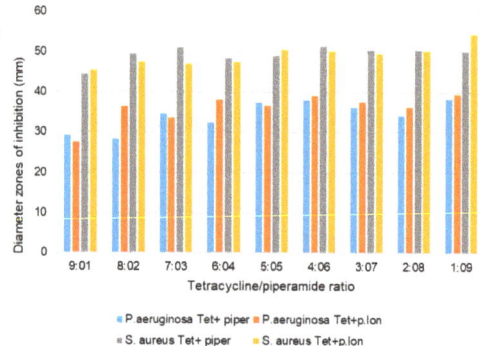

Figure 3. Inhibition zone diameters (mm) of the antibacterial effects of piperine and piperlongumine combined at various ratios with tetracycline against *S. aureus* and *P. aeruginosa*, using the agar diffusion method. The inhibition zone diameters (mm) are the means of three replicates ($n = 3$). P.lon, piperlongumine; tet, tetracycline; piper, piperine.

The MICs of the various combinations were evaluated (Table 2) to obtain the values used in calculating the FIC indices.

Table 2. Minimum inhibitory concentrations (MIC, µg/mL) of piperine and piperlongumine combined at various ratios with rifampicin (rifam), tetracycline (tetracy), itraconazole (itracon) against *S. aureus*, *P. aeruginosa*, and *C. albicans*.

Ratio of Antibiotics/Compound	S. aureus	P. aeruginosa	C. albicans
Rifam + piperine 1:9	7.8	15.6	NP*
Rifam + piperine 3:7	1.9	15.6	NP*
Rifam + piperine 5:5	3.9	62.5	NP*
Rifam + Piperine 7:3	1.9	62.5	NP*
Rifam + piperine 9:1	7.8	15.6	NP*
Rifam + piperlongumine 1:9	7.8	31.2	NP*
Rifam + piperlongumine 3:7	125	15.6	NP*
Rifam + piperlongumine 5:5	3.9	15.6	NP*
Rifam + piperlongumine 7:3	62.5	15.6	NP*
Rifam + piperlongumine 9:1	62.5	7.8	NP*
Tetracy + piperine 1:9	7.8	62.5	NP*
Tetracy + piperine 3:7	3.9	31.2	NP*
Tetracy + piperine 5:5	0.97	15.6	NP*
Tetracy + piperine 7:3	1.9	7.8	NP*
Tetracy + piperine 9:1	7.8	7.8	NP*
Tetracy + piperlongumine 1:9	31.2	31.2	NP*
Tetracy + piperlongumine 3:7	3.9	7.8	NP*
Tetracy + piperlongumine 5:5	3.9	15.6	NP*
Tetracy + piperlongumine 7:3	1.9	7.8	NP*
Tetracy + piperlongumine 9:1	62.5	7.8	NP*

Table 2. Cont.

Ratio of Antibiotics/Compound	S. aureus	P. aeruginosa	C. albicans
Itracon + piperine 1:9	NP *	NP *	3.9
Itracon + piperine 3:7	NP *	NP *	3.9
Itracon + piperine 5:5	NP *	NP *	7.8
Itracon + piperine 7:3	NP *	NP *	7.8
Itracon + piperine 9:1	NP *	NP *	15.6
Itracon + piperlongumine 1:9	NP *	NP *	31.2
Itracon + piperlongumine 3:7	NP *	NP *	7.8
Itracon + piperlongumine 5:5	NP *	NP *	7.8
Itracon + piperlongumine 7:3	NP *	NP *	3.9
Itracon + piperlongumine 9:1	NP *	NP *	31.2
Piperine only	3.9	15.6	7.8
Piperlongumine only	15.6	31.2	3.9
Rifampicin only	1.97	0.48	NP *
Tetracycline only	0.97	0.97	NP *
Itraconazole only	NP *	NP *	15.6

The MIC values represent the means of triplicates. Only five combinations were tested for MIC. *, not performed.

Rifampicin and tetracycline were combined at various ratios with piperine and piperlongumine and tested against *S. aureus*. For piperlongumine, a synergistic effect was observed at a ratio of 5:5 with rifampicin against this bacterium (Table 3). This result demonstrates that the pharmacological interaction between a bioactive compound and a conventional antimicrobial can be affected by the ratio and concentration at which the two are combined. However, antagonistic interactions were observed between piperlongumine and tetracycline at all the combination ratios tested against this bacterium (Table 3).

Table 3. Antimicrobial synergistic activity of piperine and piperlongumine against *S. aureus*, *P. aeruginosa*, and *C. albicans*.

Ratio	FIC Index		
	S. aureus	P. aeruginosa	C. albicans
Rifam + piperine 1:9	5.9 (AT)	33.5 (AT)	NP *
Rifam + piperine 3:7	0.2 (S)	33.5 (AT)	NP *
Rifam + piperine 5:5	3.9 (AT)	8.0 (AT)	NP *
Rifam + piperine 7:3	1.2 (I)	5.0 (AT)	NP *
Rifam + piperine 9:1	12.6 (AT)	0.4 (S)	NP *
Rifam + piperlongumine 1:9	4.4 (AT)	66.0 (AT)	NP *
Rifam + piperlongumine 3:7	39.0 (AT)	33.0 (AT)	NP *
Rifam + piperlongumine 5:5	0,5 (S)	1.5 (I)	NP *
Rifam + piperlongumine 7:3	17.0 (AT)	2.0 (I)	NP *
Rifam + piperlongumine 9:1	17.0 (AT)	1.0 (I)	NP *
Tetracy + piperine 1:9	10.0 (AT)	68.0 (AT)	NP *

Table 3. Cont.

Ratio	FIC Index		
	S. aureus	P. aeruginosa	C. albicans
Tetracy + piperine 3:7	4.5 (AT)	32.0 (AT)	NP *
Tetracy + piperine 5:5	0.3 (S)	0.7 (A)	NP *
Tetracy + piperine 7:3	2.4 (AT)	0.7 (A)	NP *
Tetracy + piperine 9:1	12.1 (AT)	1.5 (I)	NP *
Tetracy + piperlongumine 1:9	34.1 (AT)	33.1 (AT)	NP *
Tetracy + piperlongumine 3:7	4.1 (AT)	8.2 (AT)	NP *
Tetracy + piperlongumine 5:5	1.1 (I)	2.5 (AT)	NP *
Tetracy + piperlongumine 7:3	0.9 (A)	1.5 (I)	NP *
Tetracy + piperlongumine 9:1	48.9 (AT)	1.5 (I)	NP *
Itracon + piperine 1:9	NP *	NP *	0.8 (A)
Itracon + piperine 3:7	NP *	NP *	1.2 (I)
Itracon + piperine 5:5	NP *	NP *	4.0 (AT)
Itracon + piperine 7:3	NP *	NP *	3.0 (AT)
Itracon + piperine 9:1	NP *	NP *	4.0 (AT)
Itracon + piperlongumine 1:9	NP *	NP *	10.1 (AT)
Itracon + piperlongumine 3:7	NP *	NP *	0.7 (A)
Itracon + piperlongumine 5:5	NP *	NP *	1.3 (I)
Itracon + piperlongumine 7:3	NP *	NP *	1.0 (I)
Itracon + piperlongumine 9:1	NP *	NP *	12.0 (AT)

The activity is expressed as the fractional inhibition concentration (FIC) index, which is calculated from the MIC of the various piperamide/antimicrobial combinations. The FIC index interactions were defined as: FICI ≤ 0.5, (S) synergy; >0.5 to ≤1.0, (A) additive; >1.0 to ≤2.0, (I) indifferent; and >2.0, (AT) antagonistic [26]. *, not performed.

3. Discussion

3.1. Antibacterial Synergistic Effects of Piperine and Piperlongumine against S. aureus

For piperine, the FIC index value of rifampicin and piperine against *S. aureus* in this study showed synergistic interaction at a ratio of 3:7 (Table 3). A synergistic effect was observed between piperine and rifampicin and between piperine and tetracycline, as shown in Table 3. Rifampicin is an antibiotic that is often used in the treatment of systemic bacterial infections in antimicrobial therapy, and this antibiotic is characterized by numerous adverse effects when used consecutively for 10–14 days [29,30]. A formulation containing a fixed-dose combination of rifampicin and piperine (rifampicin 200 mg + piperine 10 mg) has been approved in India to minimize the adverse effects associated with the use of conventional rifampicin in the antimicrobial treatment against *Mycobacterium tuberculosis* [30]. Our results show here that piperine could be a compound leading to the discovery of new antibacterial drugs with minimum adverse effects. We observed that piperine and piperlongumine are capable of improving the effectiveness of rifampicin and tetracycline. We suggest, therefore, that dosages of combinations of these bioactive compounds with antibiotics could be a better option for the treatment of bacterial infections than the conventional antibiotics which often show problems with multidrug-resistant pathogens. Our study demonstrates that a combination of antibacterial (rifampicin and tetracycline) with piperamide compounds (piperine and piperlongumine) could lead to minimal systemic toxicity to normal cells during antimicrobial treatments.

3.2. Antibacterial Synergistic Effects of Piperine and Piperlongumine against P. aeruginosa

Preliminary agar diffusion assays performed individually with piperamides and antibiotics against *P. aeruginosa* (Table 1) showed that the inhibition zone diameters of tetracycline, rifampicin, piperine, and piperlongumine were 34.6 mm, 30.3 mm, 14.4 mm, and 11.5 mm, respectively. When the MIC of the various combinations was determined, the FIC index calculations showed mainly antagonistic interactions between the piperamides and the antibiotics against *P. aeruginosa*, with the exception of the 9:1 ratio of the piperine/rifampicin combination, which showed synergistic activity (Table 3). *P. aeruginosa* is a Gram-negative pathogenic bacterium that causes systemic infections in immunocompromised individuals and is often associated with antibacterial resistance [31]. For piperlongumine, no synergistic effect was observed in any of the antibiotic combinations (rifampicin and tetracycline) against *P. aeruginosa*, although additive and antagonistic interactions were observed. The results of tetracycline/piperlongumine and rifampicin/piperlongumine combinations tested at various ratios demonstrated no synergistic effects between tetracycline and piperlongumine as well as between rifampicin and piperlongumine against *P. aeruginosa*. These results suggest that piperine and piperlongumine may not improve the effectiveness of tetracycline against *P. aeruginosa* infections. Indeed, appropriate measures should be taken to avoid too heavy a consumption of herbal drugs or foods rich in piperine and piperlongumine when undergoing antimicrobial treatment with tetracycline against diseases caused by *P. aeruginosa*.

For piperine, a synergistic interaction with rifampicin was observed for a rifampicin/piperine combination at a ratio of 9:1 against *P. aeruginosa*, while antagonistic or additive interactions were observed for the other combinations tested. Piperine was previously tested for its immunomodulatory activity in enhancing the efficacy of rifampicin in a murine model of *M. tuberculosis* infection, thereby acting in synergy with rifampicin to improve its therapeutic efficacy [32]. However, the synergistic efficacy recorded in our study for a rifampicin/piperine combination showed that the efficacy could be influenced by the ratio of the combination, i.e, the synergistic, additive, or antagonistic interactions were greatly dependent on the ratio between rifampicin and piperine.

3.3. Antifungal Synergistic Effects of Piperine and Piperlongumine against C. albicans

When preliminary agar diffusion assays were performed singly on the piperamides and itraconazole against *C. albicans*, the inhibition zone diameters of piperine, piperlongumine, and itraconazole were 16.5 mm, 18.2 mm, and 15.2 mm, respectively (Table 1). The results of the FIC index evaluations of the various combinations showed additive or antagonistic interactions (Table 3). No synergistic effects were recorded in our study against *C. albicans*. *C. albicans* is an opportunistic pathogen that is responsible for most yeast infections in humans [33]. These results demonstrate that piperine and piperlongumine cannot improve the effectiveness of itraconazole, and thus herbal formulations made from these bioactive compounds should be avoided while undergoing treatments for yeast infections.

4. Materials and Methods

4.1. Sources of Antibiotics and Commercial Compounds

Analytical-grade commercial piperlongumine ($\geq$ 97.0% purity) and piperine ($\geq$ 97.0% purity) were purchased from TCI Europe N.V. (Zwijndrecht, Belgium). Tetracycline hydrochloride (Sigma-Aldrich, St. Louis MO, USA), rifampicin (Sigma-Aldrich), and itraconazole (Sigma-Aldrich) were the antibiotics used in the investigation. The selection of tetracycline, rifampicin, and itraconazole was based on their activity against bacterial and fungal strains in a previous study [34]. *S. aureus* American Type Culture Collection ATCC 25923, *P. aeruginosa* ATCC 27853, and *C. albicans* ATCC 10231 cultures used in this investigation were obtained from the Division of Pharmaceutical Biosciences, Faculty of Pharmacy, University of Helsinki, Finland. The bacterial strains were selected because they are significant human pathogens capable of causing life-threatening nosocomial infections [35,36], while *C. albicans*, on the other hand, causes fungal diseases in humans [37].

4.2. Preparation of Piperine, Piperlongumine, and Antimicrobials

Each of the commercial piperamides (piperine and piperlongumine) was prepared to a final concentration of 5 mg/mL (stock solution) in 70% ethanol and tested in the initial screening. An initial stock solution of 5 mg/mL was prepared for each of the antibiotics (tetracycline, rifampicin, and itraconazole). Piperine and piperlongumine were also prepared in combination with tetracycline, rifampicin, or itraconazole at various ratios according to the method of Van Vuuren et al. [10]. The combinations/dilutions were prepared at nine different ratios of 1:9, 2:8, 3:7, 4:6, 5:5, 6:4, 7:3, 8:2, 9:1 as follows: rifampicin/piperlongumine, rifampicin/piperine, tetracycline/piperlongumine, tetracycline/piperine, itraconazole/piperine, and itraconazole/piperlongumine.

4.3. Agar Disk-Diffusion Method

The agar disk-diffusion method was applied for the initial screening of the nine combination ratios according to the method of the Clinical and Laboratory Standards Institute [38]. Sterile Petri dishes (Ø = 14 cm, VWR International Oy, Helsinki, Finland) were used for the screening. For the antibacterial screening against *S. aureus* and *P. aeruginosa*, 25 mL of sterile base agar (Antibiotic agar No. 2, Difco, VWR) was applied as a bottom layer into the sterile Petri dishes, using a sterile serological pipet (Falcon; BDLabware Europe) and allowed to solidify. Thereafter, 25 mL of isosensitest agar (OXOID, ThermoFisher Scientific, Waltham, MA, USA) was applied as the top layer. For the antifungal screening, 25 mL of sterile base agar (Antibiotic agar No. 2, Difco VWR) was applied as a bottom layer into the sterile Petri dishes and 25 mL of Saboraud agar (OXOID, ThermoFisher Scientific, Basingstoke, United Kingdom) was applied as the top layer. The agar in the Petri dishes was allowed to solidify and then stored at +4 °C. The screening was initiated with the inoculation of the bacterial strains or *C. albicans* onto solid nutrient or Saboraud agar slants that were incubated overnight for the bacterial strains and 48 h for the fungus at +37 °C. Viable bacterial and fungal cultures from the agar slants were used to prepare an inoculum for the test. Bacterial and fungal specimens from the agar slants were transferred into 2 mL of a 0.9% (*w/v*) sodium chloride (NaCl) solution in a sterile glass tube, using a sterile inoculation loop. In all, 1 mL of the suspension was transferred into another sterile glass tube, and the absorbance was measured at 625 nm (UV–Visible Spectrophotometer, Pharmacia LKB-Biochrom 4060; Pfizer Inc., New York, NY, USA). The other milliliter of the suspension (sterile part) was diluted with the 0.9% NaCl solution so that the absorbance at 625 nm became 0.1 (this suspension contained approximately 1.5×10^8 colony-forming units (CFUs)/mL). In all, 200 µL of this diluted bacterial or fungal suspension were spread evenly on each Petri dish and left to dry for several seconds with the lid open. A sterile cork borer (11 mm diameter) was used to make six equidistant holes on the agar surface of the Petri dishes. A total of 200 µL of the 5 mg/mL concentration of each of the piperamides and 200 µL of the 10 mg/mL antimicrobial were carefully pipetted into the holes; 70% ethanol was used as the solvent control. The first screening of the combined samples was done in the same manner as described above for the agar diffusion method, and the various inhibition zones were recorded. The Petri dishes were transferred to the cold room and incubated at +4 °C for 1 h. Thereafter, they were incubated at +37 °C, overnight for the bacterial strains and 48 h for the fungal strain. The diameters of the zones of inhibition were measured with a caliper under a Petri dish magnifier and expressed as the mean of the diameters of three replicates ± the standard error of the mean (SEM).

4.4. Microdilution Method for Minimum Inhibitory Concentration Estimation

The MIC was estimated for the five best combinations of each piperamide/antimicrobial. The MIC was taken as the lowest concentration of the piperamide/antimicrobial resulting in the inhibition of at least 90% of the growth of the bacterial or fungal strain. The MIC values were determined using a microdilution turbidimetric broth method based on the guidelines of the Clinical and Laboratory Standards Institute [38]. For MIC evaluation, two-fold serial dilutions from 2500 to 9.75 µg/mL were prepared in sterile Mueller–Hinton broth (bacterial strains) and Saboraud broth (*C. albicans*) for each of the piperamide/antimicrobial combinations. The commercially pure compounds, piperine and piperlongumine (5 mg/mL concentrations in 70% ethanol), were two-fold serially diluted in Mueller–Hinton broth for the bacterial strains and Saboraud broth for the fungal strain. Tetracycline, rifampicin, and itraconazole were similarly diluted in Mueller–Hinton broth or Saboraud broth from 125 to 0.48 µg/mL, respectively; 96-well microtiter plates (Nunc, Nunclone; Nalge Nunc International, Roskilde, Denmark) were used for the tests. The bacterial or fungal cultures were inoculated in 5 mL of Mueller–Hinton broth and grown for 24 h at +37 °C for the bacterial strains or in 5 mL of Saboraud broth and grown for 48 h at +37 °C for *C. albicans* before the test. Absorbance of 1 mL of the overnight bacterial culture was measured for turbidity at 625 nm, using a UV–Visible Spectrophotometer type 1510 (ThermoFisher Scientific). The absorbance was adjusted to 0.1 at 625 nm (approximately 1.0×10^8 CFUs/mL). A total of 100 µL of this suspension $A_{625} = 0.1$ was further diluted a hundredfold to obtain a working suspension or inoculum containing 1.0×10^6 CFUs/mL. In all, 100 µL of this inoculum and 100 µL of each of the piperamide/antimicrobial combinations and solvent controls were introduced into the 96-well microtiter plates. Each well therefore contained 5×10^5 CFUs/mL. The growth control (GC) wells contained only the bacterial suspension, and the test (T) wells contained the piperamide/antimicrobial + bacterial suspension. Moreover, negative control wells were prepared for each piperamide/antimicrobial combination ratio tested, and these wells contained the piperamide/antimicrobial combinations at different ratios and the broth only. The microwell plates were incubated for 24 h in an incubator coupled to a shaker at +37 °C. The turbidity of the wells at 620 nm was recorded using a Victor 1420 spectrophotometer (PerkinElmer (Wallac Oy), Turku, Finland). The tests were done in triplicate, and the percentage growth was expressed as the mean of these triplicates ± the SEM.

4.5. Fractional Inhibitory Concentration Index

The FIC index was used to estimate the synergy [5,26]. For the FIC index calculation, the MIC values of five combinations of each piperamide/antimicrobial at different ratios were used to calculate FIC (A) and FIC (B), using the equation below:

The FIC values were calculated as follows:

$$FIC(A) = \frac{MIC\ value\ of\ combined\ piperamide\ and\ antimicrobial}{MIC\ value\ of\ antimicrobial\ alone}$$
$$FIC(B) = \frac{MIC\ value\ of\ combined\ piperamide\ and\ antimicrobial}{MIC\ value\ of\ piperamide\ alone}$$
$$FIC\ index = FIC(A) + FIC(B)$$

A FIC index value ≤ 0.5 was interpreted as synergy. The FIC index was calculated on the basis of the above-mentioned equation, in which the FIC index = X + Y and the interactions are defined as: FIC index ≤ 0.5, synergy; > 0.5 to ≤ 1.0, additive; > 1.0 to ≤ 2.0, indifferent; and > 2.0, antagonistic [26].

5. Conclusions

Piperine and piperlongumine are possible antibiotic adjuvants that should be applied in drug discovery for use as effective antibacterial treatments. The synergistic efficacy of piperlongumine and piperine in combination with rifampicin has shown that these two piperamides are bioactive scaffolds that could aid in fighting against multidrug-resistant pathogens, thereby improving the effectiveness of rifampicin in the treatment of infectious diseases. Our results show that the synergistic efficacy of piperamide compounds is dependent on the concentration and ratio of the combination. This indicates that the use of piperine and piperlongumine may minimize the adverse effects associated with conventional tetracycline and rifampicin and improve the effectiveness of these antibiotics. However, the antagonistic effects observed with the commercial compounds/antibiotics used against *P. aeruginosa* in this study demonstrate that appropriate caution should be taken to avoid the consumption of herbal drugs made from *Piper* species during antibacterial treatment therapies against *P. aeruginosa* infections. We suggest that piperine and piperlongumine could be considered as therapeutic bioactive compounds for antibacterial drug discovery. Further studies should be conducted on the mode of activity of the synergistic interaction between piperamides and antibiotics.

Author Contributions: Conceptualization, E.E.M., H.V., and Y.H.; methodology, E.E.M. and M.S.; formal analysis, E.E.M., Y.H., and M.S.; resources, H.V.; writing — original draft preparation, E.E.M. and M.S.; supervision, Y.H. and H.V.; project administration, H.V.

Funding: This research received no external funding.

Acknowledgments: The authors are grateful to the Faculty of Pharmacy, Division of Pharmaceutical Biosciences, University of Helsinki, for supporting this work and providing the materials used for the experiments.

Conflicts of Interest: The authors declare no conflicts of interest.

References

1. Brown, G.D.; Denning, D.W.; Gow, N.A.; Levitz, S.M.; Netea, M.G.; White, T.C. Hidden killers: human fungal infections. *Sci. Transl. Med.* **2012**, *4*, rv13–rv165. [CrossRef]
2. Mulholland, E.K.; Adegbola, R.A. Bacterial infections–a major cause of death among children in Africa. *N. Engl. J. Med.* **2005**, *352*, 75–77. [CrossRef]
3. Wisplinghoff, H.; Bischoff, T.; Tallent, S.M.; Seifert, H.; Wenzel, R.P.; Edmond, M.B. Nosocomial bloodstream infections in US hospitals: analysis of 24,179 cases from a prospective nationwide surveillance study. *Clin. Infect. Dis.* **2004**, *39*, 309–317. [CrossRef]
4. Kourtesi, C.; Ball, A.R.; Huang, Y.Y.; Jachak, S.M.; Vera, D.M.A.; Khondkar, P.; Tegos, G.P. Suppl 1: Microbial efflux systems and inhibitors: approaches to drug discovery and the challenge of clinical implementation. *Open Microbiol. J.* **2013**, *7*, 34. [CrossRef]
5. Abreu, A.C.; Coqueiro, A.; Sultan, A.R.; Lemmens, N.; Kim, H.K.; Verpoorte, R.; Choi, Y.H. Looking to nature for a new concept in antimicrobial treatments: Isoflavonoids from *Cytisus striatus* as antibiotic adjuvants against MRSA. *Sci. Rep.* **2017**, *7*, 3777. [CrossRef]
6. Subramani, R.; Narayanasamy, M.; Feussner, K.D. Plant-derived antimicrobials to fight against multi-drug-resistant human pathogens. *3 Biotech.* **2017**, *7*, 172. [CrossRef]
7. Alviano, D.S.; Alviano, C.S. Plant extracts: search for new alternatives to treat microbial diseases. *Curr. Pharm. Biotechnol.* **2009**, *10*, 106–121. [CrossRef]
8. Hemaiswarya, S.; Kruthiventi, A.K.; Doble, M. Synergism between natural products and antibiotics against infectious diseases. *Phytomedicine* **2008**, *15*, 639–652. [CrossRef]
9. Lambert, R.J.W. Susceptibility testing: inoculum size dependency of inhibition using the Colworth MIC technique. *J. Appl. Microbiol.* **2000**, *89*, 275–279. [CrossRef]
10. Van Vuuren, S.F.; Suliman, S.; Viljoen, A.M. The antimicrobial activity of four commercial essential oils in combination with conventional antimicrobials. *Lett. Appl. Microbiol.* **2009**, *48*, 440–446. [CrossRef]
11. Yang, S.K.; Low, L.Y.; Yap, P.S.X.; Yusoff, K.; Mai, C.W.; Lai, K.S.; Lim, S.H.E. Plant-derived antimicrobials: Insights into mitigation of antimicrobial resistance. *Rec. Nat. Prod.* **2018**, *12*, 295–316. [CrossRef]
12. Mgbeahuruike, E.E.; Yrjönen, T.; Vuorela, H.; Holm, Y. Bioactive compounds from medicinal plants: focus on *Piper* species. *S. Afr. J. Bot.* **2017**, *112*, 54–69. [CrossRef]
13. Biavatti, M.W. Synergy: an old wisdom, a new paradigm for pharmacotherapy. *Braz. J. Pharm. Sci.* **2009**, *45*, 371–378. [CrossRef]
14. Tegos, G.; Stermitz, F.R.; Lomovskaya, O.; Lewis, K. Multidrug pump inhibitors uncover remarkable activity of plant antimicrobials. *Antimicrob. Agents Chemother.* **2002**, *46*, 3133–3141. [CrossRef]
15. Piska, K.; Gunia-Krzyżak, A.; Koczurkiewicz, P.; Wójcik-Pszczoła, K.; Pękala, E. Piperlongumine (piplartine) as a lead compound for anticancer agents–Synthesis and properties of analogues. *Eur. J. Med. Chem.* **2018**, *156*, 13–20. [CrossRef]

16. Naika, R.; Prasanna, K.P.; Ganapathy, P.S. Antibacterial activity of piperlongumine an alkaloid isolated from methanolic root extract of *Piper Longum* L. *Pharmacophore.* **2010**, *1*, 141–148.
17. Karsha, P.V.; Lakshmi, O.B. Antibacterial activity of black pepper (*Piper nigrum* Linn.) with special reference to its mode of action on bacteria. *Indian J. Nat. Prod. Resour.* **2010**, *1*, 213–215.
18. Scott, I.M.; Puniani, E.; Jensen, H.; Livesey, J.F.; Poveda, L.; Sánchez-Vindas, P.; Arnason, J.T. Analysis of Piperaceae germplasm by HPLC and LCMS: a method for isolating and identifying unsaturated amides from *Piper* spp extracts. *J. Agric. Food Chem.* **2005**, *53*, 1907–1913. [CrossRef]
19. Adesina, S.K.; Adebayo, A.S.; Gröning, R. New constituents of *Piper guineense* fruit and leaf. *Die Pharmazie.* **2003**, *58*, 423–425. [CrossRef]
20. Mirza, Z.M.; Kumar, A.; Kalia, N.P.; Zargar, A.; Khan, I.A. Piperine as an inhibitor of the MdeA efflux pump of *Staphylococcus aureus*. *J. Med. Microbiol.* **2011**, *60*, 1472–1478. [CrossRef]
21. Stavri, M.; Piddock, L.J.; Gibbons, S. Bacterial efflux pump inhibitors from natural sources. *J. Antimicrob. Chemother.* **2006**, *59*, 1247–1260. [CrossRef] [PubMed]
22. Philipova, I.; Valcheva, V.; Mihaylova, R.; Mateeva, M.; Doytchinova, I.; Stavrakov, G. Synthetic piperine amide analogs with antimycobacterial activity. *Chem Biol. Drug Des.* **2018**, *91*, 763–768. [CrossRef] [PubMed]
23. Chavarria, D.; Silva, T.; Magalhães e Silva, D.; Remião, F.; Borges, F. Lessons from black pepper: piperine and derivatives thereof. *Expert Opin. Ther. Pat.* **2016**, *26*, 245–264. [CrossRef] [PubMed]
24. Umadevi, P.; Deepti, K.; Venugopal, D.V. Synthesis, anticancer and antibacterial activities of piperine analogs. *Med. Chem. Res.* **2013**, *22*, 5466–5471. [CrossRef]
25. Dusane, D.H.; Hosseinidoust, Z.; Asadishad, B.; Tufenkji, N. Alkaloids modulate motility, biofilm formation and antibiotic susceptibility of uropathogenic *Escherichia coli*. *PLoS ONE* **2014**, *9*, e112093. [CrossRef] [PubMed]
26. Kang, H.K.; Kim, H.Y.; Cha, J.D. Synergistic effects between silibinin and antibiotics on methicillin-resistant Staphylococcus aureus isolated from clinical specimens. *Biotechnol. J.* **2011**, *6*, 1397–1408. [CrossRef]
27. Tallarida, R.J. An overview of drug combination analysis with isobolograms. *J. Pharmacol. Exp. Ther.* **2006**, *319*, 1–7. [CrossRef] [PubMed]
28. Van Vuuren, S.; Viljoen, A. Plant-based antimicrobial studies–methods and approaches to study the interaction between natural products. *Planta Med.* **2011**, *77*, 1168–1182. [CrossRef]
29. Dhingra, V.K.; Rajpal, S.; Aggarwal, N.; Aggarwaln, J.K.; Shadab, K.; Jain, S.K. Adverse drug reactions observed during DOTS. *J. Commun. Dis.* **2004**, *36*, 251–259.
30. Nageswari, A.D.; Rajanandh, M.G.; Uday, M.K.R.A.; Nasreen, R.J.; Pujitha, R.R.; Prathiksha, G. Effect of rifampin with bio-enhancer in the treatment of newly diagnosed sputum positive pulmonary tuberculosis patients: A double-center study. *J. Clin. Tuberc. Mycobac. Dis.* **2018**, *12*, 73–77. [CrossRef]
31. Wu, D.C.; Chan, W.W.; Metelitsa, A.I.; Fiorillo, L.; Lin, A.N. Pseudomonas skin infection. *American J. Clin. Dermatol.* **2011**, *12*, 157–169. [CrossRef] [PubMed]
32. Sharma, S.; Kalia, N.P.; Suden, P.; Chauhan, P.S.; Kumar, M.; Ram, A.B.; Khan, I.A. Protective efficacy of piperine against Mycobacterium tuberculosis. *Tuberculosis* **2014**, *94*, 389–396. [CrossRef] [PubMed]
33. Nobile, C.J.; Johnson, A.D. *Candida albicans* biofilms and human disease. *Annu. Rev. Microbiol.* **2015**, *69*, 71–92. [CrossRef] [PubMed]
34. Mgbeahuruike, E.E.; Fyhrquist, P.; Julkunen-Tiitto, R.; Vuorela, H.; Holm, Y. Alkaloid-rich crude extracts, fractions and piperamide alkaloids of *Piper guineense* possess promising antibacterial effects. *Antibiotics* **2018**, *7*, 98. [CrossRef] [PubMed]
35. Lister, P.D.; Wolter, D.J.; Hanson, N.D. Antibacterial-resistant Pseudomonas aeruginosa: clinical impact and complex regulation of chromosomally encoded resistance mechanisms. *Clin. Microbiol. Rev.* **2009**, *22*, 582–610. [CrossRef]
36. Rasamiravaka, T.; Labtani, Q.; Duez, P.; El Jaziri, M. The formation of biofilms by *Pseudomonas aeruginosa*: A review of the natural and synthetic compounds interfering with control mechanisms. *BioMed Res. Int.* **2015**. [CrossRef] [PubMed]

37. Brown, A.J.; Brown, G.D.; Netea, M.G.; Gow, N.A. Metabolism impacts upon Candida immunogenicity and pathogenicity at multiple levels. *Trends Microbiol.* **2014**, *22*, 614–622. [CrossRef]
38. Cockerill, F.R.; Wikler, M.; Bush, K.; Dudley, M.; Eliopoulos, G.; Hardy, D. *Performance standards for antimicrobial susceptibility testing: twenty-second informational supplement. Approved Standard—Ninth Edition*; Clinical and Laboratory Standards Institute: Wayne, PA, USA, 2012.

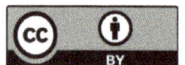

© 2019 by the authors. Licensee MDPI, Basel, Switzerland. This article is an open access article distributed under the terms and conditions of the Creative Commons Attribution (CC BY) license (http://creativecommons.org/licenses/by/4.0/).

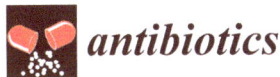

Article

Measuring Appropriate Antibiotic Prescribing in Acute Hospitals: Development of a National Audit Tool Through a Delphi Consensus

Graeme Hood [1], Kieran S. Hand [2], Emma Cramp [3], Philip Howard [4], Susan Hopkins [1] and Diane Ashiru-Oredope [1,*] on behalf of Antibiotic Prescribing Appropriateness Measures (APAM) subgroup of the national Advisory Committee on Antimicrobial Resistance, Prescribing and Healthcare Associated Infection (ARPHAI)

[1] Public Health England, London SE1 8UG, UK; graeme.hood@nhs.net (G.H.); susan.hopkins@phe.gov.uk (S.H.)
[2] University Hospital Southampton NHS Foundation Trust and School of Health Sciences, University of Southampton, Southampton SO16 6YD, UK; K.Hand@soton.ac.uk
[3] University Hospitals of Leicester NHS Trust, Leicester LE1 5WW, UK; emma.cramp@nhs.net
[4] Leeds Teaching Hospitals NHS Trust and University of Leeds, Leeds LS1 3EX, UK; Philip.howard2@nhs.net
* Correspondence: diane.ashiru-oredope@phe.gov.uk; Tel.: +44-(0)20-781-17240

Received: 6 April 2019; Accepted: 23 April 2019; Published: 29 April 2019

Abstract: This study developed a patient-level audit tool to assess the appropriateness of antibiotic prescribing in acute National Health Service (NHS) hospitals in the UK. A modified Delphi process was used to evaluate variables identified from published literature that could be used to support an assessment of appropriateness of antibiotic use. At a national workshop, 22 infection experts reached a consensus to define appropriate prescribing and agree upon an initial draft audit tool. Following this, a national multidisciplinary panel of 19 infection experts, of whom only one was part of the workshop, was convened to evaluate and validate variables using questionnaires to confirm the relevance of each variable in assessing appropriate prescribing. The initial evidence synthesis of published literature identified 25 variables that could be used to support an assessment of appropriateness of antibiotic use. All the panel members reviewed the variables for the first round of the Delphi; the panel accepted 23 out of 25 variables. Following review by the project team, one of the two rejected variables was rephrased, and the second neutral variable was re-scored. The panel accepted both these variables in round two with a 68% response rate. Accepted variables were used to develop an audit tool to determine the extent of appropriateness of antibiotic prescribing at the individual patient level in acute NHS hospitals through infection expert consensus based on the results of a Delphi process.

Keywords: Antimicrobial resistance; antibiotics; antimicrobial stewardship; inappropriate prescribing; days of therapy; Start Smart then Focus

1. Introduction

Antimicrobial resistance (AMR) is a global threat to health affecting all healthcare systems and growing at an alarming pace [1,2]. In the UK an increase in annual secondary care antibiotic consumption by 4.8% (measured as defined daily doses (DDD) of antibiotics per 1000 inhabitants per day) was reported in England between 2013 to 2017 [3]. Optimising prescribing, through the development and implementation of antimicrobial stewardship (AMS) programmes is a key area of the UK five-year AMR strategy [4]. An important element of these programmes is assessing the quality of antimicrobial prescribing. Several countries now use European Centre for Disease

Prevention and Control (ECDC) point prevalence survey (PPS) of healthcare-associated infections and antimicrobial use protocol to identify targets for quality improvement and evaluate antimicrobial stewardship programmes [5]. Surveillance data collected via PPS provide useful information for assessment of the burden of antimicrobial prescribing, however, the method has limited capacity to assess the appropriateness of prescribing in the absence of more complete individual patient-level clinical data [6]. An adaptation of the ECDC point prevalence survey tool was developed by infection experts in Australia to better measure prescribing quality; this tool performed well in validation, inter-rater reliability testing, and user feedback [7]. The Centers for Disease Control and Prevention (CDC) in the US have also published an audit tool to evaluate the quality of inpatient antibiotic prescribing with similar positive feedback [8]. These tools share common themes in their evaluation of appropriateness, such as use of individual patient clinical data and indication to aid the auditor's judgement of appropriateness. Two important limitations of existing audit protocols remain evident: Firstly, application of a broad definition of inappropriateness that includes a range of prescribing quality indicators (such as prompt intravenous-to-oral switch and appropriate dosing) that do not predict overall consumption of antibiotics; and secondly, an inability to specifically quantify the scale of inappropriate prescribing directly resulting from unnecessary doses administered. An ability to quantify the proportion of antimicrobial consumption that is unnecessary will allow healthcare organisations and governments to determine targets for a reduction in antimicrobial consumption. This will limit avoidable selection pressure for AMR and can be achieved without compromising patient safety. In addition, whilst PPS can provide a rich data source due to the fact they require a point-in-time assessment, it is not possible to measure the total duration of antibiotic use for patients assessed as part of a PPS. The national audit tool designed for NHS hospitals described in this report aims to support a focussed patient-level assessment of the appropriateness of antibiotic prescribing in secondary care.

It is not currently possible to estimate with any certainty the proportion of antimicrobial prescribing in English hospitals that is inappropriate, as electronic prescribing data directly linking hospital prescriptions to clinical data are still not widely available. A key study aim was to develop and validate a patient-level audit tool that could support estimation of the number of days of antibiotic therapy that auditors considered non-essential and therefore potentially avoidable. The proportion of inappropriate antibiotic prescribing can be represented as non-essential days of therapy (DOTs) expressed as a percentage of total days of therapy. The goal of the audit tool was to collate variables that would support assessment of those aspects of prescribing most relevant for selection pressure and resistance. If successful, this would allow the UK to potentially set goals for reduction of antibiotic consumption in hospitals that are safe and achievable. A secondary aim included creating an audit tool that helped minimise subjectivity in order to standardise the assessment of appropriateness by prompting auditors to consider certain critical information in order to support their decision.

2. Results

2.1. Defining Appropriateness

Defining the gold standard for appropriate antibiotic prescribing is challenging due to the inherently subjective nature of evaluating quality in prescribing. An initial list was compiled to incorporate elements of high-quality prescribing identified by opinion leaders in the field, the UK Government Scientific Advisory Committee on Antimicrobial Prescribing, Resistance and Healthcare Associated Infection (APRHAI) and a workshop including 22 infection experts convened to define appropriate antibiotic prescribing. The collated list (Table 1) sets out many elements of antibiotic prescribing that may be considered in an assessment of appropriateness.

Table 1. Elements of antibiotic prescribing in hospitals relevant for evaluating appropriateness [9–29].

Prescribing Elements (Potential Audit Variables)	Comments	Selected for Audit
START SMART		
No antibiotic if not indicated (no reasonable evidence of infection)	Unnecessary antibiotic exposure selects for avoidable resistance [9–11].	√
Indication documented	Good practice for continuity of care but of uncertain relevance to resistance.	√
Appropriate specimens taken for microscopy, culture, and sensitivity (MC&S)—blood cultures and suspected site of infection	Important for establishing evidence of infection and for targeting appropriate therapy but requires manual audit and >50% of cultures are negative [12,13].	√
No allergy or contra-indication to treatments	Important patient safety consideration but not relevant for resistance.	×
Prompt administration of first dose	Important patient safety consideration in cases of severe sepsis but of uncertain relevance to resistance. Already captured by national sepsis audits.	×
Treatment regimen adequate to cover most likely pathogens	Meta-analysis of RCTs reports increased risk of mortality if initial regimen inadequate [14]. Relevance to resistance uncertain.	√*
Treatment regimen not unnecessarily broad spectrum	Indiscriminate use of critical broad-spectrum agents unnecessarily selects for resistance [15–17].	√*
No redundant agents in treatment regimen	Unnecessary antibiotic exposure selects for avoidable resistance [9–11].	√
Treatment regimen compliant with local/national guideline or justified deviation	Validity dependent upon quality of local guideline. Relevance to resistance uncertain.	×
Treatment regimen cost-effective	Not relevant to resistance.	×
No underdosing	Limited evidence from modeling suggests that low doses may select resistance in pneumococci [18] but underdosing unlikely to be a problem in NHS hospitals due to pharmacist and nurse intervention.	×
No overdosing	Important patient safety consideration but likely to reduce rather than increase risk of selecting resistance [19–24].	×
Correct route of administration	Relevant for efficacy, length of stay, and risk of line infection but of uncertain relevance to resistance.	×
Prompt appropriate source control	Subjective assessment. Of uncertain relevance to resistance.	×
No missed doses or delayed doses	Of uncertain relevance to selection of resistance.	×
Therapeutic drug monitoring (TDM) for narrow therapeutic index drugs	Important primarily for patient safety (but also for efficacy); of uncertain relevance to resistance.	×
THEN FOCUS		
Prompt discontinuation of antibiotics if alternative diagnosis established and infection excluded	There is RCT evidence that unnecessary continuation selects for multi-resistant organisms [25–27].	√
Appropriate broadening of spectrum in response to MC&S results	This may necessitate an increase in broad-spectrum agent use if indicated by MC&S results. Failure to adjust ineffective treatment to MC&S results is associated with a higher risk of mortality [27].	√*
Appropriate narrowing of spectrum in response to MC&S results	Evidence largely from observational studies suggests that de-escalation to narrow-spectrum agents is safe when patients are improving clinically and a plausible pathogen has been identified [28].	√*
Prompt referral to outpatient parenteral antibiotic therapy OPAT services for suitable patients	Relevant for length of stay and risk of healthcare-associated infection (HCAI) but of uncertain relevance to resistance.	×
Prompt switch from IV to oral route of administration when safe and effective	Relevant for length of stay and risk of line infection but of uncertain relevance to resistance.	×
Antibiotic plan documented in the notes	Good practice for continuity of care but of uncertain relevance to resistance.	×
No unjustified prolonged duration of treatment	There is evidence from RCTs and observational studies that unnecessarily prolonged duration selects for multi-resistant organisms [25,26,29]. Can only be audited at the end of therapy.	√

* Prescribing elements relating to antibiotic spectrum; deprioritised for audit tool prototype

It could reasonably be argued that each of these elements is relevant to efficacy, safety, and improving patient outcomes, and critical to the assessment of appropriateness of prescribing. However, the APRHAI committee took a view that improvement in performance against certain elements would be less likely to impact upon the overall consumption of antibiotics and, consequently, would be less likely to impact upon antibiotic resistance. Three aspects were therefore given ultimate priority as most relevant to identifying avoidable selection of resistance within the UK hospital setting:

- Prescribing an antibiotic for a patient in the absence of (documented) evidence of bacterial infection.
- Prescribing a critical broad-spectrum antibiotic to patients in the absence of a (documented) rationale.
- Continuing an antibiotic prescription beyond the course length recommended in local or national guidelines, in the absence of a (documented) rationale.

2.2. Initial Draft of Audit Tool

A consensus emerged from the one-day workshop that existing antibiotic prescribing guidelines for acute hospitals often do not suggest clinical thresholds for initiating or stopping antibiotics. This means there is a lack of consistency between hospitals in assessing whether antibiotics are indicated and for how long. There was also general agreement that antibiotic consumption data alone were not sufficient to determine the proportion of prescribing that is inappropriate. This was further complicated by the failure of hospital-level antibiotic consumption data to account for patient acuity and hospital case mix. The workshop group arrived at the conclusion that an individual patient audit by an infection specialist was required to establish with greater certainty the current proportion of prescribing that is inappropriate. This process was anticipated to be less vulnerable to case mix or speciality bias. It was agreed that a patient-level audit tool would be sent for expert elicitation via a Delphi process.

2.3. Round 1 Delphi

The response rate to the initial survey was 100% (19/19), taking on average 32 minutes to complete. Of the first-round responders, 42% (8/19) were specialist antimicrobial pharmacists, 21% (4/19) were infectious disease doctors or medical microbiologists, 16% (3/19) were general medical doctors, and the remaining 21% (4/19) were antimicrobial stewardship nurses. The majority (14/19) of participants in round one had over five years' experience and practice in antimicrobial stewardship and infection. When asked what proportion of inpatients prescribed antibiotics should be audited to provide reasonable confidence of the overall assessment of the appropriateness of antibiotic prescribing in secondary care, 79% (15/19) expressed the view that either 5–10% or 10–25% of inpatients on antibiotics would be an adequate sample size to represent the entire hospital patient population. The panel members were also asked at what frequency would it be necessary and reasonable to repeat an audit assessing appropriate antibiotic prescribing; 89% (17/19) indicated annually and 11% (2/19) stated every three years would be sufficient. Twenty-three of the 25 variables were scored as relevant or highly relevant for assessing appropriateness for one or more of the main decision points (Supplementary Materials, Table S1) and were therefore accepted following Round 1. One variable, "documentation of pre-72-hour review", was rejected by the expert panel in Round 1 as not relevant to the assessment of appropriateness at any of the main decision time points. A neutral consensus was reached by the expert panel for the variable "presenting complaint"; this was subsequently rescored in the second round. The first variable was renamed to "review of antibiotic prescription within 72 h" to remove the requirement for formal documentation of the review and presented for scoring in the second round. The project team was reluctant to remove this variable due to the potential value it brings in predicting unnecessarily prolonged treatment courses.

2.4. Round 2 Delphi

Out of the nineteen respondents (from Round 1) who were invited to participate in Round 2 the response rate was 68% (13/19). The same distribution of healthcare professionals participated in Round 2 with 69% (9/13) having over 5 years' experience and practice in antimicrobial stewardship and infection. The neutral variable "presenting complaint" was rescored, with 85% (11/13) of respondents indicating this was considered relevant to assessing appropriate prescribing. A consensus was reached when the expert panel members were asked to score the renamed variable "review of antibiotic prescription within 72 h" with this being accepted by the panel (Figure 1).

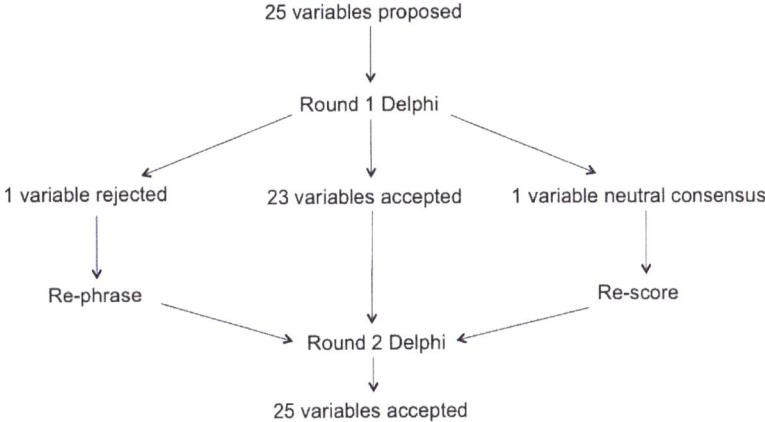

Figure 1. Overall Delphi results.

The majority (9/13) of respondents reported that there were local guidance or supportive tools available to help clinicians stop antibiotic therapy safely. Where not available, three of the four respondents agreed that such guidance would be helpful.

2.5. Feasibility

Eight of the 19 original panel members agreed that the audit tool was fit for purpose, 32% (6/19) expressed a neutral view, and 5 panel members disagreed (5/19) including one panel member stating they were unable to assess this question. The participants were asked if the time taken to complete the audit tool is a worthwhile investment of NHS resources for the benefit of patient safety and public health, with 43% (8/19) agreeing that it is, 21% (4/19) having a neutral view, 26% (5/19) disagreeing, and 10% (2/19) being unable to assess this.

3. Discussion

An audit tool consisting of 25 variables to support assessment of the appropriateness of antibiotic prescribing in secondary care has been developed. The prototype audit tool was reviewed by 19 multi-disciplinary infection specialist health professionals through a two stage modified Delphi process and all 25 variables were accepted by specialists as relevant or very relevant to the aim of the audit following rewording of just one variable.

The response rate of participants within the Delphi process was seen to reduce between rounds one and two. A systematic review of 31 studies indicated that the median response rate of a Delphi process does reduce by 2% from the first to the last round of Delphi processes [30], however even with reminder e-mails our response reduced by 32% from round one to two, so this could be interpreted as introducing potential bias. The Delphi process occurred during winter months which can operationally be a busy time for NHS hospitals. This could have been a contributing factor in the reduced response rate seen over the two rounds.

The inclusion of acuity scores within the audit tool was to help support the auditor in assessing appropriateness of antibiotics by highlighting the severity of the acute health status which could be as a result of a likely infection. The supportive use is important as a low acuity score does not rule out infection, but merely indicates no severe or deteriorating condition or a lesser probability of organ failure. Evidence from a multi-centre study of adult emergency departments in the UK reported a positive predictive value for National Early Warning Score (NEWS) ≥3 of 20% for mortality or ICU admission [31]. It was therefore considered reasonable to assess what proportion of patients treated with antibiotics either have NEWS ≥3 or localised evidence of infection at an anatomical site. An abbreviated version of the Sequential Organ Failure Assessment (SOFA) score, quick SOFA (qSOFA), was assessed in almost 75,000 adult patients hospitalised with suspected infection [32]. The predictive validity of the qSOFA score for in-hospital mortality was found to be statistically greater than the SOFA or systemic inflammatory response syndrome (SIRS) scores, supporting its use as a prompt to consider possible sepsis [32]. Applying qSOFA score ≥2 during emergency department or ward stay as a prediction tool for in-hospital all-cause mortality had a negative predictive value of 97% in adult patients with clinical suspicion of infection in a recent multi-centre study including 27 French emergency departments [33]. A qSOFA score at a threshold of 2 or more may be considered by some clinicians to be a reasonable tool for differentiating patients in whom immediate broad-spectrum antibiotics are justified, given the associated in-hospital mortality of 24% [33].

During the second round of the Delphi process the panel did not accept that formal documentation of a pre-72-hour review was relevant. The panel did however accept that whether a pre-72-hour review took place was relevant, irrespective of documentation (e.g., prescription changed but no corresponding entry in the medical notes) for the purposes of assessing appropriateness of antibiotic prescribing. In the absence of a pre-72-hour review, it is likely that patients for whom diagnostic tests support an alternative diagnosis to infection are likely to continue antibiotics longer than necessary. This variable is also important due to the potential value it brings to predicting unnecessarily prolonged treatment courses, and it is part of ongoing quality improvement work within English hospitals, so the indicator was reworded for Round 2. Secondary healthcare quality improvement work within England has focussed on reducing total antibiotic consumption as well as obtaining evidence of antibiotic review within 72 h of commencing an antibiotic [34].

The addition of separate questions to explore individual views on inappropriate prescribing within secondary care was used as it was not possible to estimate a sample size, because the proportion of non-essential DOTs was unknown. Delphi participants were asked what proportion of patients on antibiotics required auditing to give them assurance on appropriateness of antibiotic prescribing for their hospital.

The expert panel members were invited to estimate the feasibility and likely value of the audit tool; this saw 26% of the expert panel disagreeing with statements that the audit tool was fit for purpose or a worthwhile investment of NHS resources. This finding was surprising given the high degree of consensus over the relevance of individual variables for supporting the assessment of appropriateness and was not explored in more detail. It may reflect a perception of futility that a simple audit tool could not sufficiently capture the complexity of an episode of infection to enable a reproducible assessment of appropriateness. A pilot study of the audit tool to test the reliability of the instrument is clearly a prerequisite before more widespread adoption.

3.1. Study Strengths and Limitations

Strengths of this project include the development of an audit tool through a consensus of a multi-disciplinary team of experienced infection specialists working in hospital clinical practice. The authors believe the developed audit tool is the first of its kind internationally that can specifically quantify the scale of inappropriate prescribing directly resulting from unnecessary doses being administered. The audit tool was designed to minimise the burden of data collection by limiting the items of data collected to only those considered relevant or highly relevant to the specific aim of evaluation of appropriateness of prescribing at three critical prescribing decision time points. The audit tool also narrows the focus of the audit to evaluate only those elements of prescribing associated with unnecessary antibiotic doses and therefore likely to be most relevant to the selection of resistant microorganisms: whether an antibiotic is indicated at the start of treatment, whether treatment beyond 72 h is justified, and whether treatment beyond a standard course length is appropriate.

The potential to collect more detailed clinical information to explore the subjective decision that the auditors would take was advantageous. Standardisation of the assessment process may be aided by the inclusion of objective variables to capture evidence of infection or sepsis, along with markers of severity including qSOFA score, NEWS, C-reactive protein (CRP), and white blood cell count.

The potential limitations of the audit tool include the time needed to collect data and risk of subjectivity in assessment which are inherent limitations of this approach, however a balance is struck between the value of detailed patient-level data to robustly answer the important question of appropriateness set against the use of a standardised data collection tool to minimise variability in assessment. There was also limited opportunity for experts to consider variables not included in the tool, such as medical imaging and urine dipstick tests. Presenting an increased number of potentially relevant variables such as antibiotic dose and route of administration may have provided greater opportunity to discriminate between the perceived value of different variables for estimating non-essential doses. Whilst a relatively small sample of experts participated in the Delphi process, an important limitation, it is worth noting that 22 experts participated in the workshop to define appropriate antibiotic prescribing and develop the initial audit tool cascaded for the Delphi consensus. Subsequent piloting of the audit tool will need to include ongoing evaluation of the strengths and weakness of the tool and inform iterative improvements. The minor changes to the audit tool as a result of this Delphi process provide reassurance that extensive revision of the tool was not required, however a higher number of experts participating would have provided greater assurance of a reliable rating for each of the variables assessed.

Since admission and discharge dates were not included in the tool it was not possible to determine at which point during their admission a patient receives antibiotics and therefore whether a patient is receiving treatment for a healthcare-associated infection or community-acquired infection unless this is stated explicitly by the auditor. This was identified by the project team as a priority to capture in future versions of the audit tool.

The use of a web-based Delphi process limited opportunity for qualitative feedback from a face-to-face discussion and may have contributed to the lower response rate for Round 2. The selection of expert panel members was via national infection networks and only one healthcare professional also participated in the previous workshop that convened to define appropriate prescribing. To help reduce potential bias, all participants were blinded to who participated in the expert panel with individual correspondence being sent.

The use of the developed audit tool is for active treatment and does not assess long-term and peri-operative surgical prophylaxis antibiotics. An adaptation could be made to the audit tool in order to assess these groups of patients. Finally, the developed audit tool was prioritised for antibacterial agents only but could also be adapted for antifungal and antiviral agents.

3.2. Future Work

Piloting the audit tool within NHS hospitals to assess usability and operability is the next step. This would also provide additional insight and development of the tool and mitigate against the limitations of the small consensus panel. The resource burden of data collection and whether there is variation between hospitals that use electronic systems or paper-based processes needs to be quantified. Although it is anticipated that the use of electronic systems should be faster than paper-based prescribing, ease of access to information for each variable may vary. Piloting the audit tool within 5 to 10 hospitals could provide a preliminary assessment of non-essential days of antibiotic therapy prescribed to inform the sample size calculation for a definitive study. Recruiting a mixture of hospital types (teaching, district and specialist) will be important to assess the practicality of the developed audit tool. The balance between the amount of information being collected with the time taken to collect the data in a busy operational hospital will be crucial.

4. Materials and Methods

4.1. Part 1: Development of the Audit Tool

Evidence synthesis of published literature and international guidance contributed to the development of the initial prototype audit tool to try and quantify and identify inappropriate antimicrobial prescribing. The initial prototype audit tool then underwent preliminary feasibility testing at one acute teaching hospital in Southampton, England. This was conducted by a specialist pharmacist supported by a medical microbiologist, with a focus on evaluating the operability of the audit tool. After a subgroup of the UK government APRHAI scientific advisory committee drafted standards to define appropriate prescribing in secondary care a finalised prototype audit tool was created [4]. The subgroup discussed aspects of auditing including frequency, intensity, resourcing, and mechanism of data collection including feedback and reporting processes.

To elicit further expert opinion, a one-day workshop was held on 6 March 2017 with infection experts including secondary care clinicians (10/22), pharmacists (9/22), a nurse, an academic, and a medical director to explore views on the appropriateness of prescribing within hospitals. The project team including two pharmacists of the antimicrobial resistance programme at Public Health England and three national antimicrobial pharmacists met to discuss the workshop findings and updated the audit tool accordingly. Elements of the audit tool that were intended to support the assessment of appropriateness of antimicrobial prescribing were termed "variables" for the purposes of the validation process. The selection of variables to include in the audit tool was based on discussions within the antibiotic prescribing quality subgroup of APRHAI, iterative e-mail feedback from co-authors, and prototype audit tool testing in Southampton.

To support the auditor in their assessment of the severity of infection and deterioration as a result of a likely infection the National Early Warning Score (NEWS) and quick sequential organ failure assessment (qSOFA) score were incorporated into the audit tool [32,35]. A threshold NEWS value of 3 or above has been proposed as a suitable trigger to systematically screen for sepsis or septic shock in patients with suspected infection in a United States Emergency Department (ED) population with a reported negative predictive value of 99.5 (95% CI 97.8–99.9) [36].

4.2. Part 2: Validation of the Audit Tool

Between October and December 2017, a RAND-modified Delphi process was conducted to validate each individual variable within the audit tool. A multi-disciplinary expert panel of infection and public health specialists was recruited via e-mail through national infection and microbiology networks and asked to assess the relevance of each variable against a five-point Likert Scale [37]. The relevance was assessed in relation to three main decision time points during a course of antibiotic therapy:

- Initiation (was the antibiotic indicated and necessary at the start date?);
- Early post prescription review (was the antibiotic continued after infection was ruled out?);
- End of therapy (was the antibiotic continued beyond the standard duration?).

Non-essential days of antibiotic therapy were included with potential reasons as follows: (1) antibiotic not indicated/unnecessary at start date; (2) unexplained continuation of antibiotic after infection ruled out; and (3) unexplained continuation of antibiotic beyond standard duration. The standard duration was defined by individual hospitals as identified in local antibiotic guidelines. A separate questionnaire was sent to the Delphi participants to explore individual views on inappropriate prescribing within secondary care.

The expert panel participated in two rounds. Invitation via e-mail was sent to 19 participants before the first round. The online survey SelectSurvey.net was used in each Delphi round with participant reminder e-mails sent periodically. The results were discussed within the project team after the first round and the aggregated scores were shared with the participants prior to the second round. Each of the 25 variables was assessed for its relevance against the three main decision time points.

Qualitative feedback was reviewed by one project team member and common themes reported for discussion with the full project team. The threshold for accepting a variable was met if the median score was "relevant" or "very relevant" for assessing appropriateness at any one of the three decision time points. A variable was rejected if the median score for all three of the critical decision points was "irrelevant" or "very irrelevant" with a neutral score being rescored in the second round to provide a definitive response. The rewording of questions between each round occurred by the project team and was presented to the participants from Round 1 for Round 2. After completing both rounds of the Delphi process the accepted variables were incorporated into a finalised audit tool (Supplementary Materials, Figure S1).

4.3. Statistics

Data were summarised using non-parametric descriptive statistics which are considered suitable to measure consensus and stability in Delphi studies [38] and due to the number of Delphi participants. The median and percentage "relevant" and "highly relevant" responses for each of the variables in relation to each decision time point was calculated using univariate analysis.

5. Conclusions

In summary, the RAND-modified Delphi process has provided face validity of this audit tool and selection of critical variables that can be used to support the assessment of inappropriate antibiotic prescribing. The feedback from expert panel members helped shape development of the audit tool and provides an important endorsement from practising healthcare professionals within and outside the NHS. This audit methodology will help hospitals identify the location, extent, and nature of inappropriate antibiotic prescribing and provide evidence to drive local antimicrobial stewardship and focus targeted training to specific areas of improvement.

Supplementary Materials: The following are available online at http://www.mdpi.com/2079-6382/8/2/49/s1. Figure S1: Assessing appropriateness of antibiotic therapy–final national audit tool for pilot. Table S1: Round 1 Delphi results

Author Contributions: Conceptualization, D.A.-O., G.H., K.S.H.; data curation, G.H.; formal analysis, G.H.; methodology, G.H., K.S.H., and D.A.-O.; project administration, G.H.; supervision, D.A.-O; validation, K.S.H., E.C., and D.A.-O.; writing—original draft, G.H.; writing—review & editing, G.H., K.S.H., E.C., P.H., S.H., and D.A.-O.

Funding: This research received no external funding and was conducted by Public Health England

Acknowledgments: The authors would like to thank all the expert panel members who participated in the Delphi process who contributed to the development of the audit tool: Janet Appleton, Druin Burch, Kay Cawthron, Abid Hussain, Conor Jamieson, David Jenkins, Alasdair MacGowen, Sanjay Patel, Neil Powell, Jacqueline Sneddon, Adel Sheikh, Paul Wade, Laura Whitney, Antony Zorzi, James Hatcher, Enrique Castro-Sanchez, Emily Bennett, Cairine Gormley and Tania Misra.

Conflicts of Interest: The authors declare no conflict of interest.

References

1. WHO Antimicrobial Resistance. Available online: http://www.who.int/mediacentre/factsheets/fs194/en/ (accessed on 17 January 2019).
2. Review on Antimicrobial Resistance. Available online: https://amr-review.org/background.html (accessed on 17 January 2019).
3. English Surveillance Programme for Antimicrobial Utilisation and Resistance (ESPAUR) Report 2018. Available online: https://assets.publishing.service.gov.uk/government/uploads/system/uploads/attachment_data/file/759975/ESPAUR_2018_report.pdf (accessed on 22 March 2019).
4. English Surveillance Programme for Antimicrobial Utilisation and Resistance (ESPAUR) Report 2017. Available online: https://assets.publishing.service.gov.uk/government/uploads/system/uploads/attachment_data/file/656611/ESPAUR_report_2017.pdf (accessed on 18 January 2019).

5. Point Prevalence Survey of Healthcare-Associated Infections and Antimicrobial Use in European Acute Care Hospitals Surveillance Report 2011–2012. Available online: https://ecdc.europa.eu/sites/portal/files/media/en/publications/Publications/healthcare-associated-infections-antimicrobial-use-PPS.pdf (accessed on 18 January 2019).
6. Kieran, J.A.; O'Doherty, R.G.; Hudson, B. ESAC point prevalence methodology to assess antimicrobial consumption and quality of prescribing in an Australian setting. *Med. J. Aust.* **2011**, *194*, 103–104.
7. James, R.; Upjohn, L.; Cotta, M.; Luu, S.; Marshall, C.; Buising, K.; Thursky, K. Measuring antimicrobial prescribing quality in Australian hospitals: Development and evaluation of a national antimicrobial prescribing survey tool. *J. Antimicrob. Chemother.* **2015**, *70*, 1912–1918. [CrossRef] [PubMed]
8. Spivak, E.S.; Cosgrove, S.E.; Srinivasan, A. Measuring appropriate antimicrobial use: Attempts at opening the black box. *Clin. Infect. Dis.* **2016**, *63*, 1639–1644. [PubMed]
9. Lopez-Lozano, J.M.; Monnet, D.L.; Yague, A.; Burgos, A.; Gonzalo, N.; Campillos, P.; Saez, M. Modelling and forecasting antimicrobial resistance and its dynamic relationship to antimicrobial use: A time series analysis. *Int..J Antimicrob. Agents* **2000**, *14*, 21–31. [CrossRef]
10. Tacconelli, E.; Cataldo, M.A.; De Pascale, G.; Manno, D.; Spanu, T.; Cambieri, A.; Antonelli, M.; Sanguinetti, M.; Fadda, G.; Cauda, R. Prediction models to identify hospitalized patients at risk of being colonized or infected with multidrug-resistant Acinetobacter baumannii calcoaceticus complex. *J. Antimicrob. Chemother.* **2008**, *62*, 1130–1137. [CrossRef] [PubMed]
11. Tacconelli, E.; De Angellis, G.; Cataldo, M.A.; Mantengoli, E.; Spanu, T.; Pan, A.; Corti, G.; Radice, A.; Stolzuoli, L.; Antinori, S.; et al. Antibiotic usage and risk of colonization and infection with antibiotic-resistant bacteria: A hospital population-based study. *Antimicrob. Agents Chemother.* **2009**, *53*, 4264–4269. [CrossRef] [PubMed]
12. Braykov, N.P.; Morgan, D.J.; Schweizer, M.L.; Usian, D.Z.; Kelesidis, T.; Weisenberg, S.A.; Johannsson, B.; Young, H.; Cantey, J.; Scrinivason, A.; et al. Assessment of empirical antibiotic therapy optimisation in six hospitals: An observational cohort study. *Lancet Infect. Dis.* **2014**, *14*, 1220–1227. [CrossRef]
13. De Sousa, A.G.; Fernandes Junior, C.J.; Santos, G.P.D.; Laselva, C.R.; Polessi, J.; Lisboa, L.F.; Akamine, N.; Silva, E. The impact of each action in the Surviving Sepsis Campaign measures on hospital mortality of patients with severe sepsis/septic shock. *Einstein* **2008**, *6*, 323–327.
14. Paul, M.; Shani, V.; Muchtar, E.; Kariv, G.; Robenshtok, E.; Leibovici, L. Systematic review and meta-analysis of the efficacy of appropriate empiric antibiotic therapy for sepsis. *Antimicrob. Agents Chemother.* **2010**, *54*, 4851–4863. [CrossRef] [PubMed]
15. Harris, A.D.; Perencevich, E.; Roghmann, M.C.; Morris, G.; Kaye, K.S.; Johnson, J.A. Risk factors for piperacillin-tazobactam-resistant Pseudomonas aeruginosa among hospitalized patients. *Antimicrob. Agents Chemother.* **2002**, *46*, 854–858. [CrossRef]
16. Lai, C.C.; Wang, C.Y.; Chu, C.C.; Tan, C.K.; Lu, C.L.; Lee, Y.C.; Huang, Y.T.; Lee, P.I.; Hsueh, P.R. Correlation between antibiotic consumption and resistance of Gram-negative bacteria causing healthcare-associated infections at a university hospital in Taiwan from 2000 to 2009. *J. Antimicrob. Chemother.* **2011**, *66*, 1374–1382. [CrossRef]
17. Pakyz, A.L.; Oinonen, M.; Polk, R.E. Relationship of carbapenem restriction in 22 university teaching hospitals to carbapenem use and carbapenem-resistant Pseudomonas aeruginosa. *Antimicrob. Agents Chemother.* **2009**, *53*, 1983–1986. [CrossRef]
18. Opatowski, L.; Mandel, J.; Varon, E.; Boelle, P.Y.; Temime, L.; Guillemot, D. Antibiotic dose impact on resistance selection in the community: A mathematical model of beta-lactams and Streptococcus pneumoniae dynamics. *Antimicrob. Agents Chemother.* **2010**, *54*, 2330–2337. [CrossRef]
19. Guillemot, D.; Carbon, C.; Balkau, B.; Geslin, P.; Lecoeur, H.; Vauzelle-Keroedan, F.; Bouvenot, G.; Eschwege, E. Low dosage and long treatment duration of beta-lactam: Risk factors for carriage of penicillin-resistant Streptococcus pneumoniae. *JAMA* **1998**, *279*, 365–370. [CrossRef]
20. Handel, A.; Margolis, E.; Levin, B.R. Exploring the role of the immune response in preventing antibiotic resistance. *J. Theor. Biol.* **2009**, *256*, 655–662. [CrossRef]
21. Martinez, M.N.; Papich, M.G.; Drusano, G.L. Dosing regimen matters: The importance of early intervention and rapid attainment of the pharmacokinetic/pharmacodynamic target. *Antimicrob. Agents Chemother.* **2012**, *56*, 2795–2805. [CrossRef]

22. Olofsson, S.K.; Cars, O. Optimizing drug exposure to minimize selection of antibiotic resistance. *Clin. Infect. Dis.* **2007**, *45* (Suppl. 2), S129–S136. [CrossRef]
23. Schrag, S.J.; Pena, C.; Fernandez, J.; Sanchez, J.; Gomez, V.; Perez, E.; Feris, J.M.; Besser, R.E. Effect of short-course, high-dose amoxicillin therapy on resistant pneumococcal carriage: A randomized trial. *JAMA* **2001**, *286*, 49–56. [CrossRef]
24. Tam, V.H.; Louie, A.; Deziel, M.R.; Liu, W.; Drusano, G.L. The relationship between quinolone exposures and resistance amplification is characterized by an inverted U: A new paradigm for optimizing pharmacodynamics to counterselect resistance. *Antimicrob. Agents Chemother.* **2007**, *51*, 744–747. [CrossRef]
25. Singh, N.; Rogers, P.; Atwood, C.W.; Wagener, M.M.; Yu, V.L. Short-course empiric antibiotic therapy for patients with pulmonary infiltrates in the intensive care unit. A proposed solution for indiscriminate antibiotic prescription. *Am. J. Respir. Crit. Care Med.* **2000**, *162*, 505–511. [CrossRef]
26. Chastre, J.; Wolff, M.; Fagon, J.Y.; Chevret, S.; Thomas, F.; Wermert, D.; Clementi, E.; Gonzalez, J.; Jusserand, D.; Asfar, P.; et al. PneumA trial group. comparison of 8 vs 15 days of antibiotic therapy for ventilator-associated pneumonia in adults: A randomized trial. *JAMA* **2003**, *290*, 2588–2598. [CrossRef]
27. Palacios-Baena, Z.R.; Gutierrez-Gutierrez, B.; De Cueto, M.; Viale, P.; Venditti, M.; Hernandez-Torres, A.; Oliver, A.; Martinez-Martinez, L.; Calbo, E.; Pintado, V.; et al. REIPI/ESGBIS/INCREMENT Group. Development and validation of the INCREMENT-ESBL predictive score for mortality in patients with bloodstream infections due to extended-spectrum-beta-lactamase-producing Enterobacteriaceae. *J. Antimicrob. Chemother.* **2017**, *72*, 906–913.
28. Schuts, E.C.; Hulscher, M.E.; Mouton, J.W.; Verduin, C.M.; Stuart, J.W.T.C.; Overdiek, H.W.P.M.; van der Linden, P.D.; Natsch, S.; Hertogh, C.M.P.M.; Wolfs, T.F.W.; et al. Current evidence on hospital antimicrobial stewardship objectives: A systematic review and meta-analysis. *Lancet Infect. Dis.* **2016**, *16*, 847–856. [CrossRef]
29. Marra, A.R.; de Almeida, S.M.; Correa, L.; Silva, M., Jr.; Martino, M.D.; Silva, C.V.; Cal, R.G.; Edmond, M.B.; dos Santos, O.F. The effect of limiting antimicrobial therapy duration on antimicrobial resistance in the critical care setting. *Am. J. Infect. Control.* **2009**, *37*, 204–209. [CrossRef]
30. Boulkedid, R.; Abdoul, H.; Loustau, M.; Sibony, O.; Alberti, C. Using and reporting the delphi method for selecting healthcare quality indicators: A systematic review. *PLoS ONE* **2011**, *6*, e20476. [CrossRef]
31. Corfield, A.R.; Lees, F.; Zealley, I.; Houston, G.; Dickie, S.; Ward, K.; McGuffie, C. Utility of a single early warning score in patients with sepsis in the emergency department. *Emerg. Med. J.* **2014**, *31*, 482–487. [CrossRef]
32. Seymour, C.W.; Liu, V.X.; Iwashyna, T.J.; Iwashyna, T.; Brunkhorst, F.M.; Rea, T.D.; Scherag, A.; Rubenfeld, G.; Kahn, J.M.; Shankar-Hari, M.; et al. Assessment of clinical criteria for sepsis: For the third international consensus definitions for sepsis and septic shock (Sepsis-3). *JAMA* **2016**, *315*, 762–774. [CrossRef]
33. Freund, Y.; Lemachatti, N.; Krastinova, E.; Van Laer, M.; Claessens, Y.-E.; Avonso, A.; Occelli, C.; Feral-Pierssens, A.-L.; Truchot, J.; Ortega, M.; et al. Prognostic accuracy of sepsis-3 criteria for in-hospital mortality among patients with suspected infection presenting to the emergency department. *JAMA* **2017**, *317*, 301–308. [CrossRef]
34. NHS England National CQUIN Templates 2016/17. Available online: https://www.england.nhs.uk/nhs-standard-contract/cquin/cquin-16-17/ (accessed on 18 January 2019).
35. National Early Warning Score (NEWS): Standardising the Assessment of Acute Illness Severity in the NHS. Report of a Working Party. Available online: https://www.rcplondon.ac.uk/projects/outputs/national-early-warning-score-news (accessed on 18 January 2019).
36. Keep, J.W.; Messmer, A.S.; Sladden, R.; Burrell, N.; Pinate, R.; Tunnicliff, M.; Glucksman, E. National early warning score at Emergency Department triage may allow earlier identification of patients with severe sepsis and septic shock: A retrospective observational study. *Emerg. Med. J.* **2016**, *33*, 37–41. [CrossRef]
37. Vagias, W.M. *Likert-Type Scale Response Anchors*; Clemson International Institute for Tourism & Research Development, Department of Parks, Recreation and Tourism Management, Clemson University: Clemson, SC, USA, 2006.
38. Holey, E.A.; Feeley, J.L.; Dixon, J.; Whittaker, V.J. An exploration of the use of simple statistics to measure consensus and stability in Delphi studies. *BMC Med. Res. Methodol.* **2007**, *7*, 52. [CrossRef]

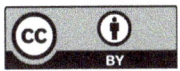

© 2019 by the authors. Licensee MDPI, Basel, Switzerland. This article is an open access article distributed under the terms and conditions of the Creative Commons Attribution (CC BY) license (http://creativecommons.org/licenses/by/4.0/).

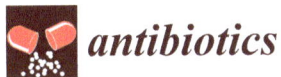

Review

Actinomycete-Derived Polyketides as a Source of Antibiotics and Lead Structures for the Development of New Antimicrobial Drugs

Helene L. Robertsen and Ewa M. Musiol-Kroll *

Interfakultäres Institut für Mikrobiologie und Infektionsmedizin, Eberhard Karls Universität Tübingen, Auf der Morgenstelle 28, 72076 Tübingen, Germany; helene.robertsen@biotech.uni-tuebingen.de
* Correspondence: ewa.musiol@biotech.uni-tuebingen.de

Received: 27 August 2019; Accepted: 10 September 2019; Published: 20 September 2019

Abstract: Actinomycetes are remarkable producers of compounds essential for human and veterinary medicine as well as for agriculture. The genomes of those microorganisms possess several sets of genes (biosynthetic gene cluster (BGC)) encoding pathways for the production of the valuable secondary metabolites. A significant proportion of the identified BGCs in actinomycetes encode pathways for the biosynthesis of polyketide compounds, nonribosomal peptides, or hybrid products resulting from the combination of both polyketide synthases (PKSs) and nonribosomal peptide synthetases (NRPSs). The potency of these molecules, in terms of bioactivity, was recognized in the 1940s, and started the "Golden Age" of antimicrobial drug discovery. Since then, several valuable polyketide drugs, such as erythromycin A, tylosin, monensin A, rifamycin, tetracyclines, amphotericin B, and many others were isolated from actinomycetes. This review covers the most relevant actinomycetes-derived polyketide drugs with antimicrobial activity, including anti-fungal agents. We provide an overview of the source of the compounds, structure of the molecules, the biosynthetic principle, bioactivity and mechanisms of action, and the current stage of development. This review emphasizes the importance of actinomycetes-derived antimicrobial polyketides and should serve as a "lexicon", not only to scientists from the Natural Products field, but also to clinicians and others interested in this topic.

Keywords: actinomycetes; bioactivity; antimicrobials; polyketides; polyketide synthases; biosynthesis

1. Introduction

More than 70 years has passed since the discovery of the first antibiotics from actinomycetes. Although some of the high G+C (bacteria with high guanine- (G) and cytosine- (C) content in their genomes) [1,2], Gram-positive bacteria of the order *Actinomycetales* and their products have been studied in depth, they remain one of the most important sources of secondary metabolites, including the naturally-derived antimicrobial drugs (e.g., β-lactams, tetracyclines, rifamycins, macrolides, aminoglycosides, and glycopeptides). In the past, the producers of valuable bioactive compounds were mainly isolated from soil samples and either directly or indirectly, using culture filtrates or extracts, subjected to susceptibility testing (diffusion method) (Figure 1). Recent advances in different disciplines of science, such as robotics [3], biology [4], chemistry [5–7], genetics [8], and/or bioinformatics [9] has extended the spectrum of methodology applied to the isolation and identification of actinomycetes and the produced metabolites. In addition to technical innovations which, for example, enable sampling of unexplored and difficult to access environments, Next Generation Sequencing Technologies (NGST) and genome mining facilitate accurate and cost-effective sequencing of actinomycetes genomes and a fast identification of genes encoding the proteins of the secondary metabolite biosynthetic machineries (biosynthetic gene clusters, BGCs). In the past two decades, hundreds of actinomycetes genomes have been sequenced and many of them have been fully annotated. The analysis of the data has demonstrated that a significant portion of the BGCs are associated with polyketide synthase (PKS) and nonribosomal peptide synthetase (NRPS) pathways, indicating that polyketides, nonribosomal peptides, and their hybrid compounds are the major secondary metabolites of actinomycetes [10,11]. The biosynthesis of both, polyketides and nonribosomal peptides, involves multifunctional megaenzymes referred as PKSs and NRPSs, respectively (Section 2). Despite the fact that polyketides are assembled according to a similar biosynthetic principle, a wide variety of chemical structures are found in the producer strains. This structural diversity is mainly accomplished through the different architecture and specificity of the PKSs, variation of the building blocks for the polyketide chain biosynthesis, and post-PKS modification reaction. Consequently, it is expected that the chemical arsenal provided by polyketide pathways encompasses molecules targeting various cellular compartments or interacting with distinct sites of the same target. Indeed, polyketide drugs such as erythromycins and rifamycins have a different mode of action. The antimicrobial drug-target interactions and their effects are well described [12–14]. In general, the four major mode of actions (MOAs) include interference with cell wall synthesis (e.g., penicillins), interference with nucleic acid synthesis (e.g., rifamycins), inhibition of metabolic pathways (e.g., sulfonamides), and inhibition of protein synthesis (e.g., erythromycins) [15,16]. A fifth MOA has been identified for the polymyxins and colistin, which disrupts the bacterial cell membranes by increasing membrane permeability [17].

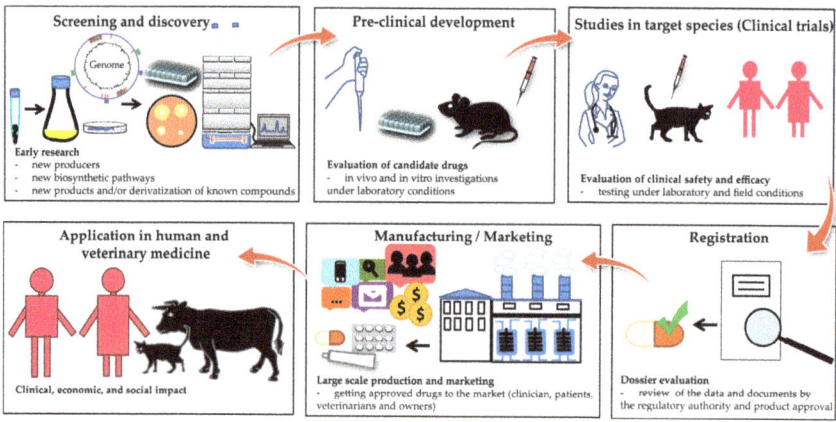

Figure 1. The process of drug development.

Based on the success of antimicrobial drugs during the "Golden Age" of antibiotic discovery (1940s–1960s) some experts were confident that "the tide had turned" in the war against pathogens causing severe infections. However, microbes develop the ability to resist the effects of an antibiotic whenever the dose of the drug is too low to eliminate the whole population of the pathogen (minimum bactericidal concentration (MBC)) and thus, antibiotic resistance developed shortly after the drugs were applied [18–24]. Resistance to antibiotics arises from chromosomal mutations or acquisition of genetic elements encoding resistance genes (horizontal gene transfer). Several resistance mechanisms have been reported [25–27]. The most frequent resistance mechanisms are exported through the efflux pumps, degradation or inactivation of an antibiotic, and modification or alteration of the cellular target of the antibiotic [15,28]. Furthermore, the overuse and misuse of antimicrobial drugs have promoted and accelerated the spreading of antibiotic resistance (e.g., methicillin-resistant *Staphylococcus aureus* (MRSA) and vancomycin-resistant *enterococci* (VRE)). New resistance mechanisms are constantly being reported, and transmission elements are identified on a regular basis [29]. According to the World Health Organisation (WHO), antimicrobial resistance is widely regarded as one of the greatest global challenges to humanity (estimated 10 million lives a year by 2050) [30]. Thus, guidelines and initiatives are being put forward in order to limit the further spread of antimicrobial resistance [31]. Some of these initiatives include the development of vaccines, faster diagnostic tests to ensure appropriate antibiotic administration, and immune-based therapies [32]. These measures could provide promising solutions for prevention of infections however, once infection occurs in a human host, antibiotics remain the choice of treatment for bacterial and fungal infections. Therefore, the need for new antibiotic classes and improvement of the old compounds remain more important than ever. Unfortunately, discovery of novel antibiotic classes is halted by the low return on investment, forcing companies to abandon their discovery platforms. According to an issue brief of The Pew Charitable Trusts from March 2019 [33], out of the roughly 38 companies currently invested in antibiotic clinical development, only four of these are multinational pharmaceutical companies. Furthermore, 90% of the current products in development are studied by small pharmaceutical or biotech companies, which are ill-equipped to deal with the expense of possible setbacks, delays or even rejections, which are often faced in clinical trials [34].

Since polyketide-derived antimicrobials have had a historical significance in human therapy, this group of compounds remain important for continuation of research aiming at: the identification of new structures and activities, the biosynthesis and/or chemical semi-synthesis for discovery of novel derivatisation routes, and finally, at understanding of resistance mechanisms to overcome this obstacle.

In this review, we focus on the therapeutically relevant polyketide drugs which were derived from actinomycetes. We describe compounds active against microbial pathogens, including pathogenic fungi and bacteria, their biosynthesis in the natural producer, and the most recent results on production optimization and derivatisation attempts. This review should serve as a "lexicon" of actinomycetes-derived antimicrobial polyketides, not only to scientists from the Natural Products field, but also to clinicians and others interested in this topic.

2. The Biosynthetic Assembly Lines

The biosynthesis of polyketides and nonribosomal peptides requires the PKS and NRPS enzymatic machineries. PKSs are grouped into type I, II, and III, and can be iterative (type I, II, III) or modular (type I) [35–39]. The diverse polyketide assembly lines have been previously reviewed [7,40–43]. Here, we introduce types of PKSs that are represented in this review.

The modular type I PKSs can give rise to large, complex polyketides. A "minimal PKS module" is composed of three essential domains; the acyltransferase (AT), the ketosynthase (KS), and the acyl carrier protein (ACP). The AT domain selects and loads the building blocks onto the activated ACPs, while the KS domain catalyses the decarboxylative Claisen-like condensation of the newly loaded unit and the already existing polyketide chain. The β-keto-processing of the generated chain is accomplished by optional domains, such as the ketoreductase (KRs), the dehydratases (DHs) and/or the enoyl reductases (ERs). The final chain termination and release of the polyketide intermediate from the PKS is facilitated by the thioesterase (TE) domain, often found as the "last domain" in the multimodular PKS.

Type II iterative PKSs are responsible for the biosynthesis of aromatic polyketides [44–46]. The overall architecture of this type of PKSs appears simpler than the one of complex modular PKSs, as they only require the presence of three enzymes, the KS_α, KS_β (also referred to as chain elongation factor (CLF)), and an ACP. During elongation, a thioester is bound to the ACP while the $KS_\alpha KS_\beta$ complex orchestrates chain extension with malonyl-CoA units exclusively. The BGCs of type II PKSs often contain additional genes encoding cyclases (CYCs) and KRs, which act as chaperones and reductive enzymes to ensure the correct cyclisation of the polyketide precursor, respectively. Finally, the presence of aromatases (AROs) leads to the biosynthesis of aromatic ring systems. The iterative type I PKS [47,48] work in a similar fashion as the iterative type II PKSs [44]. However, the bacterial iterative type I PKSs only facilitate the biosynthesis of small aromatic polyketides [35,49].

NRPSs display a similar architecture to modular type I PKSs and function in an analogous manner [39,50]. The selection and loading of the building blocks (proteinogenic or non-proteinogenic amino acids) onto peptidyl carrier proteins (PCPs) of NRPSs is catalysed by an adenylation (A) domain, resulting in an amino acid–PCP–thioester. A condensation (C) domain attaches the amino acid to the so-far synthesised peptide (chain elongation). Modifications, such as epimerisation or N-methylation at the peptide chain may occur due to the activity of the optional epimerisation (E) and methyltransferase (MT) domain, respectively. The peptide chain is released from the NRPS by a TE domain. In the case of hybrid PKS/NRPS structures [51], the transfer of the growing precursor chain between the different megaenzymes might require additional enzymes. However, this remains speculative and requires deeper investigation.

3. Clinically-Relevant Polyketide Derived Antibiotics

3.1. Erythromycin and Derivatives

The history of the macrolide erythromycin began in 1949 with a soil sample, collected in Iloilo City, (Iloilo, Philippine Islands) by Dr. Abelardo Aguilar, who sent the sample to Lilly Research Laboratories, where the soil-dwelling bacterium *Saccharopolyspora erythraea* (formerly known as *Streptomyces erythreus*) and the antibiotic erythromycin were isolated [52]. Inspired by the name of the place from which the soil sample was collected, erythromycin was launched by Eli Lilly Co. in 1952 as Ilosone (also Ilotycin) (Table 1) for treatment of respiratory tract infections, skin infections, and Legionnaire's disease.

The antibiotic erythromycin is composed of a 14-membered lactone, erythronolide B, to which two deoxysugars L-mycarose and α-D-desosamine are attached [53,54] (Figure 2). The BGC of erythromycin remains one of the most-studied in terms of the type I PKS [55–58]. The precursor erythronolide B is generated by the modular type I deoxyerythronolide B synthase (DEBS), composed of the three enzymes DEBS 1–3, encoded by the genes *eryAI–eryAIII* (Figure S1). The PKS complex contains six modules, which are responsible for the initial loading of propionyl-CoA, the six steps of chain elongation with methylmalonyl-CoA as extender units, modification of the growing polyketide chain by reductive domains, and finally chain release and cyclization by the TE domain in DEBS 3 [57,59,60]. The hydroxylation of the released aglycone is catalysed by the cytochrome P450 enzyme EryF, resulting in the intermediate erythronolide B. The glycosyltransferases EryBV and EryCII/EryCIII attach the sugar structures, derived from thymidine diphosphate (TDP)-L-mycarose and TDP-D-desosamine, which leads to the production of erythromycin D. Erythromycin D is further converted to erythromycin B or C, which are the substrates for erythromycin A. Erythromycin B is formed whenever the methyltransferase EryG is acting on erythromycin D. In the case where the molecule erythromycin D is modified by the monooxygenase EryK, erythromycin C is produced as an intermediate.

Although the strain produces a mixture of erythromycins, erythromycin A was the most abundant and biologically active compound [61]. Erythromycin shows activity against many Gram-positive and some Gram-negative bacteria, including *Haemophilus influenzae*, *S. aureus*, *Streptococcus pyogenes*, *Streptococcus pneumoniae*, *Legionella pneumophila*, *Neisseria gonorrhoeae*, and *Mycoplasma pneumonia* [61,62]. The antibiotic interacts with the large 50S subunit of the prokaryotic ribosomes and inhibits the protein biosynthesis [63,64]. More specifically, the antibiotic binds to the exit tunnel and blocks its large subunit whereby the elongation of the nascent peptide chain is stalled. This stalling leads to the premature dissociation of the peptidyl-transfer RNA (tRNA) from the ribosome [64,65]. As the inhibition occurs directly after initiation of protein synthesis, the nascent polypeptide chain remains short, however, the length size is determined by binding of the macrolide structure to the complex. Consequently, the size and conformation of erythromycin play a crucial role in the bioactivity of the molecule [66]. In case of erythromycin A, binding to the 50S subunit leads to dissociation and accumulation of peptidyl-tRNAs with six, seven, or eight amino acid residues. This accumulation causes depletion of the free tRNA pool, whereby protein biosynthesis is inhibited [65].

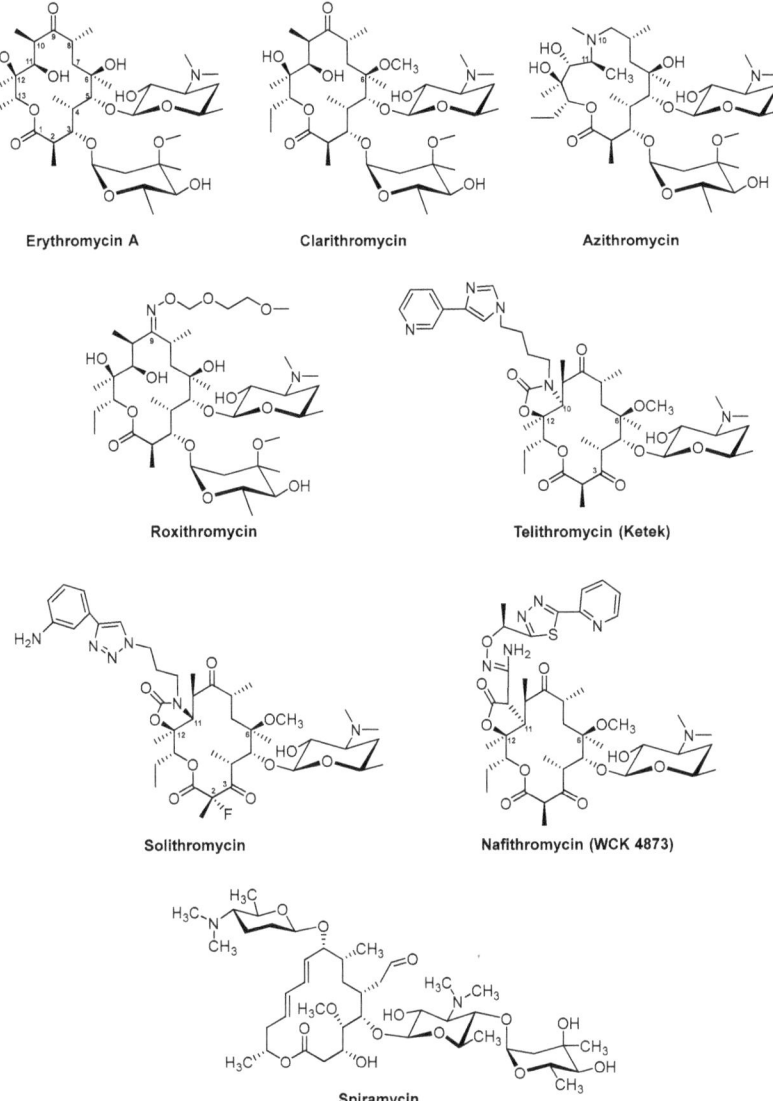

Figure 2. Structures of the two natural substances erythromycin A and spiramycin, and the semi-synthetic derivatives of erythromycin, including clarithromycin, azithromycin, roxithromycin, telithromycin (Ketek), solithromycin, and nafithromycin.

Table 1. Examples of actinomycetes-derived antimicrobial polyketide drugs.

Compound Class	Natural Product (NP) or Synthetic (S)	Compound Name	Trade Names	Original Producer Strain/Origin	Target/MOA	Most Relevant References
Erythromycin and related compounds	NP	Erythromycin A	Ilosone	*Saccharopolyspora erythraea*	Prokaryotic 50S ribosomal subunit	[52,55,58,61]
		Oleandomycin	Sigmamycin (with tetracycline)	*Streptomyces antibioticus*		[67–69]
		Spiramycin	Rovamycine	*Streptomyces ambofaciens*		[70–72]
	S	Clarithromycin	Biaxin	Erythromycin A derivative		[62,73–75]
		Roxithromycin	—			[76,77]
		Azithromycin	Zithromax	Erythromycin A (azalide)		[62,78,79]
		Telithromycin	Ketek	Erythromycin A (ketolide)		[80–82]
		Solithromycin	Solithera, CEM-101, T-4288			[83,84]
		Nafithromycin	WCK 4873			[83–85]
Tylosin and derivatives	NP	Tylosin A	Tylocine, Tylan	*Streptomyces fradiae*	Prokaryotic 50S ribosomal subunit	[86–89]
	S	Tilmicosin	Pulmotil, Micotil, Tilmovet	Tylosin A		[90,91]
		Tildipirosin	Zuprevo			[92,93]
		Tulathromycin	Draxxin			[94]
		Gamithromycin	Zactran			[95,96]
Monensin A	NP	Monensin A	Coban, Rumensin, Monensin	*Streptomyces cinnamonensis*	Ionophore (transport of Na$^+$ ions)	[97–100]
Tiacumicin B	NP	Tiacumicin B	Dificid	*Dactylosporangium aurantiacum* subsp. *hamdenensis*	RNA polymerase σ factor	[101–104]

Table 1. Cont.

Compound Class	Natural Product (NP) or Synthetic (S)	Compound Name	Trade Names	Original Producer Strain/Origin	Target/MOA	Most Relevant References
Rifamycin and derivatives	NP	Rifamycin SV	Aemcolo, Relafalk	Amycolatopsis mediterranei	Bacterial DNA–dependent RNA synthesis	[105–109]
	S	Rifampicin	Rifadin, Rimactane	Rifamycin SV		[106,110,111]
	S	Rifabutin	Mycobutin	Rifamycin SV		[112–114]
	S	Rifapentine	Priftin	Rifamycin SV		[115]
	S	Rifamixin	Normix, Rifacol, Xifacan	Rifamycin SV		[116–118]
	NP	Kanglemycin A	–	Nocardia mediterranei var. kanglensis		[119,120]
Tetracyclines	NP	Oxytetracycline	Terracycline	Streptomyces rimosus	Prokaryotic 30S ribosomal subunit	[121–124]
	NP	Chlortetracycline	Aureomycin	Streptomyces aureofaciens		[123,125,126]
		Doxycycline	Vibramycin	Chlortetracycline		[123,127,128]
		Minocycline	Minocin	Oxytetracycline		[129–131]
	S	Tigecycline	Tygacil	Minocycline		[132–135]
	S	Omadacycline	Nuzyra	Minocycline		[133,136–138]
		Eravacycline	Xerava	Fully synthetic		[139–141]
		Sarecycline	Seysara	Tetracycline		[127,133,142]
		TP-271	TP-271	Fully synthetic		[143–145]
Pristinamycins and derivatives	NP	Pristinamycin I$_A$/II$_A$ (PI$_A$ and PII$_A$)	Pyostacine	Streptomyces pristinaespiralis	Prokaryotic 50S ribosomal subunit	[146–149]
	S	Quinupristin (30%)/Dalfopristin (70%)	Synercid	PI$_A$ and PII$_A$ derivatives		[150–153]
	S	Linopristin (30%)/Flopristin (70%)	NXL-103	PI$_A$ and PII$_A$ derivatives		[154,155]
Nystatin and derivative	NP	Nystatin A1	Mycostatin, Nystop	Streptomyces noursei	Lipid receptor (ergosterol)	[156–159]
	NP	BSG005	–	Streptomyces noursei GG5073SP		[160,161]
Amphotericin	NP	Amphotericin B	Fungizone, Amphocin	Streptomyces nodosus		[162–165]
Pimaricin/Natamycin	NP	Natamycin	Natacyn, E235	Streptomyces natalensis		[166–169]

In order to improve the chemical, microbiological, and pharmacokinetic properties of macrolides, a lot of effort was put into the production of semi-synthetic and synthetic derivatives [63,170,171]. Some of the most successful semi-synthetic derivatives produced from erythromycin include the 14-membered clarithromycin and roxithromycin and the nitrogen-containing 15-membered azithromycin (Figure 2) [73,74]. Clarithromycin (trade name: Biaxin, Table 1) and roxithromycin (not commercially available, Table 1) were discovered in the 1980s in screening programs aiming at identification of erythromycin A variants with improved acidic stability and oral availability [74,75,172]. The pharmacokinetic profiles of erythromycin A and clarithromycin (6-O-methylerythromycin A derivative, Taisho Pharmaceutical Co.) are similar however, due to the methylation in clarithromycin, the antibiotic displays an increased and more stable absorption [62]. At a Croatian pharmaceutical company PLIVA, chemists succeeded in producing a range of novel erythromycin derivatives based on chemical modification of an erythromycin A oxime. One of the analogues was roxithromycin which contains a N-oxime side chain on the macrolactone ring [76,77,172]. However, since the general pharmacokinetic properties of roxithromycin are similar to those of erythromycin A, the search for more active and stable derivatives continued and ultimately, azithromycin (trade name: Zithromax, Table 1), which was the first azalide, was discovered [172,173]. Azithromycin (also CP 62,993 or XZ-450) differed from the other erythromycin derivatives due to its nitrogen-containing macrolactone ring [78,172,173]. In addition to its high stability and sustained tissue concentrations, azithromycin also had an extended activity spectrum, covering both Gram-positive and Gram-negative bacteria associated with respiratory tract infections [62,78,79,172]. Interestingly, azithromycin was the first derivative identified with a MOA different to that of erythromycin. Similar to other macrolides, azithromycin binds to the 50S ribosomal subunit. However, instead of one molecule, as it is the case for example for erythromycin, two molecules of azithromycin bind simultaneously to the 50S ribosomal subunit [174].

Another class of interesting semi-synthetic erythromycin A derivatives are the ketolides, which were developed as a part of a rational drug design approach [80,81,175]. Telithromycin (also HMR 3647) (Figure 2, Table 1), with the trade name Ketek, was the first ketolide introduced into clinical practice. The main difference between ketolides and other semi-synthetic erythromycin A derivatives is the exchange of the mycarose sugar moiety with a 3-keto group. Furthermore, telithromycin contains a large aromatic N-substituted carbamate side chain to which an imidazo-pyridyl group is attached at position C11/C12 of the aglycone structure [175]. Telithromycin was not only more stable than some of the other semi-synthetic erythromycin A derivatives under acidic conditions, the ketolide also retained activity against erythromycin resistance isolates of *S. aureus* and *S. pneumonia* [80]. It was suggested that the exchange of the sugar with a 3-keto group is the reason for the lack of macrolide–lincosamide–streptogramin B (MLS$_B$) resistance against ketolides [176]. Furthermore, telithromycin binds to prokaryote ribosomes with ten-times higher affinity than erythromycin A [177]. Unfortunately, shortly after its introduction into the clinics, severe side effects were reported ("Ketek effects"). These included visual disturbance and hepatic failure [82]. As the reports of fatal liver failures in patients receiving Ketek increased, the US Food and Drug Administration (FDA) withdrew the approval of the drug for simple infections in 2007 [73].

Since many pharmaceutical companies were in possession of large macrolide and ketolide libraries, screening for novel macrolide drug candidates continued. Two novel ketolides, solithromycin (trade names: CEM-101 and T-4288) and nafithromycin (trade name: WCK 4873) were identified and used for treatment of community-acquired bacterial pneumonia (CABP) (Figure 2, Table 1) [73,83,84]. Solithromycin is metabolically stable and shows potency against CABP-associated bacteria and the Gram-negative pathogen *N. gonorrhoeae*, which is the causative agent of gonorrhea. However, the future of solithromycin is currently less certain. Despite promising phase III study results, the US FDA rejected the approval of the drug for treatment of CABP in 2016, stating their concerns for the lack of sufficient safety studies addressing the risk of hepatotoxicity [34].

At present, nafithromycin is the only ketolide in global clinical development [85]. The compound has been enrolled in a phase II clinical study for treatment of CABP. The structure of nafithromycin

(Figure 2) differs from other ketolides. Instead of a carbamate at position C11/C12, nafithromycin contains a lactone group. In addition, the backbone of the side chain is differentiated by amino group and methyl group substituents. Finally, the side chain is attached at another position of the pyridine [73].

Erythromycin remains one of the best-studied 14-membered macrolides however, other naturally occurring macrolide antibiotics have been reported. These include oleandomycin (*Streptomyces antibioticus*, 1954), megalomicin (*Micromonospora megalomicea*, 1968), and pikromycin (*Streptomyces venezuelae*, 1951) [67,178,179], of which only oleandomycin made it into the clinics. Oleandomycin displays lower in vitro activity against *S. aureus* and *Streptococcus* spp. than erythromycin A [180]. However, scientists working at Charles Pfizer and Company claimed that the derivative sigmamycin (Table 1), a 2:1 mixture of tetracycline and oleandomycin, showed synergic effect on 22 *S. aureus* isolates, which were otherwise resistant to the two individual antibiotics [68]. Since other groups failed to reproduce the original findings, sigmamycin was removed from the market in the early 1970s [69].

Another naturally occurring macrolide is the 16-membered spiramycin (trade name: Rovamycin) (Figure 2, Table 1), which was discovered in 1954 from culture of *Streptomyces ambofaciens*, [70,71,181]. This was just two years after the discovery of erythromycin and due to a number of studies reporting better in vitro antimicrobial activity of erythromycin A compared to spiramycin, the latter never made it to clinical development in the US [72]. Although spiramycin is not commercially available in the US, pregnant women, suspecting an infection with the protozoan parasite *Toxoplasma gondii*, can request spiramycin for free from the US FDA after a consultation. The details are described in other comprehensive reviews [182,183].

Macrolide antibiotics such as erythromycin and its derivatives remain some of the most successful antibiotics in human therapy [73]. In addition to their application in treatment of common respiratory, genital, and skin infections, the overall properties of erythromycin and its derivatives still favour their use. These properties include, but are not limited to, good oral availability, narrow spectrum of activity, and a strong safety profile [73]. Furthermore, this compound class represents a safe and efficient alternative to patients suffering from allergies to penicillins [184].

3.2. Tylosin

The antibiotic tylosin (Figure 3, Table 1) was discovered in a preliminary screening by Denny and Bohrer in 1959 (Washington Research Laboratory, Washington, DC, USA) and later produced by Eli Lilly and Company in Indianapolis, Indiana (trade names: Tylocine, Tylan, tylosin tartrate) [86,185–188]. Tylosin was obtained from a fermentation culture of *Streptomyces fradiae* which was originally isolated from a soil sample collected in Thailand [86,189]. The compound is also produced by other streptomycetes strains such as *Streptomyces rimosus* [190] and *Streptomyces hygroscopicus* [191], however, *S. fradiae* remains the preferred choice for industrial fermentation of tylosin.

The naturally-derived tylosin is a mixture of the four 16-membered macrolide antibiotics tylosin A, B, C, and D [86,188,192–195]. Although tylosin A is found in highest concentration in the mixture (80–90%), tylosin B (desmycosin), tylosin C (macrocin), and tylosin D (relomycin) are also believed to contribute to the overall bioactivity of tylosin [195]. The structure of tylosin A (Figure 3) is a 16-atom polyketide lactone with the three deoxyhexose sugars D-mycaminose, mycinose (6-deoxy-D-allose), and L-mycarose attached [87].

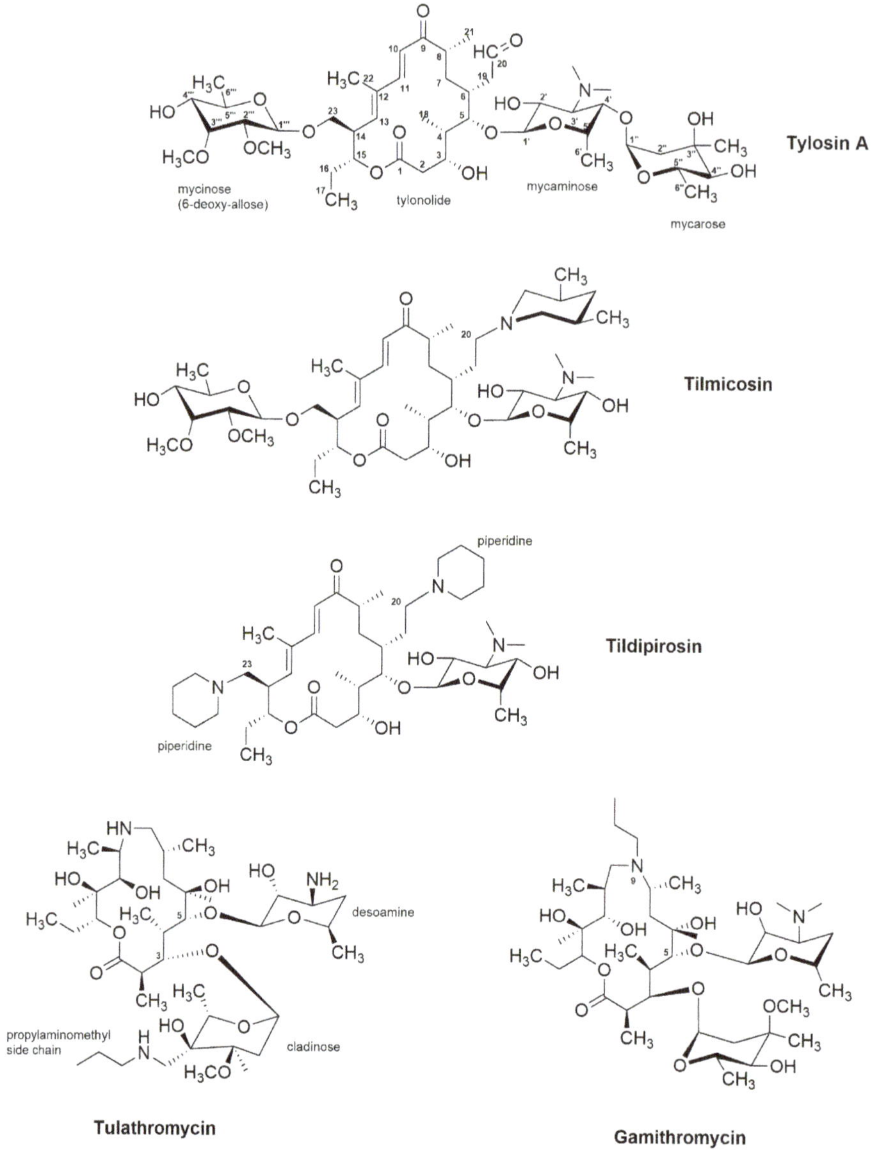

Figure 3. Structures of tylosin A and the four semi-synthetic derivatives tilmicosin, tildipirosin, tulathromycin, and gamithromycin.

The biosynthetic pathway of tylosin has been studied in detail [87,196–200]. With a size of ~85 kb, the tylosin (*tyl*) gene cluster occupies 1% of the entire genome of *S. fradiae*. Sequencing of the *tyl* gene cluster has revealed 13 genetic loci, *tylA* through *tylM*. These genes encode the PKS megaenzyme complex (TylGI–TylGV) for the assembly and cyclization of the precursor tylactone (Figure S2), proteins responsible for the biosynthesis of mycaminose, mycarose, and mycinose, hydroxylases, a methyltransferase, a reductase, and finally proteins involved in resistance and regulation. The biosynthesis of the tylosin polyketide chain is initiated by the loading of methylmalonyl-CoA to the first module in TylGI. The polyketide chain is extended by the attachment of four methylmalonyl-CoA, two malonyl-CoA, and one ethylmalonyl-CoA [88,201–204]. The TE-catalysed release of the aglycone and cyclisation of the structure yields the 16-atom tylactone, which is further modified at C20 and C23 by the two cytochrome P450 hydroxylases TylI and TylHI, respectively. The resulting intermediate tylonolide is then glycosylated through the attachment of the deoxyhexose sugars D-mycaminose, mycinose, and L-mycarose by TylMII, TylN, and TylCV, respectively [87,199,200,205] (Figure S2). Finally, to yield tylosin A, TylE and TylF modify the mycinose through the O-methylation of the C2''' and C3''' positions in the sugar. The remaining genes found in the *tyl* gene clusters encode ancillary proteins (crotonyl-CoA carboxylase/reductase (CCR), MetK, and, MetF), regulators (TylP, TylS, TylQ, TylU, TylR (TylT)), and proteins involved in resistance (TlrB–TlrD) [87].

Similar to other macrolides, tylosin inhibits protein biosynthesis in prokaryotes by binding to the large 50S subunit [88,89,185]. Poulsen et al. have shown that the disaccharide D-mycaminosyl-L-mycarose at the C5-atom in tylosin affects the binding of the molecule to the ribosome complex [206]. As opposed to erythromycin A (Figure 2), in which tri- and tetrapeptides are still released from the ribosome upon binding of the macrolide, for tylosin the C5-disaccharide extends binding of the macrolide to the ribosome, only allowing formation of dipeptides [206,207].

The antibiotic tylosin is approved exclusively for veterinary use. It is applied to treat leptospirosis, mycoplasmosis, and respiratory tract infection, caused by Gram-positive bacteria, including *Streptococcus* spp., *Staphylococcus* spp., *Clostridium perfringens*, and *Mycoplasma* spp. [208]. Historically, tylosin has been used as feed additive for cattle to prevent the development of liver abscesses and for swine as a growth promoter.

Tylosin remains a valuable antibiotic for use in veterinary medicine. However, derivatives of the native compound have been introduced in clinical practice as well. One such molecule is the semi-synthetic derivative tilmicosin, which has an extended antimicrobial spectrum compared to tylosin [90,91]. Tilmicosin displayed activity against *Pasteurella multocida* and *Pasteurella haemolytica*, and is important for treatment of bacterial pneumonia in young cattle. In addition, tilmicosin has shown improved activity against *P. multocida* in chickens. Tilmicosin is available under different trade names (Table 1), including Pulmotil and Micotil (Elanco Animal Health (https://www.elanco.com/), previously owned by Eli Lilly Company) and as Tilmovet (Huvepharma (https://www.huvepharma.com/)). Other semi-synthetic tylosin derivatives, which have been approved for treatment of respiratory diseases in animal production, include the 16-membered macrolide tildipirosin (trade name: Zuprevo) and the two 15-membered macrolides, tulathromycin (trade name: Draxxin), as well as gamithromycin (trade name: Zactran) (Figure 3, Table 1) [92–95].

In most cases, the 16-membered macrolides have less in vivo efficacy than the 14- and 15-membered macrolides. This is due to the fact that the side chains are metabolised and the generated products have a decreased activity compared to 14- and 15-membered macrolides.

3.3. Monensins

The polyether ionophore monensin A (Figure 4, Table 1) (trade names: Coban, Rumensin, and Monensin) is another example of antibiotics being particularly important for veterinary medicine. The compound was identified in fermentation cultures of *Streptomyces cinnamonensis* and reported for the first time in 1967 as monensic acid by the Lilly Research Laboratories and the Department of Biochemistry of Indiana University School of Medicine [96,209]. In the natural producer, a mixture of monensin-like agents (monensin A, B and C) is synthesised, however, monensin A is the main constituent of this product (Figure 4). Monensin A is composed of five rings to which seven methyl, one ethyl, one carboxyl, and one hydroxyl group are attached [96]. Monensin B and C vary from monensin A by their side groups. In monensin B, the ethyl group on C16 is replaced by a methyl group, whereas in monensin C the methyl group at C2 is replaced by an ethyl group [210–212]. The carboxyl and hydroxyl groups can interact through hydrogen bonds, whereby a pseudocyclic conformation of monensin is formed (Figure 4). This results in an oxygen-containing center, which is selective for cations. Due to these conformational changes of monensin, an exterior composed of alkyl groups, which render the molecule hydrophobic and capable of passing the lipid bilayer of cell membranes, is built. The ionophore monensin A is able to bind monovalent metal cations such as Li^+, Na^+, K^+, Rb^+, Cs^+, and Ag^+. However, the compound prefers sodium cations for the formation of the ion–ionophore complex, which facilitates cation transport across cell membranes. This disturbs the natural Na^+/K^+ concentration gradient in Gram-positive bacteria causing death of the cell [97,210,213–216].

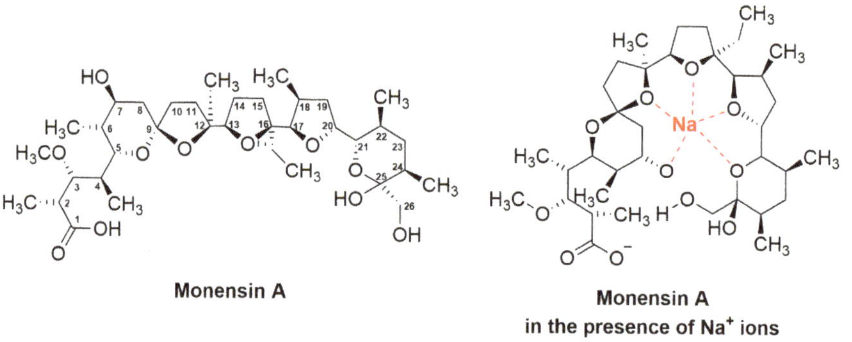

Figure 4. The structures of monensin A and monensin A in complex with sodium (Na^+) ion.

The genome sequencing of the producer and understanding the biosynthetic pathway of monensin have been crucial for optimizing the production of monensin in *S. cinnamonensis*. Sequence analysis of the 97 kb BGC of monensin (*mon*) has revealed a modular type I PKS, encoded by the genes *monAI–monAVIII* [98,217] (Figure S3). The first step in the assembly of the polyketide backbone is the loading of the "initiation module" of MonAI with malonate, which is derived from a malonyl-CoA starter unit. Twelve "downstream" extension modules in the PKS complex MonAI–AVIII catalyse the loading and condensation of additional four acetate, one butyrate, and seven propionate molecules, leading to the biosynthesis of the monensin polyketide chain. Since no TE domain is present in MonAVII, the release of the monensin intermediate must be facilitated by TEs acting in *trans*. Originally, it was assumed that either MonAIX and/or MonAX, which show homology to TEs involved in rifamycin, tylosin, and erythromycin biosynthesis [98], catalyse this reaction. Later, the enzyme MonCII, previously assigned as an epoxide hydrolase, was proposed as a putative novel TE, which might be responsible for the release of the monensin polyketide chain from the PKS assembly line [218]. The additional genes found in the *mon* gene cluster encode enzymes involved in isomerisation, epoxidation (MonCI), hydroxylation (MonBI, MonBII, and MonD), and methylation (MonE) of the structure to the final product monensin A [98,219]. Finally, the *mon* gene cluster includes three regulator genes, *monH*, *monRI*, and *monRII*, and the gene *monT*, which encodes an efflux protein, believed to confer self-resistance to the host [98,217,220,221].

Monensin A is used as a coccidiostat (inhibitor of coccidiosis) in poultry and as a non-hormonal growth promoter for cattle in the beef and dairy industry [97,210]. In addition, it was suggested that monensin A might also improve food metabolism in ruminants. Therefore, the feed additive Rumensin, which contains 6.6% monensin, was introduced for cattle to improve the composition of the intestinal bovine microbiota, reducing lactic acid formation, and ultimately leading to faster growth of cattle [99].

In 1971, monensin A was the first ionophore to be approved as a veterinary medicine. Two additional ionophore antibiotics lasalocid and salinomycin have subsequently been approved. Lasalocid, originally identified from fermentation broth of *Streptomyces lasaliensis*, was introduced in 1977 as a coccidiostat for poultry (trade name: Avatec) and later in 1982 as growth promoter for cattle (trade name: Bovatec). Salinomycin (trade name: Bio-Cox), produced by *Streptomyces albus*, received its approval as a coccidiostat for chickens in 1983 [210,222–224].

Given the nature of their applications, ionophore antibiotics have been subjected to increased concerns with regards to the association between their misuse as feed additives and development of resistance. However, studies on ionophore resistance in ruminal bacteria indicate that instead of resistance occurring as a result of mutations or horizontal gene transfer, it is more a matter of physiological selection [225]. Since ionophore antibiotics are restricted to only a few animal species and have never been used in human medicine, it appears that the risk of cross-resistance is rather low. Little is known about resistance development in bacteria subjected to ionophores. Based on in vitro and in vivo experiments several ionophore resistance mechanisms have been suggested. Those include the hypothesis of a proton-translocating enzyme which might counteract ionophore-dependent ion flux [226,227], the cell wall model of ionophore resistance [228–230], and the theory of extracellular polysaccharides (biofilm) [225], such as glycocalyx produced by ruminal bacteria. As no clear indications of resistance development and spreading have been reported, it is likely that the use of ionophore antibiotics as feed additives will continue [225].

3.4. Tiacumicin

In the 1980s, scientists working at Abbott Laboratories were screening soil samples for novel microbes with antimicrobial activities. In a soil sample from Hamden, Connecticut, USA, the novel Gram-positive bacterium *Dactylosporangium aurantiacum* subsp. *hamdenensis* subsp. Nov. AB718C-41 (NRRL 18085) was isolated based on its activity against MRSA. After scaling up the production, six novel compounds were isolated known collectively as the tiacumicins [100,231]. Structure elucidation of the tiacumicins further revealed a shared 18-membered macrolactone, which differed between the analogues based on the types of modification to the macrocyclic ring and the number and esterification pattern of the sugar groups attached. Out of the six compounds produced, tiacumicin B (Figure 5) was found in largest quantities [100].

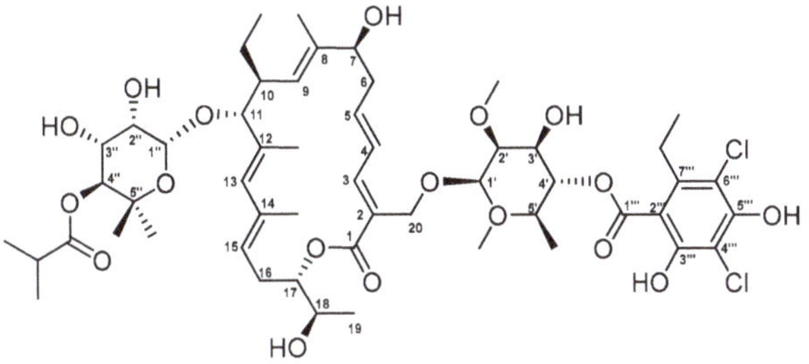

Tiacumicin B

Figure 5. Structure of tiacumicin B.

The tiacumicin (*tia*) biosynthetic gene cluster of the original producer strains *D. aurantiacum* subsp. *hamdenensis* NRRL 18,085 was elucidated by Xiao and co-workers in 2011 based on sequence analysis and gene knockout studies [101]. The data revealed the presence of 50 open reading frames (ORFs) spanning an 110,663 bp DNA region. Additional sequence analysis has shown that 31 of the originally identified 50 ORFs are directly involved in tiacumicin biosynthesis. The remaining 83 kb DNA region includes genes encoding enzymes responsible for polyketide backbone assembly, sugar biosynthesis, glycosylation, halogenation, methylation, hydroxylation, epoxidation, and resistance determinants. The four genes *tiaA1* through *tiaA4* encode the multimodular type I PKS responsible for the assembly of the central aglycone tiacumicinone (Figure S4) [101,232]. After loading of the starter unit propionate, additional three malonates, four methylmalonates, and one ethylmalonate are condensed to the polyketide chain. Several genes are encoded in the *tia* BGC, which could provide the precursors for the polyketide. The synthesis of isobutyryl-CoA, propionyl-CoA, and acyl-CoA might be catalysed by TiaC and TiaD. Furthermore, the propionyl-CoA carboxylase encoded by *tiaL* might catalyse the formation of methylmalonyl-CoA from propionyl-CoA, and the CCR encoded by *tiaK* could be responsible for provision of the ethylmalonyl-CoA subunit [233]. Upon reaching the TE domain in module eight of TiaA4, the polyketide chain is released and cyclised, yielding the tiacumicinone precursor (Figure S4). An additional TE TiaE, which shows homology to the type II TE NysE involved in nystatin biosynthesis, is found in the *tia* BGC. Since these type II TEs are believed to act as repair enzymes, removing aberrant PKS precursors, TiaE has been hypothesized to have a similar role in *tia* biosynthesis [101,234]. Tiacumicinone undergoes several modifications including C18 and C20 hydroxylations, which are catalysed by the two cytochrome P450 enzymes TiaP1 and TiaP2, respectively, and the attachment of the rhamnose sugars at position C11 and C20, catalysed by the two glycosyltransferases TiaG1 and TiaG2 (Figure S4). The sugars are further modified. First, to yield the final 4-*O*-isobutyryl-5-methyl-β-rhamnose at position C11, the sugar C-methyltransferase TiaS2 and O-acyltransferase TiaS6 incorporate the methyl and isobutyryl moieties, respectively. The sugar at C20 also undergoes several modifications. The synthesis of the homo-orsellinic moiety is believed to be catalysed by an iterative type I PKS TiaB based on a propionyl-CoA starter unit and three malonyl-CoA extender units [101]. The transfer of the aromatic moiety to the C20 sugar could then be facilitated by the acyltransferase encoded by *tiaF* (Figure S4). Further modifications to the sugar are achieved by the actions of TiaS5, responsible for the 2'-*O*-methyltransferase reaction leading to 2-*O*-methyl-β-rhamnose and, finally, the dihalogenase TiaM, which is responsible for attachment of two chlorine atoms to the homo-orsellinic acid. Within the *tia* cluster, genes encoding proteins putatively involved in regulation and resistance are also found. This includes the putative LuxR class regulator TiaR1 and the putative ArsR family transcriptional regulator TiaR2, of which only the function of TiaR2 has been experimentally verified [101]. Since the Δ*tiaR2* mutant strain produced slightly higher levels of tiacumicin than the wild type strain, the regulator might act as negative regulator in *tia* biosynthesis. TiaT1 through TiaT4 show homology to membrane proteins and ATP-binding cassette (ABC) transporter and therefore, have been hypothesized to be involved in export of tiacumicin. However, genetic and biochemical studies are necessary to clarify their role in the biosynthesis of tiacumicin [101].

Coincidentally, in the same year as the tiacumicins were discovered and reported, a Japanese group, led by Satoshi Omura, reported the discovery of the antibiotics clostomicins, produced by *Micromonospora echinospora* subsp. *armenica* subsp. Nov [235]. Structure comparisons not only revealed tiacumicin B and clostomicin B_1 to be identical, but also that a third antibiotic, lipiarmycin A3, discovered in 1975 from culture of *Actinoplanes deccanensis* A/10655, shared the same structure [231,236]. Ultimately, only tiacumicin B went through to further clinical studies. Although originally identified for its activity against MRSA, promising in vivo potency against *Clostridioides* (formerly *Clostridium*) *difficile* in animal models directed the development of tiacumicin B towards a narrow spectrum antibiotic for treatment of clostridia [233]. The antibiotic was approved by FDA in 2011 under the generic name fidaxomicin and trade name Dificid (Table 1) for treatment of *C. difficile* infections (CDI), which remains one of the main causes of hospital-acquired diarrhoea [233]. At the time, Dificid was regarded as an alternative to vancomycin, which was used to treat CDI. One of the major drawbacks of vancomycin is its broad-spectrum and bacteriostatic activity which promote reoccurrence of CDI. In contrast, fidaxomicin is a bactericidal, narrow-spectrum antibiotic and has been found to not only reduce recurrence of CDI but also promote survival of commensal gut microbes and prevent the development of colitis [102,237]. In addition, fidaxomicin is administered orally with no reports of resistance development in *C. difficile* isolates. In a recent US-based national survey, 1889 *C. difficile* isolates were collected from the stool of patients infected with the pathogen over the period of 2013 to 2016. The isolates were screened for susceptibility against fidaxomicin and showed that fidaxomicin MIC_{50} (maximum inhibitory concentration of an antibiotic, at which 50% of the isolates are inhibited) and MIC90 (maximum inhibitory concentration of an antibiotic, at which 90% of the isolates are inhibited) values toward *C. difficile* had not changed over the time period [238]. However, the fact that fidaxomicin was only recently introduced to the clinics stresses the need for continuous surveillance [238].

Recently, the MOA of tiacumicin B has been further clarified based on the cryogenic electron microscopy (cryo-EM) structure of *Mycobacterium tuberculosis* RNA polymerase (RNAP) holoenzyme in complex with lipiarmycin A3 [103]. Although the target of fidaxomicin was already known to be the bacterial RNAP [239], the recent findings could show the binding of the antibiotic to be specific for the RNAP clamp. Upon binding of fidaxomicin, the RNAP is trapped in an open-clamp conformation, which prevents the simultaneous engagement of the −10 and −35 elements needed for transcription initiation. Furthermore, since the binding sites of fidaxomicin do not overlap with those of other known RNAP inhibitors, including rifamycin and sorangicin, the risk of cross-resistance is lowered [103].

At the moment, fidaxomicin is the only substance approved for human therapy within the tiacumicin-like compounds. However, the advanced information on the structure activity relationship (SAR) of fidaxomicin might trigger a more rational structure-based design of drug analogues in the future [103].

The knowledge obtained from studies on the *tia* gene cluster aided the design of a dihalogenase-deficient Δ*tiaM* mutant strain, which produced 14 tiacumicin congeners of which 11 were novel derivatives [240]. Based on minimum inhibitory concentration (MIC) tests, tiacumicin congener 3 displayed higher potency against *Bacillus thuringiensis* (MIC = 0.5 µg/mL), *Micrococcus luteus* (MIC = 1 µg/mL), and *Enterococcus faecelis* (MIC = 4 µg/mL) compared to all other congeners and the parent compound tiacumicin B. Interestingly, in addition to its lack of chlorine atoms, congener 3 contained a propyl group on the aromatic ring. The four-fold antibacterial activity increase of congener 3 compared to tiacumicin B was putatively assigned to the structural change in the aromatic ring. In the future, this knowledge could provide the foundation for further gene manipulations, which would result in generation of novel tiacumicin derivatives with improved antibacterial activities [240]. Furthermore, these derivatives might also provide more cost-effective alternatives to fidaxomicin, the price of which remains a major point of criticism [241].

3.5. Rifamycin and Derivatives

Rifamycins (Figure 6) belong to the class of ansamycin antibiotics. This group of compounds is distinguished by a cyclic structure bridged at two nonadjacent positions by an aliphatic chain [104,105]. This basket or handle-like architecture gave rise to the naming ansamycins (Latin: ansa = handle). Ansamycins comprise a range of different substances. In the following, we cover rifamycin and its derivatives, which collectively belong to the group of naphtalenes-ansamycins.

The history of this class of compounds started in 1959 with the isolation of the naturally-derived rifamycins, a complex mixture of several congeners produced by *Streptomyces mediterranei* [106]. More detailed studies on morphology, cell wall composition, and phage susceptibility resulted in re-classification of the strain, first as *Nocardia mediterranei*, and later as *Amycolatopsis mediterranei* [105,242]. Structure elucidation has revealed common architectures of the complex of rifamycins, which include a 17-membered aliphatic chain and a C–O bond linking the benzene ring to the chain [243] (Figure 6). In the initial attempts to separate and isolate each of the congeners from the fermentation broth of *A. mediterranei*, only rifamycin B, which constitutes 5–10% of the mixture, could be purified [244]. Since the substance was the least active congeners in the mixture, further studies were necessary to identify the more potent substances. One of the breakthroughs came with the elucidation of four additional rifamycin intermediates, including rifamycin S, L, O, and SV [105,245,246].

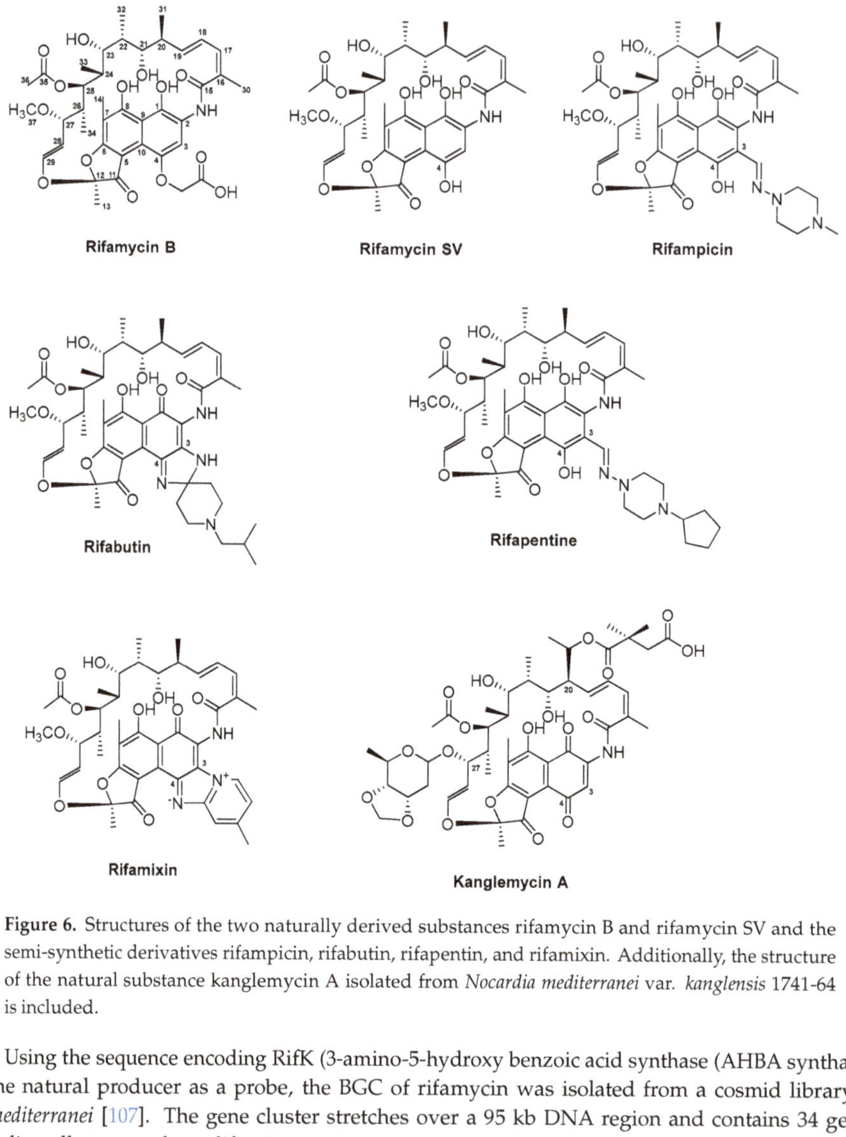

Figure 6. Structures of the two naturally derived substances rifamycin B and rifamycin SV and the semi-synthetic derivatives rifampicin, rifabutin, rifapentin, and rifamixin. Additionally, the structure of the natural substance kanglemycin A isolated from *Nocardia mediterranei* var. *kanglensis* 1741-64 is included.

Using the sequence encoding RifK (3-amino-5-hydroxy benzoic acid synthase (AHBA synthase)) in the natural producer as a probe, the BGC of rifamycin was isolated from a cosmid library of *A. mediterranei* [107]. The gene cluster stretches over a 95 kb DNA region and contains 34 genes encoding all structural, modification, resistance, export, and regulatory elements. The assembly of the polyketide chain is governed by the modular type I PKS, encoded by the five genes *rifA* through *rifE* (Figure S5). Since the loading module within RifA contains domains with homology to A and T domains of NRPSs, the rifamycin assembly line is a hybrid PKS/NRPS [247]. The starter and extender units involved in the formation of the polyketide has been identified [248]. This includes the atypical starter unit AHBA, of which biosynthesis is orchestrated by enzymes encoded by *rifG* through *rifN*. The shikimate-related pathway of aromatic biosynthesis leading to the formation of AHBA was elucidated based on gene inactivation and heterologous expression [248]. Upon loading of AHBA, the polyketide chain is further elongated by the ten extender modules, which facilitate the addition of eight acetate and two propionate extender units [107,108]. The rifamycin PKS does not encode a typical TE domain. Instead, downstream of *rifE*, the gene *rifF* which shares homology to an arylamine

N-acetyl-transferase is located. The role of RifF in chain release and macrolactam ring closure has been confirmed through an in-frame deletion, in which the ΔrifF mutant lost its ability to produce rifamycin B and instead accumulated shorter open-chain ketides [249]. An additional TE encoded by rifR has been identified in the rifamycin gene cluster [250]. However, since the ΔrifR and ΔrifF+ΔrifR mutants showed identical production profile, in which the same aberrant open-chain polyketides were detected, it was concluded that RifR is directly involved in the release of polyketide precursors from the assembly line. Furthermore, closer examinations of the PKS intermediates produced by the ΔrifF mutant revealed that while the tetraketide contained an unmodified aromatic chromophore, the pentaketide through the decaketide contained the bicyclic naphthoquinone moiety [251]. This indicated that naphthoquinone ring closure must occur while the polyketide chain is still attached to the PKS. This hypothesis was later confirmed based on the genetic studies of rif19, which encodes a 3-(3-hydroxyphenyl)propionate hydroxylase-like protein [252]. It was concluded that Rif19 catalyses the naphthoquinone ring closure, which occurs between module three in RifA and module four in RifB (Figure S5). Upon its release from the PKS, the polyketide precursor undergoes a series of post-modifications, including dehydrogenation at the C8 and hydroxylation of the C34, which results in the formation of one of the early intermediates in the post-modification pathway, namely rifamycin W [252,253]. The conversion of rifamycin W to rifamycin B involves the formation of the intermediate rifamycin SV (Figure S5) [105,252]. The final steps in the conversion of rifamycin SV to rifamycin B, through the intermediates rifamycin S, L, and O, have only recently been elucidated based on in vitro assays with the cytochrome P450 enzyme Rif16 and the two-subunit transketolase Rif15 (Figure S5) [254].

Additional genes encoding enzymes involved in regulation, export, and self-resistance have been identified in the rifamycin BGC. This includes the LuxR family regulator RifZ, which acts as an activator, and the TetR-family transcriptional regulator RifQ, which is a repressor of rifamycin biosynthesis in *A. mediterranei* [255–257]. The repressor RifQ is feedback-regulated by rifamycin B, the product of the rifamycin gene cluster in *A. mediterranei*. When a threshold concentration of rifamycin B is reached intracellularly, the substance interferes with the binding of RifQ to the promoter region of *rifP*, which encodes a membrane protein, whereby export of the antibiotic is initiated [258].

The importance of the rifamycins in human therapy is evident from their strong activities against a wide range of Gram-positive bacteria and to a lesser extent, some Gram-negatives. The reason for the higher MIC of Gram-negatives is most likely due to a reduced penetration of the rifamycins through the outer membranes of Gram-negatives [258]. The rifamycins remain the first-line treatment of tuberculosis (TB) caused by *M. tuberculosis* and for treatment of non-tuberculous mycobacterial infections [105,119,244]. Collectively, the rifamycins interact with the bacterial DNA-dependent RNAP whereby transcription is blocked.

As previously mentioned, rifamycin B itself displays modest bioactivity and therefore, the need for derivatisation of the scaffold is necessary to produce rifamycin analogues with improved activity and availability. In fact, from the naturally derived rifamycins, only rifamycin SV has been introduced in human therapy. With a strong bioactivity against Gram-positives, including *M. tuberculosis*, and moderate activity against some Gram-negatives [244], rifamycin SV was introduced into the clinic in 1963 as a topical and parental agent. Extensive semi-synthesis efforts on rifamycins delivered several clinically relevant compounds. Using information gained from SAR studies, the first series of rifamycin analogous were generated based on substitutions at the C3/C4 positions in the aromatic moiety of the intermediate 3-formyl rifamycin SV. One of the resulting substances, 3-(4-methyl-piperazinyl-iminomethyl) rifamycin SV, coined rifampicin (Figure 6), displayed strong bioactivity against Gram-positive bacteria, including *M. tuberculosis* and *Neisseria* species, and modest activity against Gram-negatives [105,110]. Just as importantly, rifampicin was fat-soluble and could be administered orally. Ultimately, rifampicin (trade names: Rifadin and Rimactane) (Table 1) was introduced for human therapy in 1968 in Italy and in 1971 in the US, and has since then been an important agent in treatment of TB, leprosy, and other mycobacterial infections [243]. Additionally, rifampicin has also been an important substance for determining the MOA of rifamycins. Based on the

3.3 Å crystal structure of the RNAP core of *Thermus aquaticus* complexed with rifampicin, Campbell and co-workers determined the binding of the antibiotic to the β subunit within the DNA/RNA channel. This binding resulted in the physical blockage of the channel for the elongating RNA, when the transcripts reach a size of two to three nucleotides in length [111]. Determining the MOA of rifampicin also aided in understanding the high frequency of resistance development in rifamycin sensitive microorganism. Since pathogens can develop resistance to rifampicin with a rate of 10^{-8} to 10^{-9} per cell division, the application of the antibiotic is restricted to combination therapy, in which the antimycobacterial agent isoniazid is often used together with rifampicin, or used only in severe cases of TB infection [105]. The high rate of resistance is most commonly associated with the acquisition of mutations in the *rpoB* gene, which encodes the β subunit in the RNAP, whereby the binding affinity of the enzyme to the antibiotic is lowered. The *rpoB* gene is highly conserved in prokaryotes, however, pathogens acquire different levels of mutations in their respective *rpoB* genes, and consequently the level of resistance also can vary amongst isolates. For clinical isolates of *M. tuberculosis*, the three amino acids S411, H406, and D396 (*T. aquaticus* numbering) are most often mutated. Mutations at these positions in the RNAP core influence the hydrogen bonds formed between the hydroxyl groups on C8 and C21 of rifampicin, which interact with S411 and with H406 and D396, respectively [105,111].

Additional rifamycin analogues obtained through the derivatisation efforts on rifamycin SV have made it through to the clinics (Figure 6). One of these analogues is the 3-(((4-cyclopentyl-1-piperazinyl) imino) methyl) rifamycin S, also known as rifapentine (trade name: Priftin) (Table 1). Rifapentine was discovered during the initial derivatisation efforts on the C3/C4 aromatic moiety in rifamycin SV. The analogue was approved for treatment of TB in 1998 and similar to rifampicin can be administered orally [115,259]. Unfortunately, isolates which are resistant to rifampicin display cross-resistance to rifapentine, which has limited the application of the antibiotic.

The two rifamycin analogues rifabutin (trade name: Mycobutin) and rifaximin (trade names: Normix, Rifacol, Xifaxan) were approved for human therapy in 1992 and 2004, respectively (Table 1) [243]. Rifamixin ((4-deoxy-4-methylpyrido [1),2)-1,2]imidazo-[5,4-c]rifamycin SV) is non-systemic and can reach high concentrations in the gastrointestinal (GI) tract, enabling its application for treatment of traveller's diarrhoea caused by enteropathogens, including *Escherichia coli* [116]. More recently, rifaximin has been further implicated in the treatment and prevention of various GI diseases, including inflammatory bowel diseases such as Crohn's disease and ulcerative colitis. Although the continuous administration of rifaximin has raised concerns for selection of resistance and undesirable disruption of the gut microbiota, several studies have shown that rifaximin may promote a healthy gut microbiota [117,260,261]. The beneficial effects of the antibiotic are lost quickly after the treatment with rifaximin was terminated which probably limits its application as a preventive agent for GI-associated diseases [118]. Only recently, an alternative antibiotic combination has been approved by the US FDA for the treatment of traveller's diarrhoea. The oral formulation developed at Cosmo Pharmaceuticals N.V. (Ireland) is based on the unique combination of rifamycin SV together with the MultiMatrix (MMX®) technology, which ensures colonic delivery of the antibiotic [109]. Based on in vitro studies, rifamycin SV MMX® (trade names: Aemcolo and Relafalk) (Table 1) was found to exhibit antibacterial activity against most enteropathogens associated with traveller's diarrhoea. Moreover, in later phase III clinical studies, the oral substance was well-tolerated in patients undergoing treatment and could shorten the duration of non-dysenteric traveller's diarrhoea [109].

The semi-synthetic derivative rifabutin (4-*N*-isobutylspiropiperidylrifamycin S) was approved for human therapy due to its inhibitory activity against a number of rifampicin-resistant *M. tuberculosis* clinical isolates in addition to its well-documented activity against *Mycobacterium avium* and *M. intracellulare* (also referred to as *Mycobacterium avium-intracellulare* complex (MAC)) [112,113]. MAC infection frequently occurs in patients with acquired immunodeficiency syndrome (AIDS) and when administered prophylactically as a 300 mg daily dose, rifabutin significantly reduces the incidence of MAC bacteraemia. However, due to the risk of cross-resistance between rifampicin and rifabutin in *M. tuberculosis* isolates, rifabutin is restricted to MAC patients and for newly diagnosed and multidrug-resistant TB in Europe [114].

During the derivatisation of rifamycins, modifications to the ansa bridge often led to compounds with lowered activities [262]. Recently, the natural ansamycin antibiotic kanglemycin A, which has an altered ansa chain, was found to maintain potency against rifampicin-resistant bacterial isolates, including multidrug-resistant *M. tuberculosis* (Figure 6). Kanglemycin A was originally isolated from *Nocardia mediterranei* var. *kanglensis* 1741-64 in 1988, however, the MOA of the compound was only recently elucidated. Based on the crystal structure of the RNAP-promoter complex of *Thermus thermophiles* with kanglemycin A, it became evident that the sugar (β-O-3,4-O,O'-methylene digitoxose) and acid (2,2-dimethyl succinic acid) moieties on the ansa bridge in the molecule increase the binding surface of the antibiotic with the RNAP. Furthermore, the additional interaction of the sugar group of kanglemycin A was hypothesized to limit the frequency of resistance development as this would require two simultaneous mutations in the binding pocket of the RNAP [119,120]. Although kanglemycin A (Table 1) itself has not been introduced to the clinics, its discovery might open up for future structural derivatisation efforts in which the ansa bridge might prove to be a valuable "target" for generating new synthetic ansamycin antibiotics with improved bioactivities.

3.6. Tetracyclines

The tetracycline group of antibiotics covers a variety of natural and semi-synthetic compounds. There are three naturally derived tetracyclines that have been described in detail and have formed the basis for 2nd and 3rd generation tetracycline derivatives. The three natural substances include chlortetracycline (trade names: Aureomycin, Table 1) discovered from the fermentation broth of *Streptomyces aureofaciens* in 1948 [125], oxytetracycline (trade name: Terracycline, Table 1) found in the broth of *Streptomyces rimosus* in 1950 [121], and finally tetracycline, which was discovered as a fermentation product of *Streptomyces viridofaciens* and the two aforementioned strains [263] (Figure 7). Based on the structural elucidation of the three compounds, which revealed a characteristic DCBA naphthacene tetra-cyclic core (Figure 7), the agents later became descriptively known as the tetracyclines [264]. Within the group of tetracyclines, tetracycline represents the simplest of the structures, whereas chlortetracycline and oxytetracycline contain modifications at the core cyclic structure. While chlortetracycline contains a chlorine atom at the C7 atom in ring D, oxytetracycline instead harbours a hydroxyl group at the C5 position in ring B.

The biosynthesis of chlortetracycline and oxytetracycline follows a similar logic and in the following, we focus on the biosynthetic principle of the latter compound. The BGC of oxytetracycline covers a 21.2 kb DNA region in *S. rimosus* and contains 21 ORFs encoding structural, modification, resistance, and regulatory elements [265]. The biosynthesis of oxytetracycline starts with the assembly of the polyketide precursor by the type II minimal PKS encoded by the genes *oxyA* through *oxyC* (Figure S6). More specifically, the KS_α (OxyA) and KS_β (OxyB) form the heterodimer responsible for chain elongation, while the ACP (OxyC) provides the extender units. An interesting feature of the natural tetracyclines is the unusual starter unit, malonamate, giving rise to the amide group on ring A in the naphthacene core [122,265]. The gene encoding the enzyme responsible for the provision of this starter unit has been identified as *oxyD*, which is located immediately downstream of the minimal PKS-encoding genes *oxyA* through *oxyC* in the oxytetracycline gene cluster in *S. rimosus*. The protein sequence of OxyD shows homology to the ATP-dependent class II asparagine synthases and it is believed to catalyse the transamination of malonate to yield malonamate [266]. Once attached to the minimal PKS, the malonamate is condensed with eight additional malonates, giving rise to the amidated decaketide backbone, which is released from the megaenzyme and further processed by AROs and CYCs encoded by genes in the oxytetracycline gene cluster (Figure S6). Based on the heterologous expression of the extended minimal PKS of oxytetracycline (OxyABCD) in *Streptomyces coelicolor* CH999, three enzymes have been identified and assumed to play a role in the correct cyclisation of the polyketide precursor [267]. This includes the NADPH-dependent KR OxyJ, which catalyses the

C9 reduction in ring D, the two-component CYC/ARO OxyK which is responsible for closing the first ring (ring D), and the CYC OxyN, catalysing the ring closure of the second ring (ring C). An additional putative CYC, encoded by *oxyI*, has been identified in the oxytetracycline gene cluster, however, since the heterologous expression of OxyABCDJKNI displayed a profile similar to that of OxyABCDJKN, it was concluded that OxyI is not directly involved in cyclisation of the third or fourth ring (ring B and A, respectively). Instead, closing of these two rings is believed to occur spontaneously [268].

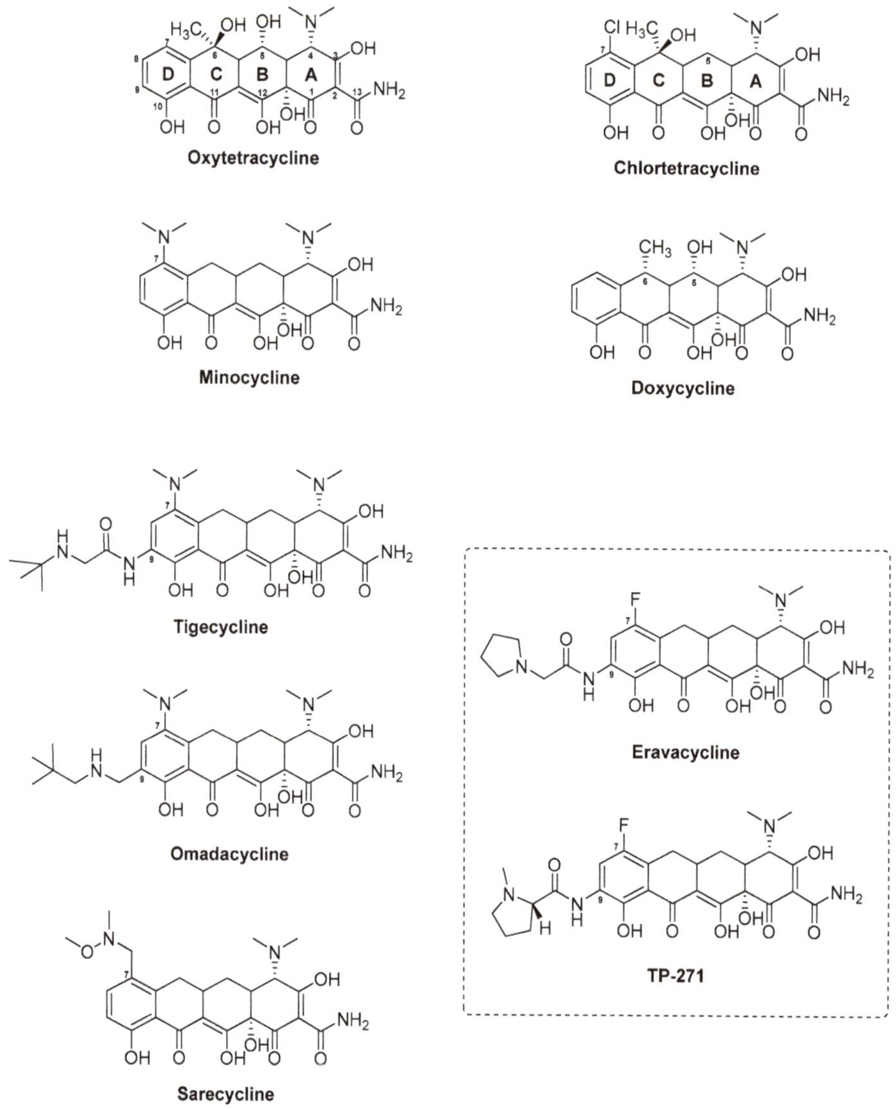

Figure 7. Structures of the naturally derived chlortetracycline and oxytetracycline and their semi-synthetic derivatives doxytetracycline, minocycline, tigecycline, omadacycline, and sarecycline. Eravacycline and TP-271 are fully synthetic tetracycline analogues.

Upon ring closure, the stable intermediate pretetramid is formed, which undergoes a series of modification reactions, of which the actual sequence remains to be clarified [269] (Figure S6). The modification of pretetramid involves a C6 methylation in ring C, which is catalysed by the S-adenosyl methionine (SAM)-dependent methyltransferase OxyF, yielding the intermediate 6-methylpretetramide. In the next step, the dihydroxylation of C4 and C12a in ring A, yielding the substance 4-keto-anhydrotetracycline, is catalysed by the two oxygenases OxyL and OxyE. While OxyL can give rise to both hydroxylations, OxyE only catalyses the addition of the hydroxyl group at the C4 position. The reason for the extra function of OxyE seems to be a matter of increasing the rate of the enzymatic reaction [268]. The further conversion of 4-keto-anhydrotetracycline is achieved first by the actions of the aminotransferase OxyQ, yielding the intermediate 4-amino-anhydrotetracycline, which then serves as a substrate for the SAM-dependent methyltransferase OxyT, catalysing a N,N-dimethylation that gives rise to anhydrotetracycline. The final enzymatic reactions leading to formation of oxytetracycline from anhydrotetracycline was recently elucidated by Wang and co-workers (Figure S6) [270]. In this study, OxyS was confirmed to catalyse the two sequential hydroxylations of C6 and C5 in ring C and B, respectively. Furthermore, OxyR was shown to act as a F_{420}-dependent reductase, which is responsible for the final C5a–C11a reduction affording oxytetracycline (Figure S6). In the case of chlortetracycline, an additional gene, *ctcP*, encoding a flavin-dependent halogenase, has been identified in the chlortetracycline BGC in *S. aureofaciens* [126]. CtcP yields the final product chlortetracycline based on the halogenation at position C7 in ring D (Figure S6). In addition to structural and tailoring genes, the BGCs of chlortetracycline and oxytetracycline include additional genes involved in resistance (*otrA* and *otrB*) and regulation (*otcG* and *otcR*). In the case of the oxytetracycline BGC, the two genes *otrA* and *otrB*, which encode proteins responsible for host resistance, are found at the flanking regions of the actual gene cluster. Based on sequence similarity, OtrA shows homology to TetM and is believed to provide resistance to *S. rimosus* by binding the ribosome and competing with the produced oxytetracycline. OtrB encodes a membrane protein and ensures the efflux of oxytetracycline from the cell [269,271]. The genes for the regulators OtcG and OtcR are also present in the flanking regions of the oxytetracycline BGC in *S. rimosus* [269,272,273]. OtcG, is a LuxR family transcriptional activator which was shown to provide positive regulation of oxytetracycline biosynthesis since an inactivation of *otcG* resulted in a mutant strain producing 40% less oxytetracycline than the wild type strain *S. rimosus* [272]. The overexpression of *otcG* did not yield a significant increase in production of oxytetracycline. OtcR was assigned to a *Streptomyces* antibiotic regulatory protein (SARP) activator of the oxytetracycline in *S. rimosus* [273]. Since a deletion of *otcR* completely abolished oxytetracycline production in the producer strain, the authors tested whether its overexpression would result in increased yields of the antibiotic. Indeed, the introduction two additional copies of *otcR*, under the control of a SF14 promoter, in *S. rimosus* increased the yields of oxytetracycline to 6.24 g/L (6.49 times higher than the yields of the parental strain) [273].

Tetracyclines are broad-spectrum antibiotics with activities against a range of microorganisms, including Gram-positive and Gram-negative bacteria, chlamydiae, mycoplasmas, and protozoan parasites [123]. They act as bacteriostatic drugs by binding to the 30S subunit of the prokaryote ribosome in a reversible fashion whereby protein synthesis is inhibited [132]. Furthermore, crystal structures of tetracycline in complex with both, the 30S subunit and 70S ribosome of *Thermus thermophiles*, have expanded the knowledge of the MOA of tetracyclines [124,274]. Based on the first X-ray structure of Brodersen et al., the primary binding site of tetracycline (Tet1) was found to be located between the head and shoulder of the 30S subunit, just above the transfer RNA (tRNA) binding site. When binding the A site, tetracycline act as a physical barrier for aminoacyl-tRNA so that the peptide chain cannot be elongated and protein synthesis is stalled [123,274]. Furthermore, the oxidised hydrophilic part of the tetracyclines appear to provide the main chemical interactions with the 16S ribosomal RNA (rRNA) and therefore, they are most important for the binding [275]. Another interesting property of the tetracyclines is their ability to chelate ions (Mg^{2+}). In addition to the hydrogen bond interactions between the hydrophilic side of tetracycline and the nucleotides on the 16s rRNA, the Mg^{2+} ions, coordinated by ring A of tetracycline, seem to further strengthen the binding to the ribosome [274]. The ion chelating properties of tetracyclines also explain their broad spectrum, including activity against Gram-negatives. In order to enter the periplasm of Gram-negatives, tetracycline forms a complex with Mg^{2+} allowing the antibiotic to pass through the porins of the outer membrane. To diffuse through the cytoplasmic membrane, tetracycline dissociates from Mg^{2+} enabling its passage through to the cytosol. The chelating complex is restored inside the cytosol [132].

The emergence of tetracycline resistance in clinical isolates has led to many studies to clarify the driving forces behind it. To date, four mechanisms by which bacteria acquire resistance to tetracyclines have been identified. These include active efflux of the antibiotic, ribosomal protection proteins, antibiotic modification, and alteration of the antibiotic target site, i.e., the ribosome. More information on the basis behind these individual resistance mechanisms can be found elsewhere [123,127,132].

The discovery of the naturally derived tetracyclines immediately triggered studies on improving the overall performance of the antibiotics. This resulted in the so-called 2nd generation tetracyclines, two of which, doxycycline and minocycline (Figure 7), were marketed in 1967 and 1972, respectively [123]. The discovery of doxycycline was based on the structural observations that the C6 hydroxyl group of tetracyclines greatly impact the stability of the molecules while antibacterial properties are not affected [128]. Consequently, derivatisation at this site of the molecule was conducted. The first attempt to alter the functional group at the C6 position in oxytetracycline gave rise to 6-methylene-5-hydroxytetracycline (methacycline), which was further modified to 6-deoxy-5-hydroxytetracycline, later named doxycycline (trade name: Vibramycin, Table 1). On the other hand, minocycline was the result of studies on biogenesis mutants of *S. aureofaciens*, the producer of chlortetracycline [129]. Here, scientists working at the former Lederle Laboratories succeeded in isolating the precursor C6-demethyl-C7-chlortetracycline (demeclocycline), which gave rise to the C6-demethyl-C6-deoxytetracycline (sancycline) precursor, that ultimately was converted to the final substance 7-dimethylamino-6-demethyl-6-deoxytetracycline (minocycline, trade name: Minocin, Table 1) [130,131]. Both doxycycline and minocycline are lipophilic molecules, which allow for oral absorption and thereby extend their applicability in the human therapy. Furthermore, they display improved antibacterial activities compared to tetracycline, including potent activities against Gram-negative bacteria such as *E. coli* and *Pseudomonas aeruginosa* and against the Gram-positive bacteria *S. aureus* and *E. faecalis* [127]. The importance of their introduction in human therapy was further strengthened by their activities against tetracycline-resistant isolates.

To ensure the continuous potential of the tetracyclines, a second round of derivatisation efforts, aiming at discovering novel tetracycline analogues with activities against both susceptible and tetracycline-resistant isolates, was initiated in the 1990s [123]. These efforts gave rise to the so-called glycylcyclines, also referred to as the 3rd generation tetracyclines, including tigecycline, omadacycline, and sarecycline (Figure 7) [127,133]. Tigecycline (trade name: Tygacil) was the first of the 3rd generation tetracyclines and was the result of the derivatisation of minocycline (Table 1) [134]. Compared to its precursor, tigecycline contains a *N*-alkyl-glycylamido group at position C9 in ring D. This structural modification resulted in a ~10–100-fold improved binding of tigecycline to the ribosome when compared to tetracycline [127,134]. Based on the crystal structure of *T. thermophilus* 70S ribosome bound to tigecycline, it has been shown that while the derivative binds the 30S subunit in the same manner as tetracycline, the interaction of tigecycline with the ribosome is greatly improved based on its additional *tert*-butylglycylamido group [274]. In cell-free translation assays tigecycline was capable of retaining its binding to the ribosome in the presence of the two resistance determinants TetM and TetO, confirming the activity of the derivative against tetracycline-resistant clinical isolates, which had acquired resistance based on ribosome protection proteins [135]. Tigecycline was approved by the US FDA in 2005 [132]. The current major limitation of tigecycline is its poor oral bioavailability and consequently the antibiotic is administered intravenously, giving rise to nausea and vomiting in the majority of patients [276].

Three additional 3rd generation tetracycline analogues have been approved by the US FDA for various applications in human therapy. Two of these, omadacycline (trade name: Nuzyra) and eravacycline (trade name: Xerava), bear a C9 substitution on ring D and have been licensed as broad-spectrum antibiotics, while the third, sarecycline (trade name: Seysara), was developed specifically as a narrow-spectrum tetracycline antibiotic for treatment of acne (Table 1). Omadacycline is an aminomethylcycline derivative of minocycline, which was isolated based on its superior activity against tetracycline-susceptible and -resistant bacteria, lack of toxicity, and the oral bioavailability [136,137,264]. Additionally, omadacycline shows improved activity against Gram-positive isolates compared to tigecycline and superior activity against Gram-negatives compared to eravacycline. This improved activity is believed to be a consequence of the C7 dimethylamino group and the C9 aminomethyl moiety in ring D of the molecule, since these modifications allow the antibiotic to evade the most common resistant determinants of efflux and ribosome protection [276]. The antibiotic was approved by the US FDA in October 2018 for the treatment of acute bacterial skin/skin structure infections, caused by a variety of bacteria, including methicillin-susceptible and -resistant strains of *S. aureus*, and for treatment of CABP, caused by *S. pneumonia* and methicillin-susceptible *S. aureus* [138]. Furthermore, omadacycline is currently undergoing safety and efficacy studies for its use in treatment of uncomplicated urinary tract infections. Eravacycline, developed at Tetraphase Pharmaceuticals, Inc., varies from the other clinical available 3rd generation tetracycline analogues with its fluorine atom at the C7 position and a pyrrolidinoacetamido group on the C9 of ring D (Figure 7) [139,140]. It displays activity against both Gram-positives and Gram-negatives and has been approved by the US FDA for treatment of infections caused by multidrug-resistant microorganisms, including carbapenem-resistant *Enterobacteriaceae*, MRSA, VREs, and extended spectrum β-lactamase (ESBL)-producing *Enterobacteriaceae* [141]. Following the same logic as for tigecycline and omadacycline, the altered functional groups on this fully synthetic tetracycline derivative was designed to evade tetracycline resistance determinants, which is evident from the retained activity of eravacycline against TetM-protected *E. coli* cells tested in an in vitro transcription/translation assay [140]. An additional fully synthetic tetracycline derivative, named TP-271 (Table 1), is currently being investigated by Tetraphase Pharmaceuticals, Inc. for its activity against pathogens causing CABP, anthrax, tularemia, and bubonic plague [143,144]. Similar to eravacycline, TP-271 is TetM-insensitive and can be used as an agent for bacterial isolates with this type of acquired resistance [143]. According to the pipeline of Tetraphase Pharmaceuticals, TP-271 is currently in phase I clinical testing [145]. The latest 3rd generation tetracycline to be approved by the US FDA, is the sarecycline, an aminomethylcycline with the unique and stable methoxy(methyl)aminomethyl modification at position C7 in ring D. Unlike the other tetracyclines, sarecycline has been approved as a narrow-spectrum antibacterial agent for the treatment of moderate to severe acne vulgaris caused by *Cutibacterium acnes* (formerly *Propionibacterium acnes*). Sarecycline was developed to meet the need for a safe treatment regime against acnes vulgaris, while simultaneously limiting resistance development of *C. acnes* [142].

3.7. Streptogramins

The group of streptogramins is an important class of antibiotics given their chemical complexity and potent antibacterial activity. They are composed of a mixture of two chemically unrelated substances, known as type A and type B streptrogramins, which are produced by the same host in a 70:30 ratio, respectively [277,278]. Streptogramin A and B, produced by *Streptomyces graminofaciens*, were the first in the group of streptogramin antibiotics to be discovered and provided the name for the substance class [279]. Following their discovery in 1953, several additional streptogramins were identified, some of which include mikamycin from *Streptomyces mitakaensis* [280,281], griseoviridin and viridogrisein from *Streptomyces griseoviridis* [282], as well as virginiamycin from *Streptomyces virginiae* [283]. Out of these substances, virginiamycin has had significant impact on veterinary medicine. Since its discovery, virginiamycin (trade names: Staphylomycin and Stafac) has been used all over the world in animal production as a disease control agent and feed additive for swine, poultry, and cattle. However, due to scientific concerns of resistance transmission between animals and humans, the use of drugs containing virginiamycin as a feed additive in Europe has been forbidden since 1999 [284]. Pristinamycin (Figure 8) is a close structural relative to virginiamycin. The antibiotic was first isolated from *Streptomyces pristinaespiralis*, which produces the two substances pristinamycin II$_A$ and pristinamycin I$_A$ in the ratio 70:30 [146,147]. Within the group of streptogramins, the two natural substances virginiamycin and pristinamycin and the semi-synthetic quinupristin–dalfopristin substance mixture (trade name: Synercid) (Figure 8, Table 1) have been subject to the most studies and will be the focus of this section. Since virginiamycin and pristinamycin share a common biosynthetic logic (Figure S7), only pristinamycin with its significant role in human medicine will be described.

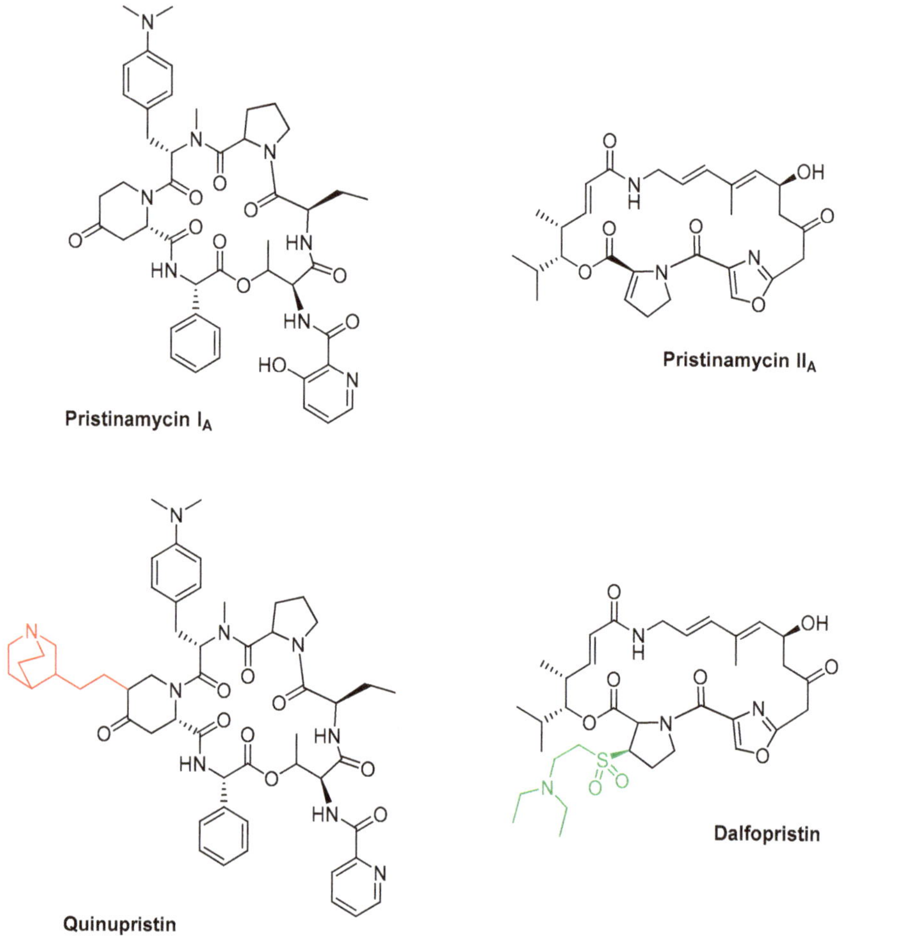

Figure 8. Structures of the two naturally derived antibiotics pristinamycin I$_A$ and pristinamycin II$_A$ and their two respective semi-synthetic analogues quinupristin and dalfopristin.

The biosynthetic gene cluster of pristinamycin remains one of the largest bacterial antibiotic clusters identified, covering a DNA region of 210 kb [148]. Within this region, 45 genes, covering a 120 kb region, are involved in the biosynthesis, regulation, and resistance of pristinamycin. Pristinamycin II is synthesised by a hybrid PKS/NRPS complex responsible for the assembly of the starter unit isobutyryl-CoA with six malonyl-CoA extender units and the amino acids glycine, serine, and proline

(Figure S7). The assembly starts at SnaE1, which ensures the successful loading of isobuturyl-CoA followed by its extension with two malonyl-CoA and glycine. The following four modules in SnaE2 and SnaE3 attach additional four malonyl-CoA extender units to the growing chain. In between the genes for the two megaenzymes SnaE2 and SnaE3, *snaG* through *snaL* are located. Together their respective enzymes are believed to be responsible for the C12 methyl group in pristinamycin II [148]. Downstream of *snaL*, the gene for the hybrid PKS/NRPS SnaE4 is located that is responsible for attachment of serine before transferring the precursor chain to the final module. The last NRPS module of SnaD, including the TE domain is responsible for the attachment of proline to the polyketide-hybrid chain and the release and cyclisation of the precursor chain. An interesting feature of the PKS is its lack of AT domains. Sequence analysis of the BGC and phylogenetic analysis of discrete ATs suggested that similar to the *trans*-AT KirCI, which is involved in kirromycin biosynthesis [285], SnaM also groups in the clade of discrete ATs of *trans*-AT-PKSs [148,286]. This indicates that SnaM might be responsible for an *in trans* loading of malonate units to assemble the pristinamycin II polyketide chain.

Pristinamycin I is synthesised from the NRPS encoded by genes *snbA*, *snbC*, and *snbDE*, which ensures the successful condensation of the four non-proteinogenic amino acids 3-hydroxypicolinic acid, L-aminobutyric acid, 4-N, N-dimethylamino-N-methyl-L-phenylalanine (DMAPA), 4-oxo-L-pipecolic acid, L-phenylglycine, and the two proteinogenic amino acids L-threonine and L-proline (Figure S7). Through the actions of the TE domain in the C-terminal of SnbDE, the precursor is released from the NRPS and cyclised. Additionally, 12 genes are involved in pristinamycin I biosynthesis through their synthesis of the amino acid precursors. This includes *hpaA* for 3-hydroxypicolinic acid, *pipA* and *snbF* for 4-oxo-L-pipecolic acid, and *papA/B/C/M* for DMAPA biosynthesis. For the non-proteinogenic amino acids, sequence analyses identified *pglA* through *pglE* to be involved in their biosynthesis [148]. Furthermore, within the 210 kb DNA region, several genes encoding regulatory elements have been identified [287,288]. Knowledge of the complex regulatory network behind pristinamycin I and II biosynthesis have fed metabolic engineering approaches in order to improve yields in the natural host [289,290]. In the study of Li and co-workers, the team systematically manipulated the cluster-situated genes *spbR* and *papR1* through *papR6* and found the best production enhancement of pristinamycin II_A when deleting either *papR3* or *papR5* and overexpressing both *papR4* and *papR6*. Surprisingly, strains overexpressing the major SARP activator PapR2 resulted in lowered pristinamycin production which could indicate a maximum threshold concentration of pristinamycin II_A in *S. pristinaespiralis* [290].

When applied separately as therapeutics, the type A and B streptogramins only provide a bacteriostatic effect. In combination, the two antibiotics act in a synergetic manner leading to a bactericidal activity against susceptible pathogens. Streptogramin antibiotics are active against a range of Gram-positive bacteria, including the severely resistant pathogens MRSA, vancomycin-resistant *S. aureus* (VRSA), *E. faecium* strains, and drug-resistant *S. pneumonia*. Activity against Gram-negative bacteria is mostly restricted to pathogens causing upper respiratory tract infection, including *H. influenza*, *Haemophilus parainfluenzae*, *M. pneumonia*, and *Moraxella catarrhalis* [150,277,278]. The synergistic activity of the type A and B streptogramins can be explained from the unique MOA, in that both antibiotics bind to the prokaryotic 50S ribosomal subunit however, at separate sites. The type A substances inhibit the early phase of protein elongation through their binding to the A and P sites on the 23S rRNA, thereby preventing the attachment of tRNA at each site [149,278]. Type B streptogramins also bind to the P site on the ribosome however, inhibit the late stage of polypeptide chain elongation by binding the exit tunnel of the ribosome. As a result, elongation of the nascent polypeptide chain is prevented and incomplete peptide chains are released from the complex. While the MOA of type B streptogramins is similar to that of erythromycin and related macrolides, the MOA for the type A streptogramins is similar to that of chloramphenicol. Furthermore, it has been shown that the binding of group A streptogramins to the P site leads to conformational changes in the subunit, which increases the affinity to the ribosome of the type B streptogramins. Even upon dissociation of the type A substances from the ribosome, the increase of ribosome affinity for type B streptogramins remains, explaining the synergetic effect of the mixture [291]. Recently, the crystal structure of the 50S ribosomal subunit from *Deinococcus radiodurans* in complex with Synercid (quinupristin/dalfopristin, Figure 8) has expanded our knowledge on the binding of streptogramins antibiotics to the ribosome [151]. Firstly, the two streptogramins share direct contact with a single nucleotide A2062 (*E. coli* numbering) through hydrophobic interactions and hydrogen bonds. This leads to conformational changes at A2062 whereby the binding of both antibiotics is strengthened. Secondly, an additional conformational change occurs when dalfopristin (type A) binds to the peptidyl transferase center (PTC) in that the universally conserved nucleotide U2585 is rotated to point away from the tunnel of the PTC. The altered conformation of U2585 in the PTC is stabilised by hydrogen bonds and might explain the post-antibiotic effect of streptogramin A antibiotics, in which protein synthesis is still inhibited after treatment with the antibiotic has been terminated [151].

To date, several resistance mechanisms against streptogramin antibiotics have been proposed. Some of these include target modification, drug inactivation, drug efflux, and impermeability [278,292]. Excellent reviews exist detailing the mode of drug resistance [292–294]. Briefly, a common resistance mechanism developed towards macrolide antibiotics is ribosomal target modification. This antibiotic resistance is encoded by the erythromycin-resistance methylase (*erm*) genes, which can mono- or dimethylate an adenosine residue of the 23S rRNA of the ribosomal 50S subunit [295]. Methylation changes the conformation of the ribosome and collectively causes resistance towards antibiotics of the MLS$_B$ group. Additionally, the pathogen can develop resistance by drug inactivation through acetyltransferases (targets type A) and hydrolases (targets type B) or by drug efflux, encoded by genes such as *msrA/B*, *mefA*, *lsa*, and *vga* [294,296,297]. Resistance against streptogramins depends on the substance type. Type B streptogramins, which shares properties with erythromycin, are classified as MLS$_B$ antibiotics, which suffer from cross-resistance between each other. Type A streptogramins instead show cross-resistance with lincosamides and pleuromutilins and group in the lincosamide–streptogramin A–pleuromutilin (LS$_A$P) antibiotics. Since bacterial isolates with lowered susceptibility towards the synergetic mixture have already been isolated, it is evident that caution should be taken when administering these drugs. In order to reduce the risk of resistance towards this important class of compounds, streptogramins are classified as drugs of last resort [278].

Due to its hydrophobic nature, pristinamycin (Table 1) is administered orally, which limits its use in paediatrics and intensive care [152,278]. To solve the issue of bioavailability, medicinal chemists employed by the French chemical and pharmaceutical company Rhône-Poulenc Rorer worked on synthesising novel pristinamycin derivatives with improved water solubility. Their attempts proved successful and in 1999 the US FDA approved the antibiotic Synercid (Table 1), which is a 70:30 mixture of the two semi-synthetic derivatives dalfopristin (type A) and quinupristin (type B), for treatment of bacteraemia caused by VRE and skin/skin structure infections caused by methicillin-susceptible *S. aureus* and *S. pyogenes* [152,153,278]. Information on the synthesis of dalfopristin and quinupristin (Figure 8) remain scarce. From the published structures, it is known that quinupristin is the result of derivatisation of pristinamycin I$_A$ at position five of the 4-oxo pipicolic acid residue and that dalfopristin is generated based on the substitution of pristinamycin II$_A$ with a 2-diethylaminoethane thiol [292].

Synercid suffers from its own limitations, including a high treatment price and the risk of infusion site thrombosis in addition to myalgias and arthralgias [154]. A more recent example of a semi-synthetic pristinamycin derivative is NXL-103 (Table 1), which is a 70:30 mixture of flopristin (type A) and linopristin (type B) [154,155]. As opposed to Synercid, NXL-103 is administered orally thereby avoiding the complication associated with intravenous therapy. Additionally, NXL-103 has been shown to possess an improved activity against multiple Gram-positive isolates when compared to Synercid [155]. With its expanded activity against clinical Gram-positive isolates such as MRSA, methicillin-resistant *Staphylococcus epidermidis*, and VRE, NXL-103 could provide an additional treatment option to the current drugs on the market. However, since the report of phase II clinical trials in 2010, to the best of our knowledge, no new information on NXL-103 exists and the drug made no progress towards its introduction into the market [154].

4. Other Clinically Relevant Polyketide-Derived Antimicrobials

4.1. Nystatin A1

The antifungal polyene macrolides are characterised by a large macrolactone ring containing 20 to 40 carbon atoms connected by a series of conjugated double bonds, an exocyclic carboxyl group, and a mycosamine sugar. Several compounds belonging to this group have been studied in detail, including candicidin, nystatin, amphotericin, and pimaricin (also referred to as natamycin) [298,299] (Figure 9). In this review, we focus on nystatin A1, amphotericin B, and pimaricin/natamycin, since these are the drugs still used in the clinic.

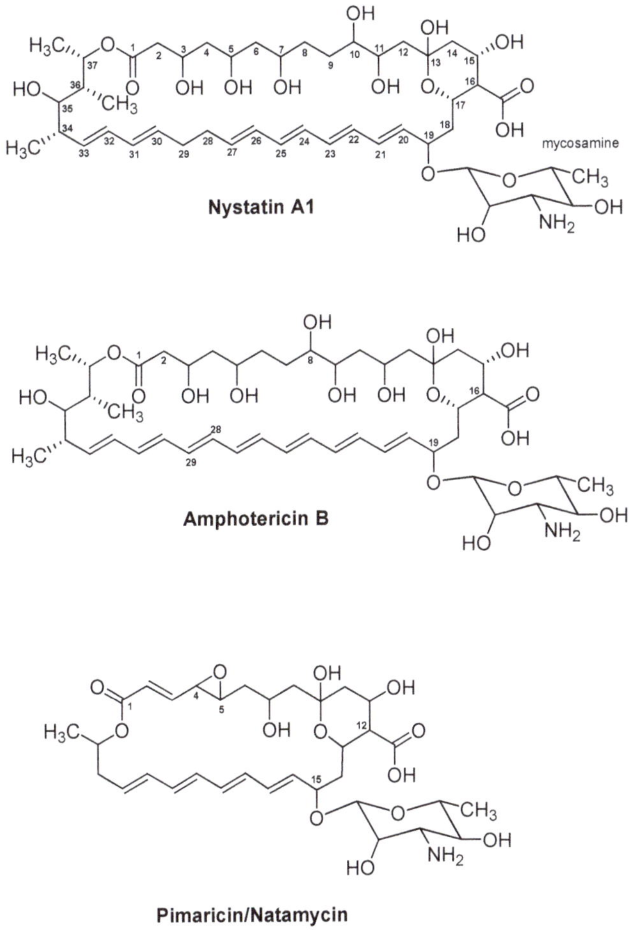

Figure 9. Structures of the three antifungal compounds nystatin A1, amphotericin B, and pimaricin (also referred to as natamycin).

The first polyene macrolide was discovered in 1950 by E.L. Hazen and R.F. Brown from the New York State Department of Health and was the initially named fungicidin [156,300]. The compound was discovered from *Streptomyces* No. 48240 isolated from a soil sample collected at a farm owned by H.

Nourse. Later, the strain was renamed *S. noursei* and the compound name changed from fungicidin to nystatin [157]. With the advances in analytical separation techniques it became evident that nystatin was a mixture of three components, namely nystatin A1, A2, and A3. Nystatin A1 was the major component in the fermentation mixture [301]. So far, *S. noursei* remains the commercial strain for production of nystatin, however, other strains, including *Streptomyces fungicidicus* ATCC 27,432 [302] and *Streptomyces albulus* ATCC 12,757 [303], have also been identified as nystatin producers.

Nystatin A1 (brand names: Mycostatin and Nystop) (Table 1) is composed of a 38-membered macrolactone ring which includes sets of two and four conjugated double bonds separated by one saturated bond (Figure 9). Similar to other polyene macrolides, nystatin contains a mycosamine sugar attached to the aglycone ring in addition to an exocyclic carboxyl group (Figure 9) [299,304].

The aglycone macrolide of nystatin (Figure 9) is assembled from one acetyl-CoA starter unit and further extended through condensation with three methylmalonyl-CoA and 15 malonyl-CoA extender units (Figure S8). The assembly of the nystatin precursor is governed by a type I PKS, composed of a total of one loading and 18 extender modules, which are all encoded in the six genes *nysA*, *nysB*, *nysC*, *nysI*, *nysJ*, and *nysK* [158]. The TE domain found at the C-terminal of module 18 in NysK is responsible for chain termination and cyclisation, forming the aglycone precursor of nystatin. Immediately downstream of *nysC*, the gene *nysE* is located. NysE displays protein similarity to TEs found in *Streptomyces venezuelae* and *Streptomyces fradiae*, however, the role of the enzyme has not been experimentally verified. It is postulated that this additional TE enzyme, like in the case of erythromycin and tylosin biosynthesis, acts as a "proof-reading" enzyme to avoid stalling at the PKS. Additional genes found in the nystatin gene cluster include the two P450 monooxygenases, encoded by *nysL* and *nysN*, which are responsible for the C10 hydroxylation and C16 methyl group oxidation, respectively. The role of NysN has been confirmed based on genetic inactivation. The $\Delta nysN$ mutant lost the ability to produce nystatin A1, and instead the analogue 16-decarboxy-16-methyl nystatin was isolated from the culture broth [160].

The biosynthesis and transfer of the mycosamine sugar to the aglycone of nystatin are carried out by three enzymes encoded by *nysDI*, *nysDII*, and *nysDIII* [158]. Specifically, the biosynthesis of the sugar is believed to be facilitated by the aminotransferase NysDII and the guanosine diphosphate (GDP)-mannose-4,6-dehydratase NysDIII, while the attachment of mycosamine at C19 of the nystatin aglycone is thought to be catalysed by the glycosyltransferase NysDI. Furthermore, it has been postulated that mycosamine is synthesised from a GDP-mannose instead of deoxythymidine diphosphate (dTDP)-glucose [298].

Two ATP-binding cassette (ABC) transporter-encoding genes *nysG* and *nysH* are located at the border of the nystatin gene cluster [305]. Since mutants in either of the two genes displayed similar phenotypes, NysG–NysH is thought to be part of the same transporter. Furthermore, four genes *nysRI* through *nysRIV* encoding regulator proteins have been identified and their role clarified in the nystatin gene cluster [299,306]. NysRIV is most likely directly controlling the expression of nystatin biosynthesis genes. More information on the regulation governing nystatin biosynthesis in *S. noursei* can be found elsewhere [299,306].

Nystatin A1 is primarily used as a topical agent e.g., in treatment of mucous membrane candidiasis caused by members of the yeast-like family *Candida* [307]. As it is the case for most polyenes, nystatin has a low water solubility and shows detectable toxicity, which restricts its application in human therapy. The explanation for the toxicity is found in the MOA shared among the polyenes. In general, the MOA of polyenes is based on their interaction with sterols in eukaryotic cell membranes, resulting in pores and increase membrane permeability for ions and small molecules, which is usually lethal for the cell [159]. Although nystatin displays a higher selectivity toward the ergosterol found in fungal cell membranes, it can also interact with the cholesterol of mammalian cells membranes, which is limiting its use for human therapy. Taken together, due to its undesired toxicity, low solubility, and lower antifungal potency than that of amphotericin B, the application of nystatin as human medicine remains restricted [160,308].

With the elucidation of the gene cluster responsible for the biosynthesis of the polyene macrolides candicidin, pimaricin, amphotericin, and nystatin it has become evident that the overall organisation of these cluster is highly similar [298]. This logic was utilised to design a polyene-specific polymerase chain reaction (PCR)-guided genome screening approach to screen for novel polyene-producing actinomycetes [309]. Using the sequence of a cytochrome P450 hydroxylase gene, which is similar between polyenes, the authors could identify and later confirm the presence of a Nystatin-like *Pseudonocardia* Polyene (NPP) gene cluster in the rare actinomycete *Pseudonocardia autotrophica* [310]. Structural analysis of NPP revealed an aglycone identical to that of nystatin however, with a modified sugar residue (a unique disaccharide moiety; mycosaminyl-(α1-4)-*N*-acetyl-glucosamine) [311]. Compared to nystatin A1, NPP A1 displayed a 300-fold increase in water solubility, 10-fold reduced hemolytic activity, but also ~50% lower antifungal activity against *Candida albicans*. The issue of lowered bioactivity was later solved through the manipulation of the ER domain in module five (ER5) of the NPP biosynthetic cluster [312]. Deleting this gene disables the reduction at the C28–C29 unsaturated bond in the aglycone of NPP A1 hence, generating a heptaene instead of the original tetraene. The new derivative NPP B1 displayed in vitro and in vivo activity against *C. albicans* and improved hemolytic activity compared to amphotericin B. However, the production yields of NPP B1 in the pathway-engineered strain (*P. autotrophica* ER5 mutant) were extremely low. In an attempt to solve this issue, the *P. autotrophica* ER5 mutant strain was subjected to *N*-methyl-*N*'-nitro-*N*-nitrosoguanidine (NTG) iterative random mutagenesis [312]. The resulting mutants were screened in zone-of-inhibition agar plug assays in which the mutant strain 3R-42 produced the largest inhibition zone. The transcriptional analysis further revealed a general up-regulation of the NPP biosynthetic genes in the 3R-42 mutant compared to the original ER5 mutant. Based on this observation, the authors introduced a second copy of each putative regulatory gene into the chromosome of the 3R-42 mutant strain and could determine a final NPP B1 production of 31.6 mg/L [312], which was a substantial increase in comparison to the 0.77 mg/L NPP B1 produced by the original ER5 mutant.

Additionally, studies on the biosynthesis of nystatin itself also open up for the discovery of novel derivatives with improved properties. In fact, based on genetic engineering of the nystatin gene cluster, Brautaset and colleagues obtained seven nystatin derivatives with altered exocyclic carboxy groups and polyol regions [160]. The mutational studies were based on the already obtained *S. noursei* mutant strain GG5073SP, in which the ER5 was deleted. This mutant produced a heptaene nystatin analogue, named S44HP. The introduction of a CL346AS mutation in the *nysN* of GG5073SP resulted in the mutant BSM1 and the isolation of a novel compound. Its structure was confirmed as 16-decarboxy-16-methyl-28,29-didehydro-nystatin (BSG005) by nuclear magnetic resonance (NMR) analysis. The authors also succeeded in generating a mutant strain, BSM3, which in addition to the mutation in *nysN* also was disrupted in the dehydratase (DH) domain in module 15, located in NysJ. The mutant strain BSM3 produced the analogue 5-oxo-5-deoxy-16-decarboxy-16-methyl-28,29-didehydro nystatin (BSG020). Both BSG005 and BSG020 display improved toxicities and comparable antifungal activities against disseminated candidiasis in a mouse model when compared to amphotericin B and thus, represent promising candidates for the development of new antifungal drugs [160]. The derivatives have not yet been introduced for human therapy however, based on information obtained from the homepage of the Swedish biotech company Biosergen AS, the company has selected the BSG005 candidate for further preclinical and clinical tests (Table 1) [161].

4.2. Amphotericin B

The antifungal polyene macrolide amphotericin B (trade names: Fungizone and Amphocin) was first discovered together with amphotericin A in the 1950s in the fermentation broth of soil-derived *Streptomyces nodosus* [162]. While amphotericin A contains a tetraene chromophore, amphotericin B possesses a heptaene (Figure 9).

The BGC of amphotericin B has been fully sequenced. The sequence analysis revealed that the cluster organisation is similar to the BGC of nystatin [313]. The polyketide chain is biosynthesised by an assembly line involving one loading (encoded by *amphA*) and 18 extension modules (encoded by the five genes *amphB*, *amphC*, and *amphI* through *amphK*) (Figure S8). Assembly of the precursor on the amphotericin PKS is initiated by the loading of a malonyl-CoA starter unit which is further elongated by additional 15 acetate and nine propionate extender units (Figure S8) [163]. In the last module, encoded by *amphK*, a TE domain is responsible for chain termination and release from the PKS. Two putative cytochrome P450 enzymes AmphL and AmphN are possibly involved in the modification of the amphotericin B structure. While AmphL most likely catalyses the C8 hydroxylation in the macrolactone, AmphN may facilitate the oxidation of the methyl group on C16 to yield a carboxyl group. Targeted deletion of *amphN* resulted in a *S. nodosus* mutant strain producing a amphotericin analogue in which the exocyclic methyl group is retained [314]. The fact that the antifungal activity of this analogue was unchanged, and the haemolytic activity reduced compared to amphotericin B, makes the derivative an interesting candidate for clinical studies.

Additional modification of amphotericin is facilitated by the glycosyltransferase, encoded by *amphDI*, which is responsible for the attachment of the mycosamine to the aglycone core of amphotericin [313,314]. The biosynthesis of the mycosamine is believed to be catalysed by a GDP-mannose-4,6-dehydratase encoded by *amphDIII*, which uses GDP-mannose derived from primary metabolism as substrate [298]. The product of the AmphDIII-catalysed dehydratase reaction is GDP-4-keto-6-deoxy-D-mannose and not GDP-3-keto-6-deoxy-D-mannose, which is the substrate recognised by the transaminase AmphDII. So far, no GDP-4-keto-6-deoxy-D-mannose-3,4-isomerase has been identified in any of the polyene gene clusters and it is hypothesised that the ketoisomerisation reaction is the result of a spontaneous, non-enzymatic reaction [298].

Export of amphotericin B has been hypothesised to be facilitated by two putative ABC transporters, encoded by *amphG* and *amphH*. The reason why two transporters are present in the gene cluster remains unknown. It has been speculated that ABC transporters can confer self-resistance of the producing host [313]. Based on the high degree of sequence similarity between nystatin and amphotericin PKS genes, it has been postulated that the genes *amphRI* through *amphRIV* are homologues of the genes *nysRI*–*nysRIV* in nystatin and encode regulatory proteins, which act in a very similar fashion [298,315].

Since its marketing in 1957, amphotericin B (Table 1) has been used as the "gold standard" for treatment of the most severe dimorphic fungal and yeast infections, caused by *Blastomyces*, *Candida*, *Cryptococcus*, and *Histoplasma* spp. [307]. The MOA of amphotericin B is identical to that of nystatin. Despite its preference for ergosterol found in fungal cellular membranes, amphotericin B also interacts to a lesser extend with the cholesterol found in mammalian cell membranes [164]. This and the side effects, including nephrotoxicity present a major limitation to the application of amphotericin B as an antibiotic for human therapy. In addition to its antifungal properties, amphotericin has also been implemented in delaying onset of prion disease in cultured cells with human immunodeficiency virus (HIV) and in inhibition of the protozoal parasite *Leishmania* [313].

Although amphotericin B shows a promising spectrum of activity and potential applications, the compound is poorly soluble in water and displays certain toxicity, which restricts its use in intravenous therapy. Consequently, only life-threatening fungal infections are treated with amphotericin B. Interestingly, despite its use as an antifungal drug for more than 40 years, reports of mycological resistance development in clinical fungi isolates against amphotericin B remain relatively scarce [316]. Nonetheless, resistance occurs, as it was demonstrated by the isolation of resistant *Candida* spp., *Fusarium* spp., and *Scedosporium apiospermum* [317]. In these fungi, drug resistance is most likely conferred by either the production of alternative ergosterols to which the amphotericin B is less efficient or simply by decreasing the ergosterol level in the fungal cell membranes. Both mechanisms reduce the potency of the antifungal drug [316].

The promising features of amphotericin B, such as broad-spectrum activity and low resistance against the compound were encouraging for numerous engineering attempts in order to improve the properties of the antifungal drug. A great improvement in the solubility of the amphotericin B was already achieved in the case of Fungizone, which is a mixture of amphotericin B and the bile acid deoxycholate [165]. Additionally, reduction in the overall toxicity of amphotericin B was further achieved through liposome encapsulation, which has resulted in the three formulations; Amphotec, AmBisome, and Abelcet [165]. Unfortunately, the reduced toxicity of the liposome-packed amphotericin B seems to come at a cost in antifungal efficiency.

The extensive investigations on amphotericin and polyene biosynthesis are of advantage for targeted engineering to increase production yields and to generate new derivatives with improved therapeutic properties. Furthermore, it should be noted that great efforts have been made in the field of semi-synthesis and several amphotericin B analogues with improved solubility and toxicity have been generated using different chemical approaches. Many of these have already been reviewed elsewhere [318]. Despite the many advances in both semi-synthesis and genetic engineering for obtaining amphotericin B analogues with improved properties, the yields of the derivatives are often very low, and to date, none of the reported amphotericin B analogues have made it through to the market. Consequently, the actinomycetes-derived substance amphotericin B remains one of the most important polyketides in the sparse portfolio of antifungal drugs. This urges the need for improved production titers in the natural producer strain. Recently, Zhang and co-workers set out to improve yields of amphotericin B in a newly isolated strain *Streptomyces* spp. ZJB 2013082, which produced the antifungal substance in low yields [319]. Using a combination of ultraviolet (UV) and NTG mutagenesis, the mutant strain N3 was isolated, which produced 1735 mg/L, a substantially increased amount of the product compared to the 56.2 mg/L obtained from the parent strain ZJB 2013082. Additionally, the N3 mutant accumulated less amphotericin A than the parent strain ZJB 2013082. This could be of industrial importance, since substance A is only allowed to account for more than five percent in the amphotericin mixture. The genome sequence of the N3 mutant is not yet published however, identification of the genomic architecture in the N3 mutant could help guide future engineering efforts to obtain a stable production host for amphotericin B.

4.3. Pimaricin/Natamycin

Pimaricin (later renamed natamycin, trade names: Natacyn and E235) (Figure 9, Table 1) was first discovered in the 1950s as the product of soil-derived *Streptomyces natalensis* isolated from the South African region of Natal [166,320]. Additional producer strains have been identified, including *Streptomyces chattanoogensis* [321,322] and *Streptomyces lydicus* [323].

The structure of pimaricin varies slightly from those of amphotericin B and nystatin A1 (Section 4.1) owing to the smaller size of the macrolactone (Figure 9). Pimaricin is composed of a 26-membered aglycone, containing four conjugated double bonds, to which the characteristic mycosamine sugar is attached at the C15 atom. The tetraene polyene further contains an exocyclic carboxyl group at C12, a functionally interestingly epoxide at C4/C5, and an internal hemiketal ring, which originates from a spontaneous cyclisation of the C9 keto group with a hydroxyl group on C13 [167].

The elucidation of pimaricin biosynthesis has relied primarily on genome sequencing and genetic studies of the two pimaricin-producer strains *S. chattanoogensis* and *S. natalensis* [320]. In the case of *S. natalensis*, an 85 kb-large genomic region containing 16 ORFs was identified from a cosmid library as the pimaricin gene cluster [167]. Pimaricin biosynthesis follows a logic, which is highly similar to that governing amphotericin B and nystatin biosynthesis. Since the gene clusters identified from *S. chattanoogensis* and *S. natalensis* are nearly identical, the following subsection will describe the studies on *S. natalensis*.

The assembly of the 26-membered lactone, termed pimaricinolide, is catalysed by a type I PKS composed of 13 (one starter and 12 extender) modules, encoded by the genes *pimS0–pimS4* (Figure S9). Chain initiation starts at PimS0 with the loading of a malonyl-CoA. Further elongation, catalysed by PimS1 through PimS4, leads to the condensation of additional 12 acetate units and one propionate unit to the growing polyketide precursor. In PimS4, the last domain, a TE, is responsible for the release and cyclisation of pimaricinolide [167]. Further examination of the pimaricin gene cluster has revealed an additional gene *pimI*, which encodes an enzyme with homology to the TE found in the candicidin gene cluster in *S. griseus* and to the TylO in the tylosin gene cluster in *S. fradiae*. It has been postulated that the additional TE in the pimaricin gene cluster helps to remove aberrant precursors from the PKS, ensuring continuous biosynthesis [167,204]. Upon its release from the PKS, pimaricinolide undergoes oxidation of the methyl group on C12 resulting in the formation of a carboxylic acid. This is catalysed by PimG, a cytochrome P450 enzyme. The resulting 12-carboxy-pimaricinolide is then glycosylated at the C15 hydroxyl group through the attachment of a mycosamine by the actions of the glycosyltransferase PimK. The final modification of the pimaricin precursor involves another cytochrome P450 (encoded by the gene *pimD*) which catalyse the oxidation leading to the spontaneous formation of an epoxy group between C4 and C5.

Sugar biosynthesis is believed to involve only two enzymes; PimJ, a GDP-mannose-4,6-dehydratase responsible for the conversion of GDP-mannose (from primary metabolism) to GDP-4-keto-6-deoxymannose, and PimC, a GDP-3-keto-6-deoxymannose aminotransferase, which synthesises GDP-mycosamine from GDP-3-keto-6-deoxymannose. Similar to what has been described for mycosamine biosynthesis in amphotericin B and nystatin, no gene encoding an enzyme responsible for the 3,4-isomerisation required for the conversion of GDP-4-keto-6-deoxymannose to GDP-3-keto-6-deoxymannose was found in the pimaricin gene cluster, and the reaction is believed to occur spontaneously [298,320].

The three gene products of *pimA*, *pimB*, and *pimH* have been putatively assigned to proteins ensuring the export of pimaricin in *S. natalensis*. While PimA and PimB group in the family of ABC transporters, PimH might encode an efflux pump [320,324]. The functions of PimA and PimB remain to be experimentally verified. For the homologues of PimA and PimB (ScnA and ScnB) in *S. chattanoogensis*, it was reported that they are involved in primary exporters of natamycin [324]. With amino acid sequence similarities of above 95% for ScnA/ScnB and PimA/PimB, it is likely that the later enzymes have a similar function and also act as primary transporters of pimaricin.

The regulatory mechanisms governing pimaricin biosynthesis has been studied in *S. natalensis* and *S. chattanoogensis*. Two transcriptional regulators PimM and PimR play an important role in pimaricin production in *S. natalensis* [325,326]. Furthermore, the amino acid exporter PimT and the putative cholesterol oxidase PimE add an extra layer of regulation to the pimaricin biosynthesis. While PimT was found to play a role in export of quorum-sensing pimaricin-inducer (PI) factor [327], PimE could act as a signalling molecule, triggering production of pimaricin in the producer in the presence of fungi [328,329]. The complex regulation cascade contains potential "targets" for engineering of the producer and increasing the production of the antifungal compound. Some of the most successful examples include overexpression of the regulator-encoding gene *scnRII* (homologue to *pimM*) in *S. chattanoogensis*, deletion of *sngR*, a γ-butyrolactone receptor-encoding gene, in *S. natalensis*, and chromosomal integration of the *Vitreoscilla* haemoglobin *vgb* gene in *S. gilvosporeus*, resulting in 460%, 460%, and 407% increase in pimaricin yields, respectively, in the mutant strains compared to wild types [320,330–332].

More than 40 years after the introduction of pimaricin to the market, it remains an important antifungal agent and it is still used in the treatment of fungal keratitis, an infection of the cornea caused primarily by filamentous fungi *Fusarium* and *Aspergillus*, and yeast-like *Candida* [168]. Due to its low water solubility and limited oral absorption, pimaricin is mainly available as a topical agent in human medicine. Recently, an antiprotozoan activity of pimaricin was detected which makes the compound attractive for potential treatment of keratitis caused by *Acanthamoeba*.

The MOA of pimaricin differs from that of nystatin and amphotericin B. While the main target of the pimaricin is ergosterol, which is the major sterol found in fungal cells membranes, pimaricin only binds to the lipid receptor. The interaction between pimaricin and ergosterol has been examined in *Aspergillus niger*, showing that upon its binding, pimaricin blocks transport of amino acids and glucose across the fungal plasma membrane, which leads to cell death [169]. Due to its specific interaction with ergosterol, the development of microbial resistance towards pimaricin is seen as posing only a minor risk [320]. This, combined with its low oral absorption, has paved the way for pimaricin as a food preservative. Sold under the label E235, pimaricin is approved as a protecting agent against yeast and mould and is used for surface treatment of hard, semi-hard, and semi-soft cheeses, and of dried, cured sausage in Europe. Other applications of pimaricin are summarised in the review by Aparicio and co-workers [320]. Additionally, pimaricin is the only antifungal agent to date, which has gained the generally regarded as safe (GRAS) status.

While pimaricin itself remains an important agent for treatment of fungal keratitis and as a food preservative, efforts to engineer strains which produce novel pimaricin analogues with improved solubility and toxicity have been undertaken. These efforts have been greatly aided by the complete genome sequencing of S. natalensis and S. chattanoogensis, both harbouring the BGC of pimaricin. Recently, Qi and co-workers could identify three novel pimaricin analogues based on a single mutation of the gene scnG in S. chattanoogensis (pimG in S. natalensis) [333], which encodes the cytochrome P450 enzyme responsible for the formation of carboxyl group at the C12 in pimaricin. Out of the three identified derivatives, 12-decarboxy-12-methyl pimaricin and 4,5-desepoxy-12-decarboxy-12-methyl pimaricin, both displayed reduced cytotoxicity compared to pimaricin. Additionally, 12-decarboxy-12-methyl pimaricin showed a two-fold increase in antifungal activity against C. albicans ATCC 14,053 compared to pimaricin. Through further biochemical and genetic analyses, 4,5-desepoxy-12-decarboxy-12-methyl pimaricin was found to be the precursor of 12-decarboxy-12-methyl pimaricin in the reaction catalysed by the C4/C5 epoxidase encoded by scnD (pimD). Therefore, to ensure the complete conversion of 4,5-desepoxy-12-decarboxy-12-methyl pimaricin into 12-decarboxy-12-methyl pimaricin, scnD was overexpressed in the $\Delta scnG$ mutant, which led to a 20% increase in production of the latter derivative. However, with an overall yield of 268 ± 10 mg/L for 12-decarboxy-12-methyl pimaricin in the best performing mutant, the needs for further engineering to optimise yields are necessary. In this case, the pathway-specific regulators PimM and PimR or the PI-factor could be the next targets for improving pimaricin derivative production [333].

5. Strategies and Tools for the Discovery of Natural Products

The emergence of antibiotic resistant microbes is alarming and underlines the urgent need for new drugs to combat the pathogens. However, the discovery and approval of new antibiotics is more difficult than expected [334–336]. Therefore, the question arises: how to improve the chances for finding new antimicrobial compounds? Recently, new approaches and advances of the existing technologies within the early stage of drug discovery and development were reported.

For natural product-derived antimicrobial compounds, the "journey" starts with the identification of the source (e.g., producer organism) and/or the bioactive molecule, responsible for the inhibition or killing of a pathogen. Already at this stage, the re-discovery rate of known structures might be reduced by taking samples and isolation of potential producers or compounds from undiscovered environments [337–343]. This is often limited by the fact that organisms originating from "extreme" habitats require special cultivation conditions and thus, many strategies were developed to overcome this barrier (e.g., co-cultivation [344–346], iChip [347–352], or combination of both [353]).

Confirmed or potential producers of new antimicrobial agents are further analysed by diverse "omics" approaches [342,354–357]. The downstream evaluation of the collected data sets using bioinformatics tools enables for example the identification of the BGC for the product of interest and/or provides an overview on the overall biosynthetic potential of target strain (genome mining) [9,358–360]. In cases where promising BGCs were identified, however, no products were found with the available fermentation and analytic methods [361–364], the expression of the clusters and production of the respective metabolite might be achieved by addition of elicitors [341,342,365–369] or the heterologous expression of the BGC in optimized hosts [370–375].

In order to improve the production of relevant products, including polyketides, molecular biology tools and methods (e.g., vectors, plasmids, recombinases, CRISPR-Cas9, promoters, and other synthetic parts as well as methods for their delivery (conjugation, protoplast transformation, and direct transformation)) are used. They play an important role for engineering of both, the natural producer and heterologous hosts. Challenges and new opportunities for the genetic manipulation of actinomycetes were recently reviewed [376–381].

Although each one of these cutting-edge technologies and approaches already contributed to the identification of new compounds, the interplay of the different disciplines will grant a better access to novel natural products with valuable bioactivities.

6. Conclusions and Outlook

Actinomycetes are one of the most prolific sources of biologically active secondary metabolites, including polyketides. In the past decades, numerous polyketide compounds were isolated and developed to highly potent antimicrobial drugs, which have saved millions of lives. However, rapid emergence of multidrug resistant pathogens is occurring worldwide which poses a severe threat to human health. This calls for the discovery and development of new antibiotics and antimicrobial strategies. Unlike drugs used in case of chronic diseases (e.g., diabetes, cardiovascular disease, cancer, arthritis, asthma), antibiotics are taken for a short period of time and thus, they are non-profitable and economically unattractive. This and several other obstacles such as high costs of the research and development and insufficient investment from stakeholders has prompted the big pharmaceutical companies to terminate the development of new antibiotics. Currently, it seems that the screening and development of new lead structures for novel antimicrobial agents is mainly conduced at public research and non-profit institutions.

The fact that many habitats around the globe are unexplored and poorly investigated for the presence of antibiotic-producing microbes, such as actinomycetes, motived researchers to collect samples from these environments and isolate the diverse producers of potentially new bioactive compounds. The valuable knowledge obtained from the investigation of the biosynthesis, regulation and natural resistance in the natural host of the old drugs as well as the recent developments within screening and isolation methods, sequencing and genome mining, and analytics potentiate the platforms for drug discovery. For example, the analysis of a relatively underexplored genus of *Actinoallomurus* led to the discovery of two new spirotetronate polyketide antibiotics NAI414-A and NAI414-B [382].

As exemplified in this review (Section 3.1), the success in derivatisation and combination of existing compound classes has enabled the continuous efficient treatment of otherwise resistant clinical isolates. In particular, the knowledge gained from detailed MOA and SAR studies of the antimicrobials have paved the way for the development of drugs with improved pharmacokinetic properties and expanded spectrum of bioactivity, compared to the original substance. In the future, semi-synthesis will continue to play an important role in drug development, of both, old and new drug candidates.

Last, but not least, support from governments and cooperation across the world e.g., public research institutions as well as United Nations organisations, the WHO, the Food and Agriculture Organization, and the inter-governmental World Organisation for Animal Health, combined with strategies offering long-term incentive for the pharmaceutical companies to reinvigorate their antimicrobial drug discovery platforms are an important political aspect that has been gaining more attention these days. The option of the US FDA to gain a fast-track approval of drug leads which can be used to treat serious or life-threatening conditions might further enhance the chances of taking on the expenses associated with drug discovery by pharmaceutical companies. The combination of all these efforts may give a competitive advantage in the never-ending race between the discovery of antimicrobials and the rise of drug resistance in pathogens.

Supplementary Materials: The following are available online at http://www.mdpi.com/2079-6382/8/4/157/s1, Figure S1: The erythromycin biosynthetic pathway, Figure S2: The tylosin biosynthetic pathway, Figure S3: The monensin biosynthetic pathway, Figure S4: The biosynthetic pathway of tiacumicin, Figure S5: The biosynthetic pathway of rifamycin, Figure S6: The biosynthetic pathway of oxytetracycline and chlortetracycline, Figure S7: The biosynthetic pathways of pristinamycin II and pristinamycin I, Figure S8: The biosynthetic pathways of nystatin and amphotericin B, Figure S9: The biosynthetic pathway of pimaricin.

Author Contributions: The review was written and edited by the authors H.R. and E.M.-K.

Funding: The authors and work in their laboratory are supported by the Eberhard Karls Universität Tübingen, the Deutsche Forschungsgemeinschaft (DFG), the Bundesministeriums für Bildung und Forschung (BMBF) (FKZ 031L 0018A, ERASysApp), the German Center for Infection Research (DZIF) (TTU 09.912), and Biovet (Sofia, Bulgaria).

Conflicts of Interest: The authors declare no conflict of interest.

Abbreviations

A	adenylation domain	MBC	minimum bactericidal concentration
ABC	ATP-binding cassette	MIC	minimum inhibitory concentration
ACP	acyl carrier protein	MLS_B	macrolide–lincosamide–streptogramin B
AHBA	3-amino 5-hydroxybenzoic acid	MOA	mode of action
ARO	aromatase	MRSA	methicillin-resistant *Staphylococcus aureus*
AT	acyltransferase	MT	methyltransferase domain
BGC	biosynthetic gene cluster	NADPH	nicotinamide adenine dinucleotide phosphate
C	condensation domain	NGST	Next Generation Sequencing Technologies
CABP	community-acquired bacterial pneumonia	NMR	nuclear magnetic resonance
CCR	crotonyl-CoA carboxylase/reductase	NRPS	nonribosomal peptide synthetase
CDI	*Clostridioides difficile* infection	NTG	N-methyl-N'-nitro-N-nitrosoguanidine
CLF	chain elongation factor	ORF	open reading frame
CoA	coenzyme A	PCP	peptidyl carrier protein
cryo EM	cryogenic electron microscopy	PCR	polymerase chain reaction
CYC	cyclase	PKS	polyketide synthase
DEBS	deoxyerythronolide B synthase	PTC	peptidyl transferase center
DH	dehydratase	RNA	ribonucleic acid
DNA	deoxyribonucleic acid	RNAP	RNA polymerase
dTDP	deoxythymidine diphosphate	rRNA	ribosomal RNA
E	epimerisation domain	SAM	S-adenosyl methionine
ER	enoyl reductase	SAR	structure activity relationship
ESBL	extended spectrum β-lactamase	SARP	*Streptomyces* antibiotic regulatory protein
FDA	Food and Drug Administration	Spp.	Species
GDP	guanosine diphosphate	TB	Tuberculosis
GI	gastrointestinal	TDP	thymidine diphosphate
Kb	kilobase	TE	Thioesterase
KR	ketoreductase	tRNA	transfer RNA
KS	ketosynthase	VRE	vancomycin-resistant *Enterococci*
LS_AP	Lincosamide–streptogramin A–pleuromutilin	VRSA	vancomycin-resistant *Staphylococcus aureus*
MAC	*Mycobacterium avium-intracellulare* complex	WHO	World Health Organisation

References

1. Mohammadipanah, F.; Dehhaghi, M. Classification and taxonomy of actinobacteria. In *Biology and Biotechnology of Actinobacteria*; Wink, J., Mohammadipanah, F., Hamedi, J., Eds.; Springer: Berlin/Heidelberg, Germany, 2017; pp. 51–77.
2. Barka, E.A.; Vatsa, P.; Sanchez, L.; Gaveau-Vaillant, N.; Jacquard, C.; Klenk, H.P.; Clément, C.; Ouhdouch, Y.; van Wezel, G.P. Taxonomy, physiology, and natural products of Actinobacteria. *Microbiol. Mol. Biol. Rev.* **2016**, *80*, 1–43. [CrossRef] [PubMed]
3. García, J.C.; Patrão, B.; Almeida, L.; Pérez, J.; Menezes, P.; Dias, J.; Sanz, P.J. A natural interface for remote operation of underwater robots. *IEEE Comput. Graph. Appl.* **2015**, *37*, 34–43. [CrossRef] [PubMed]
4. Cook, T.B.; Pfleger, B.F. Leveraging synthetic biology for producing bioactive polyketides and non-ribosomal peptides in bacterial heterologous hosts. *Medchemcomm* **2019**, *10*, 668–681. [CrossRef] [PubMed]
5. Abu-Melha, S. Design, Synthesis and DFT/DNP Modeling Study of New 2-Amino-5-arylazothiazole Derivatives as Potential Antibacterial Agents. *Molecules* **2018**, *23*, 434. [CrossRef] [PubMed]
6. Lenci, E.; Trabocchi, A. Smart Design of Small-Molecule Libraries: When Organic Synthesis Meets Cheminformatics. *ChemBioChem* **2019**, *20*, 1115–1123. [CrossRef] [PubMed]

7. Musiol-Kroll, E.; Wohlleben, W. Acyltransferases as tools for polyketide synthase engineering. *Antibiotics* **2018**, *7*, 62. [CrossRef]
8. Tong, Y.; Robertsen, H.L.; Blin, K.; Weber, T.; Lee, S.Y. CRISPR-Cas9 toolkit for Actinomycete genome editing. In *Synthetic Metabolic Pathways*; Springer: Berlin/Heidelberg, Germany, 2018; pp. 163–184.
9. Blin, K.; Shaw, S.; Steinke, K.; Villebro, R.; Ziemert, N.; Lee, S.Y.; Medema, M.H.; Weber, T. antiSMASH 5.0: Updates to the secondary metabolite genome mining pipeline. *Nucleic Acids Res.* **2019**, *47*, W81–W87. [CrossRef]
10. Komaki, H.; Sakurai, K.; Hosoyama, A.; Kimura, A.; Igarashi, Y.; Tamura, T. Diversity of nonribosomal peptide synthetase and polyketide synthase gene clusters among taxonomically close *Streptomyces* strains. *Sci. Rep.* **2018**, *8*, 6888. [CrossRef]
11. Nett, M.; Ikeda, H.; Moore, B.S. Genomic basis for natural product biosynthetic diversity in the actinomycetes. *Nat. Prod. Rep.* **2009**, *26*, 1362–1384. [CrossRef]
12. Santos, R.; Ursu, O.; Gaulton, A.; Bento, A.P.; Donadi, R.S.; Bologa, C.G.; Karlsson, A.; Al-Lazikani, B.; Hersey, A.; Oprea, T.I.; et al. A comprehensive map of molecular drug targets. *Nat. Rev. Drug Discov.* **2017**, *16*, 19. [CrossRef]
13. Wilson, D.N.; Harms, J.M.; Nierhaus, K.H.; Schlünzen, F.; Fucini, P. Species-specific antibiotic-ribosome interactions: Implications for drug development. *Biol. Chem.* **2005**, *386*, 1239–1252. [CrossRef]
14. Koehbach, J.; Craik, D.J. The Vast Structural Diversity of Antimicrobial Peptides. *Trends Pharmacol. Sci.* **2019**, *40*, 517–528. [CrossRef]
15. Tenover, F.C. Mechanisms of antimicrobial resistance in bacteria. *Am. J. Med.* **2006**, *119* (Suppl. 1), S3–S10; discussion S62–S70. [CrossRef]
16. Du Toit, A. Antimicrobials: Putting antibiotic action into context. *Nat. Rev. Microbiol.* **2016**, *14*, 725. [CrossRef]
17. Levy, S.B.; Marshall, B. Antibacterial resistance worldwide: Causes, challenges and responses. *Nat. Med.* **2004**, *10*, S122. [CrossRef]
18. Beckh, W.; Kulchar, G.V. Treatment-Resistant Syphilis: An Evaluation of the Causative Factors in Eighteen Cases. *Arch. Derm. Syphilol.* **1939**, *40*, 1–12. [CrossRef]
19. Andersson, D.I.; Nicoloff, H.; Hjort, K. Mechanisms and clinical relevance of bacterial heteroresistance. *Nat. Rev. Microbiol.* **2019**, *17*, 479–496. [CrossRef]
20. Hofer, U. The cost of antimicrobial resistance. *Nat. Rev. Microbiol.* **2019**, *17*, 3. [CrossRef]
21. Eagle, H. The binding of penicillin in relation to its cytotoxic action: II. The reactivity with penicillin of resistant variants of *Streptococci, Pneomocci*, and *Staphylococci*. *J. Exp. Med.* **1954**, *100*, 103–115. [CrossRef]
22. Stekel, D. First report of antimicrobial resistance pre-dates penicillin. *Nature* **2018**, *562*, 192. [CrossRef]
23. Frieri, M.; Kumar, K.; Boutin, A. Antibiotic resistance. *J. Infect. Public Health* **2017**, *10*, 369–378. [CrossRef]
24. Turner, N.A.; Sharma-Kuinkel, B.K.; Maskarinec, S.A.; Eichenberger, E.M.; Shah, P.P.; Carugati, M.; Holland, T.L.; Fowler, V.G., Jr. Methicillin-resistant *Staphylococcus aureus*: An overview of basic and clinical research. *Nat. Rev. Microbiol.* **2019**, *17*, 203–218. [CrossRef]
25. Blair, J.M.A.; Webber, M.A.; Baylay, A.J.; Ogbolu, D.O.; Piddock, L.J.V. Molecular mechanisms of antibiotic resistance. *Nat. Rev. Microbiol.* **2015**, *13*, 42. [CrossRef]
26. Kaur, P.; Peterson, E. Antibiotic resistance mechanisms in bacteria: Relationships between resistance determinants of antibiotic producers, environmental bacteria, and clinical pathogens. *Front. Microbiol.* **2018**, *9*, 2928.
27. Pambos, O.J.; Kapanidis, A.N. Tracking antibiotic mechanisms. *Nat. Rev. Microbiol.* **2019**, *17*, 201. [CrossRef]
28. Alanis, A.J. Resistance to antibiotics: Are we in the post-antibiotic era? *Arch. Med. Res.* **2005**, *36*, 697–705. [CrossRef]
29. Carroll, L.M.; Gaballa, A.; Guldimann, C.; Sullivan, G.; Henderson, L.O.; Wiedmann, M. Identification of Novel Mobilized Colistin Resistance Gene *mcr-9* in a Multidrug-Resistant, Colistin-Susceptible *Salmonella enterica* Serotype *Typhimurium* Isolate. *MBio* **2019**, *10*, e00853-19. [CrossRef]
30. World Health Organization. New report calls for urgent action to avert antimicrobial resistance crisis. *Joint News Release*. 29 April 2019. Available online: https://www.who.int/news-room/detail/29-04-2019-new-report-calls-for-urgent-action-to-avert-antimicrobial-resistance-crisis (accessed on 25 August 2019).
31. World Health Organization. Antibiotic Resistance. 2019. Available online: https://www.who.int/news-room/fact-sheets/detail/antibiotic-resistance (accessed on 25 August 2019).

32. Spellberg, B. The future of antibiotics. *Crit. Care* **2014**, *18*, 228. [CrossRef]
33. Pew Charitable Trusts. Tracking the Pipeline of Antibiotics in Development. 2019. Available online: http://www.pewtrusts.org/en/research-and-analysis/issue-briefs/2014/03/12/tracking-the-pipeline-of-antibiotics-in-development (accessed on 25 August 2019).
34. Owens, B. Solithromycin rejection chills antibiotic sector. *Nat. Biotechnol.* **2017**, *35*, 187–188. [CrossRef]
35. Weissman, K. Chapter 1 Introduction to Polyketide Biosynthesis. In *Methods in Enzymology*; Academic Press: Cambridge, MA, USA, 2009; Volume 459, pp. 3–16.
36. Shen, B. Polyketide biosynthesis beyond the type I, II and III polyketide synthase paradigms. *Curr. Opin. Chem. Biol.* **2003**, *7*, 285–295. [CrossRef]
37. Hertweck, C. The biosynthetic logic of polyketide diversity. *Angew. Chemie Int. Ed.* **2009**, *48*, 4688–4716. [CrossRef]
38. Ridley, C.P.; Lee, H.Y.; Khosla, C. Evolution of polyketide synthases in bacteria. *Proc. Natl. Acad. Sci. USA* **2008**, *105*, 4595–4600. [CrossRef]
39. Süssmuth, R.D.; Mainz, A. Nonribosomal peptide synthesis—Principles and prospects. *Angew. Chem. Int. Ed.* **2017**, *56*, 3770–3821. [CrossRef]
40. Challis, G.L.; Wilkinson, B. Biosynthetic assembly lines themed issue. *Nat. Prod. Rep.* **2016**, *33*, 120–121. [CrossRef]
41. Staunton, J.; Weissman, K.J. Polyketide biosynthesis: A millennium review. *Nat. Prod. Rep.* **2001**, *18*, 380–416. [CrossRef]
42. Helfrich, E.J.N.; Piel, J. Biosynthesis of polyketides by trans-AT polyketide synthases. *Nat. Prod. Rep.* **2016**, *33*, 231–316. [CrossRef]
43. Musiol, E.M.; Weber, T. Discrete acyltransferases involved in polyketide biosynthesis. *Medchemcomm* **2012**, *3*, 871–886. [CrossRef]
44. Meurer, G.; Gerlitz, M.; Wendt-Pienkowski, E.; Vining, L.C.; Rohr, J.; Hutchinson, C.R. Iterative type II polyketide synthases, cyclases and ketoreductases exhibit context-dependent behavior in the biosynthesis of linear and angular decapolyketides. *Chem. Biol.* **1997**, *4*, 433–443. [CrossRef]
45. Caffrey, P. Dissecting complex polyketide biosynthesis. *Comput. Struct. Biotechnol. J.* **2012**, *3*, e201210010. [CrossRef]
46. Chen, A.; Re, R.N.; Burkart, M.D. Type II fatty acid and polyketide synthases: Deciphering protein–protein and protein–substrate interactions. *Nat. Prod. Rep.* **2018**, *35*, 1029–1045. [CrossRef]
47. Herbst, D.A.; Townsend, C.A.; Maier, T. The architectures of iterative type I PKS and FAS. *Nat. Prod. Rep.* **2018**, *35*, 1046–1069. [CrossRef]
48. Chen, H.; Du, L. Iterative polyketide biosynthesis by modular polyketide synthases in bacteria. *Appl. Microbiol. Biotechnol.* **2016**, *100*, 541–557. [CrossRef]
49. Weber, T. Antibiotics: Biosynthesis, Generation of Novel Compounds. *Encycl. Ind. Biotechnol.* **2010**, 1–12. [CrossRef]
50. Bloudoff, K.; Schmeing, T.M. Structural and functional aspects of the nonribosomal peptide synthetase condensation domain superfamily: Discovery, dissection and diversity. *BBA Proteins Proteom.* **2017**, *1865*, 1587–1604. [CrossRef]
51. Miyanaga, A.; Kudo, F.; Eguchi, T. Protein–protein interactions in polyketide synthase–nonribosomal peptide synthetase hybrid assembly lines. *Nat. Prod. Rep.* **2018**, *35*, 1185–1209. [CrossRef]
52. McGuire, J.M.; Bunch, R.L.; Anderson, R.C.; Boaz, H.E.; Flynn, E.H.; Powell, H.M.; Smith, J.W. Ilotycin, a new antibiotic. *Antibiot. Chemother. (Northfield, Ill.)* **1952**, *2*, 281–283.
53. Wiley, P.F.; Gerzon, K.; Flynn, E.H.; Sigal, M.V., Jr.; Weaver, O.; Quarck, U.C.; Chauvette, R.R.; Monahan, R. Erythromycin. X. 1 Structure of Erythromycin. *J. Am. Chem. Soc.* **1957**, *79*, 6062–6070. [CrossRef]
54. Harris, D.R.; McGeachin, S.G.; Mills, H.H. The structure and stereochemistry of erythromycin A. *Tetrahedron Lett.* **1965**, *6*, 679–685. [CrossRef]
55. Cortes, J.; Haydock, S.F.; Roberts, G.A.; Bevitt, D.J.; Leadlay, P.F. An unusually large multifunctional polypeptide in the erythromycin-producing polyketide synthase of *Saccharopolyspora erythraea*. *Nature* **1990**, *348*, 176. [CrossRef]
56. Summers, R.G.; Donadio, S.; Staver, M.J.; Wendt-Pienkowski, E.; Hutchinson, C.R.; Katz, L. Sequencing and mutagenesis of genes from the erythromycin biosynthetic gene cluster of *Saccharopolyspora erythraea* that are involved in L-mycarose and D-desosamine production. *Microbiology* **1997**, *143*, 3251–3262. [CrossRef]

57. Donadio, S.; Staver, M.; McAlpine, J.; Swanson, S.J.; Katz, L. Modular Organization of Genes Required for Complex Polyketide Biosynthesis. *Science* **1991**, *252*, 675–679. [CrossRef]
58. Oliynyk, M.; Samborskyy, M.; Lester, J.B.; Mironenko, T.; Scott, N.; Dickens, S.; Haydock, S.F.; Leadlay, P.F. Complete genome sequence of the erythromycin-producing bacterium *Saccharopolyspora erythraea* NRRL23338. *Nat. Biotechnol.* **2007**, *25*, 447. [CrossRef]
59. Zhang, H.; Wang, Y.; Wu, J.; Skalina, K.; Pfeifer, B.A. Complete biosynthesis of erythromycin A and designed analogs using *E. coli* as a heterologous host. *Chem. Biol.* **2010**, *17*, 1232–1240. [CrossRef]
60. Weissman, K.J. Genetic engineering of modular PKSs: From combinatorial biosynthesis to synthetic biology. *Nat. Prod. Rep.* **2016**, *33*, 203–230. [CrossRef]
61. Kibwage, I.O.; Hoogmartens, J.; Roets, E.; Vanderhaeghe, H.; Verbist, L.; Dubost, M.; Pascal, C.; Petitjean, P.; Levol, G. Antibacterial activities of erythromycins A, B, C, and D and some of their derivatives. *Antimicrob. Agents Chemother.* **1985**, *28*, 630–633. [CrossRef]
62. Amsden, G.W. Erythromycin, clarithromycin, and azithromycin: Are the differences real? *Clin. Ther.* **1996**, *18*, 56–72. [CrossRef]
63. Mazzei, T.; Mini, E.; Novelli, A.; Periti, P. Chemistry and mode of action of macrolides. *J. Antimicrob. Chemother.* **1993**, *31*, 1–9. [CrossRef]
64. Vester, B.; Douthwaite, S. Macrolide resistance conferred by base substitutions in 23S rRNA. *Antimicrob. Agents Chemother.* **2001**, *45*, 1–12. [CrossRef]
65. Tenson, T.; Lovmar, M.; Ehrenberg, M. The mechanism of action of macrolides, lincosamides and streptogramin B reveals the nascent peptide exit path in the ribosome. *J. Mol. Biol.* **2003**, *330*, 1005–1014. [CrossRef]
66. Svetlov, M.S.; Plessa, E.; Chen, C.W.; Bougas, A.; Krokidis, M.G.; Dinos, G.P.; Polikanov, Y.S. High-resolution crystal structures of ribosome-bound chloramphenicol and erythromycin provide the ultimate basis for their competition. *RNA* **2019**, *25*, 600–606. [CrossRef]
67. Sobin, B.A.; English, A.R.; Celmer, W.D. PA 105, a new antibiotic. In *Antibiotics Annual*; Welch, H., Marti-Ibannez, F., Eds.; Medical Encyclopedia Inc.: New York, NY, USA, 1955; pp. 827–830.
68. English, A.R.; McBride, T.J.; Van Halsema, G.; Caklozzi, M. Biologic studies on PA 775, a combination of tetracycline and oleandomycin with synergistic activity. *Antibiot. Chemother.* **1956**, *6*, 511–522.
69. Podolsky, S.H. *The Antibiotic Era: Reform, Resistance, and the Pursuit of a Rational Therapeutics*; JHU Press: Baltimore, MD, USA, 2015; pp. 1–328.
70. Albouy, R.; Duchesnay, G.; Eloy, P.; Pestel, M.; Ravina, A.; Rey, M. A new French antibiotic: Spiramycin. *Antibiot. Annu.* **1955**, *3*, 223.
71. Kellow, W.F.; Lepper, M.H.; Plaut, S.; Rosenthal, I.M.; Spies, H.W. Spiramycin in the treatment of infection. *Antibiot. Annu.* **1955**, *3*, 658.
72. Sutherland, R. Spiramycin: A reappraisal of its antibacterial activity. *Br. J. Pharmacol. Chemother.* **1962**, *19*, 99–110. [CrossRef]
73. Fernandes, P.; Martens, E.; Pereira, D. Nature nurtures the design of new semi-synthetic macrolide antibiotics. *J. Antibiot. (Tokyo)* **2016**, *70*, 527. [CrossRef]
74. Barry, A.L.; Jones, R.N.; Thornsberry, C. In vitro activities of azithromycin (CP 62,993), clarithromycin (A-56268; TE-031), erythromycin, roxithromycin, and clindamycin. *Antimicrob. Agents Chemother.* **1988**, *32*, 752–754. [CrossRef]
75. Watanabe, Y.; Moritomo, S.; Adachi, T.; Kashimure, M.; Asaka, T. Chemical modification of erythromycin. IX. 1. *J. Antibiot. (Tokyo)* **1993**, *46*, 647–660. [CrossRef]
76. Barlam, T.; Neu, H.C. In vitro comparison of the activity of RU 28965, a new macrolide, with that of erythromycin against aerobic and anaerobic bacteria. *Antimicrob. Agents Chemother.* **1984**, *25*, 529–531. [CrossRef]
77. Jorgensen, J.H.; Redding, J.S.; Howell, A.W. In vitro *activity* of the new macrolide antibiotic roxithromycin (RU 28965) against clinical isolates of *Haemophilus influenzae*. *Antimicrob. Agents Chemother.* **1986**, *29*, 921–922. [CrossRef]
78. Mutak, S. Azalides from azithromycin to new azalide derivatives. *J. Antibiot. (Tokyo)* **2007**, *60*, 85. [CrossRef]
79. Retsema, J.; Girard, A.; Schelkly, W.; Manousos, M.; Anderson, M.; Bright, G.; Borovoy, R.; Brennan, L.; Mason, R. Spectrum and mode of action of azithromycin (CP-62,993), a new 15-membered-ring macrolide with improved potency against gram-negative organisms. *Antimicrob. Agents Chemother.* **1987**, *31*, 1939–1947. [CrossRef]

80. Bryskier, A. Ketolides—Telithromycin, an example of a new class of antibacterial agents. *Clin. Microbiol. Infect.* **2000**, *6*, 661–669. [CrossRef]
81. Ednie, L.M.; Jacobs, M.R.; Appelbaum, P.C. Comparative antianaerobic activities of the ketolides HMR 3647 (RU 66647) and HMR 3004 (RU 64004). *Antimicrob. Agents Chemother.* **1997**, *41*, 2019–2022. [CrossRef]
82. Ross, D.B. The FDA and the case of Ketek. *N. Engl. J. Med.* **2007**, *356*, 1601–1604. [CrossRef]
83. McGhee, P.; Clark, C.; Kosowska-Shick, K.M.; Nagai, K.; Dewasse, B.; Beachel, L.; Appelbaum, P.C. In vitro activity of CEM-101 against *Streptococcus pneumoniae* and *Streptococcus pyogenes* with defined macrolide resistance mechanisms. *Antimicrob. Agents Chemother.* **2010**, *54*, 230–238. [CrossRef]
84. Rodvold, K.A.; Gotfried, M.H.; Chugh, R.; Gupta, M.; Friedland, H.D.; Bhatia, A. Comparison of plasma and intrapulmonary concentrations of nafithromycin (WCK 4873) in healthy adult subjects. *Antimicrob. Agents Chemother.* **2017**, *61*, e01096-17. [CrossRef]
85. World Health Organisation. Antibacterial Agents in Clinical Development. 2018. Available online: https://apps.who.int/iris/handle/10665/275487 (accessed on 25 August 2019).
86. McGuire, J.M.; Boniece, W.S.; Higgens, C.E.; Hoehn, M.M.; Stark, W.M.; Westhead, J.; Wolfe, R.N. Tylosin, a New Antibiotic: I. Microbiological Studies. *Antibiot. Chemother.* **1961**, *11*, 320–327.
87. Cundliffe, E.; Bate, N.; Butler, A.; Fish, S.; Gandecha, A.; Merson-Davies, L. The tylosin-biosynthetic genes of *Streptomyces fradiae*. *Antonie Van Leeuwenhoek* **2001**, *79*, 229–234. [CrossRef]
88. Baltz, R.H.; Seno, E.T. Genetics of *Streptomyces fradiae* and tylosin biosynthesis. *Annu. Rev. Microbiol.* **1988**, *42*, 547–574. [CrossRef]
89. Tejedor, F.; Ballesta, J.P.G. Ribosome structure: Binding site of macrolides studied by photoaffinity labeling. *Biochemistry* **1985**, *24*, 467–472. [CrossRef]
90. Ose, E.E. In vitro antibacterial properties of EL-870, a new semi-synthetic macrolide antibiotic. *J. Antibiot. (Tokyo)* **1987**, *40*, 190–194. [CrossRef]
91. Debono, M.; Willard, K.E.; Kirst, H.A.; Wind, J.A.; Crouse, G.D.; Tao, E.V.; Vicenzi, J.T.; Counter, F.T.; Ott, J.L.; Ose, E.E.; et al. Synthesis and antimicrobial evaluation of 20-deoxo-20-(3,5-dimethylpiperidin-1-yl) desmycosin (tilmicosin, EL-870) and related cyclic amino derivatives. *J. Antibiot. (Tokyo)* **1989**, *42*, 1253–1267. [CrossRef]
92. Michael, G.B.; Eidam, C.; Kadlec, K.; Meyer, K.; Sweeney, M.T.; Murray, R.W.; Watts, J.L.; Schwarz, S. Increased MICs of gamithromycin and tildipirosin in the presence of the genes *erm (42)* and *msr(E)-mph(E)* for bovine *Pasteurella multocida* and *Mannheimia haemolytica*. *J. Antimicrob. Chemother.* **2012**, *67*, 1555–1557. [CrossRef]
93. Menge, M.; Rose, M.; Bohland, C.; Zschiesche, E.; Kilp, S.; Metz, W.; Allan, M.; Röpke, R.; Nürnberger, M. Pharmacokinetics of tildipirosin in bovine plasma, lung tissue, and bronchial fluid (from live, nonanesthetized cattle). *J. Vet. Pharmacol. Ther.* **2012**, *35*, 550–559. [CrossRef]
94. Evans, N.A. Tulathromycin: An overview of a new triamilide antimicrobial for livestock respiratory disease. *Vet. Ther.* **2005**, *6*, 83.
95. Huang, R.A.; Letendre, L.T.; Banav, N.; Fischer, J.; Somerville, B. Pharmacokinetics of gamithromycin in cattle with comparison of plasma and lung tissue concentrations and plasma antibacterial activity. *J. Vet. Pharmacol. Ther.* **2010**, *33*, 227–237. [CrossRef]
96. Agtarap, A.; Chamberlin, J.W.; Pinkerton, M.; Steinrauf, L.K. Structure of monensic acid, a new biologically active compound. *J. Am. Chem. Soc.* **1967**, *89*, 5737–5739. [CrossRef]
97. Chapman, H.D.; Jeffers, T.K.; Williams, R.B. Forty years of monensin for the control of coccidiosis in poultry. *Poult. Sci.* **2010**, *89*, 1788–1801. [CrossRef]
98. Oliynyk, M.; Stark, C.B.; Bhatt, A.; Jones, M.A.; Hughes-Thomas, Z.A.; Wilkinson, C.; Oliynyk, Z.; Demydchuk, Y.; Staunton, J.; Leadlay, P.F. Analysis of the biosynthetic gene cluster for the polyether antibiotic monensin in *Streptomyces cinnamonensis* and evidence for the role of *monB* and *monC* genes in oxidative cyclization. *Mol. Microbiol.* **2003**, *49*, 1179–1190. [CrossRef]
99. Goodrich, R.D.; Garrett, J.E.; Gast, D.R.; Kirick, M.A.; Larson, D.A.; Meiske, J.C. Influence of monensin on the performance of cattle. *J. Anim. Sci.* **1984**, *58*, 1484–1498. [CrossRef]
100. Hochlowski, J.E.; Swanson, S.J.; Ranfranz, L.M.; Whittern, D.N.; Buko, A.M.; McAlpine, J.B. Tiacumicins, A Novel Complex of 18-Membered Macrolides. *J. Antibiot. (Tokyo)* **1987**, *40*, 575–588. [CrossRef]

101. Xiao, Y.; Li, S.; Niu, S.; Ma, L.; Zhang, G.; Zhang, H.; Zhang, G.; Ju, J.; Zhang, C. Characterization of tiacumicin B biosynthetic gene cluster affording diversified tiacumicin analogues and revealing a tailoring dihalogenase. *J. Am. Chem. Soc.* **2011**, *133*, 1092–1105. [CrossRef]
102. Swanson, R.N.; Hardy, D.J.; Shipkowitz, N.L.; Hanson, C.W.; Ramer, N.C.; Fernandes, P.B.; Clement, J.J. In vitro and in vivo evaluation of tiacumicins B and C against *Clostridium difficile*. *Antimicrob. Agents Chemother.* **1991**, *35*, 1108–1111. [CrossRef]
103. Lin, W.; Das, K.; Degen, D.; Mazumder, A.; Duchi, D.; Wang, D.; Ebright, Y.W.; Ebright, R.Y.; Sineva, E.; Gigliotti, M.; et al. Structural Basis of Transcription Inhibition by Fidaxomicin (Lipiarmycin A3). *Mol. Cell* **2018**, *70*, 60–71.e15. [CrossRef]
104. Prelog, V.; Oppolzer, W. Ansamycine, eine neuartige Klasse von mikrobiellen Stoffwechselprodukten. *Helv. Chim. Acta* **1973**, *56*, 2279–2287. [CrossRef]
105. Floss, H.G.; Yu, T.W. Rifamycin mode of action, resistance, and biosynthesis. *Chem. Rev.* **2005**, *105*, 621–632. [CrossRef]
106. Sensi, P.; Margalith, P.; Timbal, M.T. Rifomycin, a new antibiotic; preliminary report. *Farm. Sci.* **1959**, *14*, 146.
107. August, P.R.; Tang, L.; Yoon, Y.J.; Ning, S.; Müller, R.; Yu, T.W.; Taylor, M.; Hoffmann, D.; Kim, C.G.; Zhang, X.; et al. Biosynthesis of the ansamycin antibiotic rifamycin: Deductions from the molecular analysis of the rif biosynthetic gene cluster of *Amycolatopsis mediterranei* S699. *Chem. Biol.* **1998**, *5*, 69–79. [CrossRef]
108. Watanabe, K.; Rude, M.A.; Walsh, C.T.; Khosla, C. Engineered biosynthesis of an ansamycin polyketide precursor in *Escherichia coli*. *Proc. Natl. Acad. Sci. USA* **2003**, *100*, 9774–9778. [CrossRef]
109. Hoy, S.M. Rifamycin SV MMX®: A Review in the Treatment of Traveller's Diarrhoea. *Clin. Drug Investig.* **2019**, *39*, 691–697. [CrossRef]
110. Maggi, N.; Pasqualucci, C.R.; Ballotta, R.; Sensi, P. Rifampicin: A new orally active rifamycin. *Chemotherapy* **1966**, *11*, 285–292. [CrossRef]
111. Campbell, E.A.; Korzheva, N.; Mustaev, A.; Murakami, K.; Nair, S.; Goldfarb, A.; Darst, S.A. Structural mechanism for rifampicin inhibition of bacterial RNA polymerase. *Cell* **2001**, *104*, 901–912. [CrossRef]
112. Della Bruna, C.; Schioppacassi, G.; Ungheri, D.; Jabès, D.; Morvillo, E.; Sanfilippo, A. LM 427, a new spiropiperidylrifamycin: In vitro and in vivo studies. *J. Antibiot. (Tokyo)* **1983**, *36*, 1502–1506. [CrossRef]
113. Brogden, R.N.; Fitton, A. Rifabutin. *Drugs* **1994**, *47*, 983–1009. [CrossRef]
114. Kunin, C.M. Antimicrobial activity of rifabutin. *Clin. Infect. Dis.* **1996**, *22*, S3–S14. [CrossRef]
115. Jarvis, B.; Lamb, H.M. Rifapentine. *Drugs* **1998**, *56*, 607–616. [CrossRef]
116. Scarpignato, C.; Pelosini, I. Rifaximin, a poorly absorbed antibiotic: Pharmacology and clinical potential. *Chemotherapy* **2005**, *51*, 36–66. [CrossRef]
117. Koo, H.L.; DuPont, H.L. Rifaximin: A unique gastrointestinal-selective antibiotic for enteric diseases. *Curr. Opin. Gastroenterol.* **2010**, *26*, 17. [CrossRef]
118. Fodor, A.A.; Pimentel, M.; Chey, W.D.; Lembo, A.; Golden, P.L.; Israel, R.J.; Carroll, I.M. Rifaximin is associated with modest, transient decreases in multiple taxa in the gut microbiota of patients with diarrhoea-predominant irritable bowel syndrome. *Gut Microbes* **2019**, *10*, 22–33. [CrossRef]
119. Mosaei, H.; Molodtsov, V.; Kepplinger, B.; Harbottle, J.; Moon, C.W.; Jeeves, R.E.; Ceccaroni, L.; Shin, Y.; Morton-Laing, S.; Marrs, E.C.L.; et al. Mode of Action of Kanglemycin A, an Ansamycin Natural Product that Is Active against Rifampicin-Resistant *Mycobacterium tuberculosis*. *Mol. Cell* **2018**, *72*, 263–274.e5. [CrossRef]
120. Peek, J.; Lilic, M.; Montiel, D.; Milshteyn, A.; Woodworth, I.; Biggins, J.B.; Ternei, M.A.; Calle, P.Y.; Danziger, M.; Warrier, T.; et al. Rifamycin congeners kanglemycins are active against rifampicin-resistant bacteria via a distinct mechanism. *Nat. Commun.* **2018**, *9*, 4147. [CrossRef]
121. Finlay, A.C.; Hobby, G.L. Terramycin, a new antibiotic. *Science* **1950**, 85–87. [CrossRef]
122. Thomas, R.; Williams, D.J. Oxytetracycline biosynthesis: Origin of the carboxamide substituent. *J. Chem. Soc. Chem. Commun.* **1983**, 677–679. [CrossRef]
123. Chopra, I.; Roberts, M. Tetracycline antibiotics: Mode of action, applications, molecular biology, and epidemiology of bacterial resistance. *Microbiol. Mol. Biol. Rev.* **2001**, *65*, 232–260. [CrossRef]
124. Brodersen, D.E.; Clemons, W.M., Jr.; Carter, A.P.; Morgan-Warren, R.J.; Wimberly, B.T.; Ramakrishnan, V. The structural basis for the action of the antibiotics tetracycline, pactamycin, and hygromycin B on the 30S ribosomal subunit. *Cell* **2000**, *103*, 1143–1154. [CrossRef]
125. Duggar, B.M. Aureomycin: A product of the continuing search for new antibiotics. *Ann. N. Y. Acad. Sci.* **1948**, *51*, 177–181. [CrossRef]

126. Zhu, T.; Cheng, X.; Liu, Y.; Deng, Z.; You, D. Deciphering and engineering of the final step halogenase for improved chlortetracycline biosynthesis in industrial *Streptomyces aureofaciens*. *Metab. Eng.* **2013**, *19*, 69–78. [CrossRef]
127. Nguyen, F.; Starosta, A.L.; Arenz, S.; Sohmen, D.; Dönhöfer, A.; Wilson, D.N. Tetracycline antibiotics and resistance mechanisms. *Biol. Chem.* **2014**, *395*, 559–575. [CrossRef]
128. Stephens, C.R.; Beereboom, J.J.; Rennhard, H.H.; Gordon, P.N.; Murai, K.; Blackwood, R.K.; von Wittenau, M.S. 6-Deoxytetracyclines. IV.1,2 Preparation, C-6 Stereochemistry, and Reactions. *J. Am. Chem. Soc.* **1963**, *85*, 2643–2652. [CrossRef]
129. McCormick, J.R.D.; Sjolander, N.O.; Hirsch, U.; Jensen, E.R.; Doerschuk, A.P. A new family of antibiotics: The demethyltetracyclines. *J. Am. Chem. Soc.* **1957**, *79*, 4561–4563. [CrossRef]
130. McCormick, J.R.D.; Hirsch, U.; Sjolander, N.O.; Doerschuk, A.P. Cosynthesis of tetracyclines by pairs of *Streptomyces aureofaciens* mutants. *J. Am. Chem. Soc.* **1960**, *82*, 5006–5007. [CrossRef]
131. Martell, M.J.; Boothe, J.H. The 6-deoxytetracyclines. VII. Alkylated aminotetracyclines possessing unique antibacterial activity. *J. Med. Chem.* **1967**, *10*, 44–46. [CrossRef]
132. Zakeri, B.; Wright, G.D. Chemical biology of tetracycline antibiotics. *Biochem. Cell Biol.* **2008**, *86*, 124–136. [CrossRef]
133. Sum, P.E.; Lee, V.J.; Testa, R.T.; Hlavka, J.J.; Ellestad, G.A.; Bloom, J.D.; Gluzman, Y.; Tally, F.P. Glycylcyclines. 1. A new generation of potent antibacterial agents through modification of 9-aminotetracyclines. *J. Med. Chem.* **1994**, *37*, 184–188. [CrossRef]
134. Petersen, P.J.; Jacobus, N.V.; Weiss, W.J.; Sum, P.E.; Testa, R.T. In vitro and in vivo antibacterial activities of a novel glycylcycline, the 9-t-butylglycylamido derivative of minocycline (GAR-936). *Antimicrob. Agents Chemother.* **1999**, *43*, 738–744. [CrossRef]
135. Bergeron, J.; Ammirati, M.; Danley, D.; James, L.; Norcia, M.; Retsema, J.; Strick, C.A.; Su, W.G.; Sutcliffe, J.; Wondrack, L. Glycylcyclines bind to the high-affinity tetracycline ribosomal binding site and evade Tet(M)-and Tet(O)-mediated ribosomal protection. *Antimicrob. Agents Chemother.* **1996**, *40*, 2226–2228. [CrossRef]
136. Nelson, M.L.; Ismail, M.Y.; McIntyre, L.; Bhatia, B.; Viski, P.; Hawkins, P.; Rennie, G.; Andorsky, D.; Messersmith, D.; Stapleton, K.; et al. Versatile and facile synthesis of diverse semisynthetic tetracycline derivatives via Pd-catalyzed reactions. *J. Org. Chem.* **2003**, *68*, 5838–5851. [CrossRef]
137. Draper, M.P.; Weir, S.; Macone, A.; Donatelli, J.; Trieber, C.A.; Tanaka, S.K.; Levy, S.B. Mechanism of action of the novel aminomethylcycline antibiotic omadacycline. *Antimicrob. Agents Chemother.* **2014**, *58*, 1279–1283. [CrossRef]
138. Dougherty, J.A.; Sucher, A.J.; Chahine, E.B.; Shihadeh, K.C. Omadacycline: A New Tetracycline Antibiotic. *Ann. Pharmacother.* **2019**, *53*, 486–500. [CrossRef]
139. Sun, C.; Wang, Q.; Brubaker, J.D.; Wright, P.M.; Lerner, C.D.; Noson, K.; Charest, M.; Siegel, D.R.; Wang, Y.M.; Myers, A.G.; et al. A robust platform for the synthesis of new tetracycline antibiotics. *J. Am. Chem. Soc.* **2008**, *130*, 17913–17927. [CrossRef]
140. Grossman, T.H.; Starosta, A.L.; Fyfe, C.; O'Brien, W.; Rothstein, D.M.; Mikolajka, A.; Wilson, D.N.; Sutcliffe, J.A. Target-and resistance-based mechanistic studies with TP-434, a novel fluorocycline antibiotic. *Antimicrob. Agents Chemother.* **2012**, *56*, 2559–2564. [CrossRef]
141. Lee, Y.R.; Burton, C.E. Eravacycline, a newly approved fluorocycline. *Eur. J. Clin. Microbiol. Infect. Dis.* **2019**, 1–8. [CrossRef]
142. Zhanel, G.; Critchley, I.; Lin, L.Y.; Alvandi, N. Microbiological profile of sarecycline, a novel targeted spectrum tetracycline for the treatment of acne vulgaris. *Antimicrob. Agents Chemother.* **2019**, *63*, e01297-18. [CrossRef]
143. Grossman, T.H.; Fyfe, C.; O'Brien, W.; Hackel, M.; Minyard, M.B.; Waites, K.B.; Dubois, J.; Murphy, T.M.; Slee, A.M.; Weiss, W.J.; et al. Fluorocycline TP-271 Is Potent against Complicated Community-Acquired Bacterial Pneumonia Pathogens. *mSphere* **2017**, *2*, e00004-17. [CrossRef]
144. Liu, F.; Myers, A.G. Development of a platform for the discovery and practical synthesis of new tetracycline antibiotics. *Curr. Opin. Chem. Biol.* **2016**, *32*, 48–57. [CrossRef]
145. Tetraphase-Pharmaceuticals. Pipeline. Available online: https://www.tphase.com/products/pipeline/ (accessed on 25 August 2019).
146. Preud'homme, J.; Tarridec, P.; Belloc, A. 90. Isolation, characterization and identification of the components of pristinamycin. *Bull. Soc. Chim. Fr.* **1968**, *2*, 585–591.

147. Celmer, W.D.; Sobin, B.A. The isolation of two synergistic antibiotics from a single fermentation source. *Antibiot. Annu.* **1955**, *3*, 437–441.
148. Mast, Y.; Weber, T.; Gölz, M.; Ort-Winklbauer, R.; Gondran, A.; Wohlleben, W.; Schinko, E. Characterization of the 'pristinamycin supercluster'of *Streptomyces pristinaespiralis*. *Microb. Biotechnol.* **2011**, *4*, 192–206. [CrossRef]
149. Cocito, C.; Di Giambattista, M.; Nyssen, E.; Vannuffel, P. Inhibition of protein synthesis by streptogramins and related antibiotics. *J. Antimicrob. Chemother.* **1997**, *39* (Suppl. A), 7–13. [CrossRef]
150. Bouanchaud, D.H. In vitro and in vivo antibacterial activity of quinupristin/dalfopristin. *J. Antimicrob. Chemother.* **1997**, *39*, 15–21. [CrossRef]
151. Harms, J.M.; Schlünzen, F.; Fucini, P.; Bartels, H.; Yonath, A. Alterations at the peptidyl transferase centre of the ribosome induced by the synergistic action of the streptogramins dalfopristin and quinupristin. *BMC Biol.* **2004**, *2*, 4. [CrossRef] [PubMed]
152. Barriere, J.C.; Bouanchaud, D.H.; Paris, J.M.; Rolin, O.; Harris, N.V.; Smith, C. Antimicrobial activity against *Staphylococcus aureus* of semisynthetic injectable streptogramins: RP 59500 and related compounds. *J. Antimicrob. Chemother.* **1992**, *30*, 1–8. [CrossRef] [PubMed]
153. Finch, R.G. Antibacterial Activity of Quinupristin/Dalfopristin. *Drugs* **1996**, *51*, 31–37. [CrossRef] [PubMed]
154. Politano, A.D.; Sawyer, R.G. NXL-103, a combination of flopristin and linopristin, for the potential treatment of bacterial infections including community-acquired pneumonia and MRSA. *Curr. Opin. Investig. Drugs (Lond. UK 2000)* **2010**, *11*, 225.
155. Noeske, J.; Huang, J.; Olivier, N.B.; Giacobbe, R.A.; Zambrowski, M.; Cate, J.H.D. Synergy of streptogramin antibiotics occurs independently of their effects on translation. *Antimicrob. Agents Chemother.* **2014**, *58*, 5269–5279. [CrossRef]
156. Hazen, E.L.; Brown, R. Fungicidin, an Antibiotic Produced by a Soil Actinomycete. *Proc. Soc. Exp. Biol. Med.* **1951**, *76*, 93–97. [CrossRef] [PubMed]
157. Hazen, E.L.; Brown, R.; Mason, A. Protective action of fungicidin (nystatin) in mice against virulence enhancing activity of oxytetracycline on *Candida albicans*. *Antibiot. Chemother. (Northfield, Ill.)* **1953**, *3*, 1125.
158. Brautaset, T.; Sekurova, O.N.; Sletta, H.; Ellingsen, T.E.; Strøm, A.R.; Valla, S.; Zotchev, S.B. Biosynthesis of the polyene antifungal antibiotic nystatin in *Streptomyces noursei* ATCC 11455: Analysis of the gene cluster and deduction of the biosynthetic pathway. *Chem. Biol.* **2000**, *7*, 395–403. [CrossRef]
159. Bolard, J. How do the polyene macrolide antibiotics affect the cellular membrane properties? *BBA Rev. Biomembr.* **1986**, *864*, 257–304. [CrossRef]
160. Brautaset, T.; Sletta, H.; Nedal, A.; Borgos, S.E.; Degnes, K.F.; Bakke, I.; Volokhan, O.; Sekurova, O.N.; Treshalin, I.D.; Mirchink, E.P.; et al. Improved antifungal polyene macrolides via engineering of the nystatin biosynthetic genes in *Streptomyces noursei*. *Chem. Biol.* **2008**, *15*, 1198–1206. [CrossRef]
161. Biosergen. BSG005 for Systemic Fungal Infections. Available online: http://biosergen.se/products-pipeline/bsg005-for-systemic-fungal-infections/ (accessed on 25 August 2019).
162. Dutcher, J.D. The Discovery and Development of Amphotericin B. *Dis. Chest* **1968**, *54*, 296–298. [CrossRef] [PubMed]
163. McNamara, C.; Crawforth, J.; Hickman, B.; Norwood, T.; Rawlings, B. Biosynthesis of amphotericin B. *J. Chem. Soc. Perkin Trans. 1* **1998**, 83–88. [CrossRef]
164. Brajtburg, J.; Powderly, W.G.; Kobayashi, G.S.; Medoff, G. Amphotericin B: Current understanding of mechanisms of action. *Antimicrob. Agents Chemother.* **1990**, *34*, 183. [CrossRef] [PubMed]
165. Clemons, K.V.; Stevens, D.A. Comparative Efficacies of Four Amphotericin B Formulations—Fungizone, Amphotec (Amphocil), AmBisome, and Abelcet—Against Systemic Murine Aspergillosis. *Antimicrob. Agents Chemother.* **2004**, *48*, 1047–1050. [CrossRef] [PubMed]
166. Struyk, A.P.; Drost, G.; Haisvisz, J.M.; van Eek, T.; Hoogerheide, J.C. Pimaricin, a new antifungal antibiotic. In *Antibiotics Annual 1957–1958*; Welch, H., Marti-Ibanez, F., Eds.; Medical Encyclopedia, Inc.: New York, NY, USA, 1958; pp. 878–885.
167. Aparicio, J.F.; Fouces, R.; Mendes, M.V.; Olivera, N.; Martín, J.F. A complex multienzyme system encoded by five polyketide synthase genes is involved in the biosynthesis of the 26-membered polyene macrolide pimaricin in *Streptomyces natalensis*. *Chem. Biol.* **2000**, *7*, 895–905. [CrossRef]
168. Ansari, Z.; Miller, D.; Galor, A. Current thoughts in fungal keratitis: Diagnosis and treatment. *Curr. Fungal Infect. Rep.* **2013**, *7*, 209–218. [CrossRef] [PubMed]

169. Te Welscher, Y.M.; van Leeuwen, M.R.; de Kruijff, B.; Dijksterhuis, J.; Breukink, E. Polyene antibiotic that inhibits membrane transport proteins. *Proc. Natl. Acad. Sci. USA* **2012**, *109*, 11156–11159. [CrossRef]
170. Ma, C.X.; Lv, W.; Li, Y.X.; Fan, B.Z.; Han, X.; Kong, F.S.; Tian, J.C.; Cushman, M.; Liang, J.H. Design, synthesis and structure-activity relationships of novel macrolones: Hybrids of 2-fluoro 9-oxime ketolides and carbamoyl quinolones with highly improved activity against resistant pathogens. *Eur. J. Med. Chem.* **2019**, *169*, 1–20. [CrossRef]
171. Ma, C.; Ma, S. Various novel erythromycin derivatives obtained by different modifications: Recent advance in macrolide antibiotics. *Mini Rev. Med. Chem.* **2010**, *10*, 272–286. [CrossRef]
172. Jelić, D.; Antolović, R. From erythromycin to azithromycin and new potential ribosome-binding antimicrobials. *Antibiotics* **2016**, *5*, 29. [CrossRef]
173. Aronoff, S.C.; Laurent, C.; Jacobs, M.R. In vitro activity of erythromycin, roxithromycin and CP 62993 against common paediatric pathogens. *J. Antimicrob. Chemother.* **1987**, *19*, 275–276. [CrossRef] [PubMed]
174. Schlünzen, F.; Harms, J.M.; Franceschi, F.; Hansen, H.A.S.; Bartels, H.; Zarivach, R.; Yonath, A. Structural basis for the antibiotic activity of ketolides and azalides. *Structure* **2003**, *11*, 329–338. [CrossRef]
175. Ackermann, G.; Rodloff, A.C. Drugs of the 21st century: Telithromycin (HMR 3647)—The first ketolide. *J. Antimicrob. Chemother.* **2003**, *51*, 497–511. [CrossRef] [PubMed]
176. Bonnefoy, A.; Girard, A.M.; Agouridas, C.; Chantot, J.F. Ketolides lack inducibility properties of MLS (B) resistance phenotype. *J. Antimicrob. Chemother.* **1997**, *40*, 85–90. [CrossRef] [PubMed]
177. Douthwaite, S. Structure-activity relationships of ketolides vs. macrolides. *Clin. Microbiol. Infect.* **2001**, *7*, 11–17. [CrossRef] [PubMed]
178. Brockmann, H.; Henkel, W. Pikromycin, ein bitter schmeckendes Antibioticum aus Actinomyceten (Antibiotica aus Actinomyceten, VI. Mitteil. *Chem. Ber.* **1951**, *84*, 284–288. [CrossRef]
179. Weinstein, M.J.; Wagman, G.H.; Marquez, J.A.; Testa, R.T.; Oden, E.; Waitz, J.A. Megalomicin, a new macrolide antibiotic complex produced by *Micromonospora*. *J. Antibiot. (Tokyo)* **1969**, *22*, 253–258. [CrossRef] [PubMed]
180. Garrod, L.P. The erythromycin group of antibiotics. *Br. Med. J.* **1957**, *2*, 57. [CrossRef] [PubMed]
181. Pinnerts-Indico, S. Une nouvelle espèce de *Streptomyces* productrice d'antibiotiques: *Streptomyces ambofaciens* n. sp. *Ann. L Inst. Pasteur* **1954**, *87*, 702–707.
182. Rubinstein, E.; Keller, N. Spiramycin renaissance. *J. Antimicrob. Chemother.* **1998**, *42*, 572–576. [CrossRef]
183. Kanfer, I.; Skinner, M.F.; Walker, R.B. Analysis of macrolide antibiotics. *J. Chromatogr. A* **1998**, *812*, 255–286. [CrossRef]
184. Washington, J.A.; Wilson, W.R. Erythromycin: A Microbial and Clinical Perspective after 30 Years of Clinical Use (Second of Two Parts). *Mayo Clin. Proc.* **1985**, *60*, 271–278. [CrossRef]
185. Papich, M.G. Tylosin. In *Saunders Handbook of Veterinary Drugs-E-Book: Small and Large Animal*; Elsevier Health Sciences: St. Louis, MO, USA, 2015; pp. 826–827.
186. Denny, C.B.; Sharpe, L.E.; Bohrer, C.W. Effects of tylosin and nisin on canned food spoilage bacteria. *Appl. Microbiol.* **1961**, *9*, 108. [PubMed]
187. Denny, C.B.; Bohrer, C.W. Effect of antibiotics on the thermal death rate of spores of food spoilage organisms. *J. Food Sci.* **1959**, *24*, 247–252. [CrossRef]
188. Hamill, R.L.; Haney, M.E., Jr.; Stamper, M.; Wlley, P.F. Tylosin, a New Antibiotic: II. Isolation, Properties, and Preparation of Pesmycosin, a Microbiologically Active Degradation Product. *Antibiot. Chemother.* **1961**, *11*, 328–334.
189. Stark, W.M.; Daily, W.A.; McGuire, J.M. A fermentation study of the biosynthesis of tylosin in synthetic media. *Sci. Rep. Ist. Super. Sanita* **1961**, *1*, 340–354. [PubMed]
190. Pape, H.; Brillinger, G.U. Metabolic products of microorganisms. 113. Biosynthesis of thymidine diphospho mycarose in a cell-free system from *Streptomyces rimosus*. *Arch. Mikrobiol.* **1973**, *88*, 25. [CrossRef]
191. Jensen, A.L.; Darken, M.A.; Schultz, J.S.; Shay, A.J. Relomycin: Flask and Tank Fermentation Studies. *Antimicrob. Agents Chemother.* **1963**, *161*, 49–53.
192. Hamill, R.L.; Stark, W.M. Macromicin, a new antibiotic, and Lactenocin, an active degradation product. *J. Antibiot. (Tokyo)* **1964**, *17*, 133–139.
193. Whaley, H.A.; Patterson, E.L.; Dornbush, A.C.; Backus, E.J.; Bohonos, N. Isolation and characterization of relomycin, a new antibiotic. *Antimicrob. Agents Chemother.* **1963**, *161*, 45.
194. Roets, E.; Beirinckx, P.; Quintens, I.; Hoogmartens, J. Quantitative analysis of tylosin by column liquid chromatography. *J. Chromatogr. A* **1993**, *630*, 159–166. [CrossRef]

195. Loke, M.L.; Ingerslev, F.; Halling-Sørensen, B.; Tjørnelund, J. Stability of tylosin A in manure containing test systems determined by high performance liquid chromatography. *Chemosphere* **2000**, *40*, 759–765. [CrossRef]
196. Cox, K.L.; Fishman, S.E.; Larson, J.L.; Stanzak, R.; Reynolds, P.A.; Yeh, W.K.; van Frank, R.M.; Birmingham, V.A.; Hershberger, C.L.; Seno, E.T. The use of recombinant DNA techniques to study tylosin biosynthesis and resistance in *Streptomyces fradiae*. *J. Nat. Prod.* **1986**, *49*, 971–980. [CrossRef]
197. Merson-Davies, L.A.; Cundiiffe, E. Analysis of five tylosin biosynthetic genes from the *tylIBA* region of the *Streptomyces fradiae* genome. *Mol. Microbiol.* **1994**, *13*, 349–355. [CrossRef] [PubMed]
198. Gandecha, A.R.; Large, S.L.; Cundliffe, E. Analysis of four tylosin biosynthetic genes from the *tylLM* region of the *Streptomyces fradiae* genome. *Gene* **1997**, *184*, 197–203. [CrossRef]
199. Fouces, R.; Mellado, E.; Diez, B.; Barredo, J.L. The tylosin biosynthetic cluster from *Streptomyces fradiae*: Genetic organization of the left region. *Microbiology* **1999**, *145*, 855–868. [CrossRef] [PubMed]
200. Stratigopoulos, G.; Cundliffe, E. Expression Analysis of the Tylosin-Biosynthetic Gene Cluster: Pivotal Regulatory Role of the *tylQ* Product. *Chem. Biol.* **2002**, *9*, 71–78. [CrossRef]
201. Baltz, R.H.; Seno, E.T. Properties of *Streptomyces fradiae* mutants blocked in biosynthesis of the macrolide antibiotic tylosin. *Antimicrob. Agents Chemother.* **1981**, *20*, 214–225. [CrossRef]
202. Rodriguez, E.; Ward, S.; Fu, H.; Revill, W.P.; McDaniel, R.; Katz, L. Engineered biosynthesis of 16-membered macrolides that require methoxymalonyl-ACP precursors in *Streptomyces fradiae*. *Appl. Microbiol. Biotechnol.* **2004**, *66*, 85–91. [CrossRef]
203. Castonguay, R.; Valenzano, C.R.; Chen, A.Y.; Keatinge-Clay, A.; Khosla, C.; Cane, D.E. Stereospecificity of ketoreductase domains 1 and 2 of the tylactone modular polyketide synthase. *J. Am. Chem. Soc.* **2008**, *130*, 11598–11599. [CrossRef]
204. Butler, A.R.; Bate, N.; Cundliffe, E. Impact of thioesterase activity on tylosin biosynthesis in *Streptomyces fradiae*. *Chem. Biol.* **1999**, *6*, 287–292. [CrossRef]
205. Butler, A.R.; Flint, S.A.; Cundliffe, E. Feedback control of polyketide metabolism during tylosin production. *Microbiology* **2001**, *147*, 795–801. [CrossRef] [PubMed]
206. Poulsen, S.M.; Kofoed, C.; Vester, B. Inhibition of the ribosomal peptidyl transferase reaction by the mycarose moiety of the antibiotics carbomycin, spiramycin and tylosin. *J. Mol. Biol.* **2000**, *304*, 471–481. [CrossRef] [PubMed]
207. Hansen, J.L.; Ippolito, J.A.; Ban, N.; Nissen, P.; Moore, P.B.; Steitz, T.A. The structures of four macrolide antibiotics bound to the large ribosomal subunit. *Mol. Cell* **2002**, *10*, 117–128. [CrossRef]
208. Lyutskanova, D.G.; Stoilova-Disheva, M.M.; Peltekova, V.T. Increase in tylosin production by a commercial strain of *Streptomyces fradiae*. *Appl. Biochem. Microbiol.* **2005**, *41*, 165–168. [CrossRef]
209. Haney, M.E.J.; Hoehn, M.M. Monensin, a new biologically active compound. I. Discovery and isolation. *Antimicrob. Agents Chemother.* **1967**, *7*, 349–352. [PubMed]
210. Łowicki, D.; Huczyński, A. Structure and antimicrobial properties of monensin A and its derivatives: Summary of the achievements. *BioMed Res. Int.* **2013**, 742149. [CrossRef]
211. Duax, W.L.; Smith, G.D.; Strong, P.D. Complexation of metal ions by monensin. Crystal and molecular structure of hydrated and anhydrous crystal forms of sodium monensin. *J. Am. Chem. Soc.* **1980**, *102*, 6725–6729. [CrossRef]
212. Barrans, Y.; Alleaume, M.; Jeminet, G. Complexe de sodium de l'ionophore monensine B monohydrate. *Acta Crystallogr. Sect. B Struct. Sci. Cryst. Eng. Mater.* **1982**, *38*, 1144–1149. [CrossRef]
213. Riddell, F.G.; Arumugam, S.; Cox, B.G. The monesin-mediated transport of Na+ and K+ through phospholipid bilayers studied by 23Na-and 39K-NMR. *BBA Biomembr.* **1988**, *944*, 279–284. [CrossRef]
214. Nakazato, K.; Hatano, Y. Monensin-mediated antiport of Na+ and H+ across liposome membrane. *BBA Biomembr.* **1991**, *1064*, 103–110. [CrossRef]
215. Sandeaux, R.; Seta, P.; Jeminet, G.; Alleaume, M.; Gavach, C. The influence of pH on the conductance of lipid bimolecular membranes in relation to the alkaline ion transport induced by carboxylic carriers grisorixin, alborixin and monensin. *BBA Biomembr.* **1978**, *511*, 499–508. [CrossRef]
216. Antonenko, Y.N.; Yaguzhinsky, L.S. The ion selectivity of nonelectrogenic ionophores measured on a bilayer lipid membrane: Nigericin, monensin, A23187 and lasalocid A. *BBA Biomembr.* **1988**, *938*, 125–130. [CrossRef]
217. Zhang, Y.; Lin, C.Y.; Li, X.M.; Tang, Z.K.; Qiao, J.; Zhao, G.R. DasR positively controls monensin production at two-level regulation in *Streptomyces cinnamonensis*. *J. Ind. Microbiol. Biotechnol.* **2016**, *43*, 1681–1692. [CrossRef] [PubMed]

218. Harvey, B.M.; Hong, H.; Jones, M.A.; Hughes-Thomas, Z.A.; Goss, R.M.; Heathcote, M.L.; Bolanos-Garcia, V.M.; Kroutil, W.; Staunton, J.; Leadlay, P.F.; et al. Evidence that a Novel Thioesterase is Responsible for Polyketide Chain Release during Biosynthesis of the Polyether Ionophore Monensin. *ChemBioChem* **2006**, *7*, 1435–1442. [CrossRef] [PubMed]
219. Hüttel, W.; Spencer, J.B.; Leadlay, P.F. Intermediates in monensin biosynthesis: A late step in biosynthesis of the polyether ionophore monensin is crucial for the integrity of cation binding. *Beilstein J. Org. Chem.* **2014**, *10*, 361–368. [CrossRef] [PubMed]
220. Lu, F.; Hou, Y.; Zhang, H.; Chu, Y.; Xia, H.; Tian, Y. Regulatory genes and their roles for improvement of antibiotic biosynthesis in *Streptomyces*. *3 Biotech* **2017**, *7*, 250. [CrossRef] [PubMed]
221. Tang, Z.K.; Li, X.M.; Pang, A.P.; Lin, C.Y.; Zhang, Y.; Zhang, J.; Qiao, J.; Zhao, G.R. Characterization of three pathway-specific regulators for high production of monensin in *Streptomyces cinnamonensis*. *Appl. Microbiol. Biotechnol.* **2017**, *101*, 6083–6097. [CrossRef] [PubMed]
222. Jiang, C.; Wang, H.; Kang, Q.; Liu, J.; Bai, L. Cloning and Characterization of the Polyether Salinomycin Biosynthesis Gene Cluster of *Streptomyces albus* XM211. *Appl. Environ. Microbiol.* **2012**, *78*, 994–1003. [CrossRef] [PubMed]
223. Migita, A.; Watanabe, M.; Hirose, Y.; Watanabe, K.; Tokiwano, T.; Kinashi, H.; Oikawa, H. Identification of a gene cluster of polyether antibiotic lasalocid from *Streptomyces lasaliensis*. *Biosci. Biotechnol. Biochem.* **2009**, *73*, 169–176. [CrossRef]
224. Roder, J.D. Ionophore Toxicity and Tolerance. *Vet. Clin. N. Am. Food Anim. Pract.* **2011**, *27*, 305–314. [CrossRef] [PubMed]
225. Russell, J.B.; Houlihan, A.J. Ionophore resistance of ruminal bacteria and its potential impact on human health. *FEMS Microbiol. Rev.* **2003**, *27*, 65–74. [CrossRef]
226. Bergen, W.G.; Bates, D.B. Ionophores: Their effect on production efficiency and mode of action. *J. Anim. Sci.* **1984**, *58*, 1465–1483. [CrossRef] [PubMed]
227. Chen, M.; Wolin, M.J. Effect of monensin and lasalocid-sodium on the growth of methanogenic and rumen saccharolytic bacteria. *Appl. Environ. Microbiol.* **1979**, *38*, 72–77. [PubMed]
228. Newbold, C.J.; Wallace, R.J.; Watt, N.D. Properties of ionophore-resistant *Bacteroides ruminicola* enriched by cultivation in the presence of tetronasin. *J. Appl. Bacteriol.* **1992**, *72*, 65–70. [CrossRef] [PubMed]
229. Callaway, T.R.; Adams, K.A.; Russell, J.B. The ability of "low G+C gram-positive" ruminal bacteria to resist monensin and counteract potassium depletion. *Curr. Microbiol.* **1999**, *39*, 226–230. [CrossRef] [PubMed]
230. Callaway, T.R.; Russell, J.B. Variations in the ability of ruminal gram-negative *Prevotella* species to resist monensin. *Curr. Microbiol.* **2000**, *40*, 185–189. [CrossRef]
231. McAlpine, J.B. The ups and downs of drug discovery: The early history of Fidaxomicin. *J. Antibiot. (Tokyo)* **2017**, *70*, 492. [CrossRef]
232. Niu, S.; Hu, T.; Li, S.; Xiao, Y.; Ma, L.; Zhang, G.; Zhang, H.; Yang, X.; Ju, J.; Zhang, C. Characterization of a Sugar-O-methyltransferase TiaS5 Affords New Tiacumicin Analogues with Improved Antibacterial Properties and Reveals Substrate Promiscuity. *ChemBioChem* **2011**, *12*, 1740–1748. [CrossRef]
233. Erb, W.; Zhu, J. From natural product to marketed drug: The tiacumicin odyssey. *Nat. Prod. Rep.* **2013**, *30*, 161–174. [CrossRef]
234. Koglin, A.; Löhr, F.; Bernhard, F.; Rogov, V.V.; Frueh, D.P.; Strieter, E.R.; Mofid, M.R.; Güntert, P.; Wagner, G.; Walsh, C.T.; et al. Structural basis for the selectivity of the external thioesterase of the surfactin synthetase. *Nature* **2008**, *454*, 907–911. [CrossRef] [PubMed]
235. Ōmura, S.; Imamura, N.; Oiwa, R.; Kuga, H.; Iwata, R.; Masuma, R.; Iwai, Y. Clostomicins, new antibiotics produced by *Micromonospora echinospora* subsp. armenica subsp. Nov. I Production, isolation and physico-chemical and biological properties. *J. Antibiot.* **1986**, *39*, 1407–1412.
236. Coronelli, C.; White, R.J.; Lancini, G.C.; Parenti, F. Lipiarmycin, a new antibiotic from *Actinoplanes*. II. Isolation, chemical, biological and biochemical characterization. *J. Antibiot. (Tokyo)* **1975**, *28*, 253–259. [CrossRef] [PubMed]
237. Louie, T.J.; Emery, J.; Krulicki, W.; Byrne, B.; Mah, M. OPT-80 Eliminates *Clostridium Difficile* and Is Sparing of *Bacteroides* Species during Treatment of *C. Difficile* Infection. *Antimicrob. Agents Chemother.* **2009**, *53*, 261–263. [CrossRef] [PubMed]

238. Thorpe, C.M.; McDermott, L.A.; Tran, M.K.; Chang, J.; Jenkins, S.G.; Goldstein, E.J.C.; Patel, R.; Forbes, B.A.; Johnson, S.; Gerding, D.N.; et al. US-based National Surveillance for Fidaxomicin Susceptibility of *Clostridioides difficile* (formerly *Clostridium*) Associated Diarrheal Isolates from 2013–2016. *Antimicrob. Agents Chemother.* **2019**, *63*, e00391-19. [CrossRef] [PubMed]
239. Talpaert, M.; Campagnari, F.; Clerici, L. Lipiarmycin: An antibiotic inhibiting nucleic acid polymerases. *Biochem. Biophys. Res. Commun.* **1975**, *63*, 328–334. [CrossRef]
240. Zhang, H.; Tian, X.; Pu, X.; Zhang, Q.; Zhang, W.; Zhang, C. Tiacumicin Congeners with Improved Antibacterial Activity from a Halogenase-Inactivated Mutant. *J. Nat. Prod.* **2018**, *81*, 1219–1224. [CrossRef] [PubMed]
241. Bartsch, S.M.; Umscheid, C.A.; Fishman, N.; Lee, B.Y. Is fidaxomicin worth the cost? An economic analysis. *Clin. Infect. Dis.* **2013**, *57*, 555–561. [CrossRef]
242. Lechevalier, M.P.; Prauser, H.; Labeda, D.P.; Ruan, J.S. Two new genera of nocardioform actinomycetes: *Amycolata* gen. nov. and *Amycolatopsis* gen. nov. *Int. J. Syst. Evol. Microbiol.* **1986**, *36*, 29–37. [CrossRef]
243. Mariani, R.; Maffioli, S.I. Bacterial RNA polymerase inhibitors: An organized overview of their structure, derivatives, biological activity and current clinical development status. *Curr. Med. Chem.* **2009**, *16*, 430–454. [CrossRef]
244. Sensi, P. History of the Development of Rifampin. *Clin. Infect. Dis.* **1983**, *5*, S402–S406. [CrossRef] [PubMed]
245. Oppolzer, W.; Prelog, V.; Sensi, P. Konstitution des Rifamycins B und verwandter Rifamycine. *Experientia* **1964**, *20*, 336–339. [CrossRef] [PubMed]
246. Lancini, G.G.; Gallo, G.G.; Sartori, G.; Sensi, P. Isolation and structure of rifamycin L and its biogenetic relationship with other rifamycins. *J. Antibiot. (Tokyo)* **1969**, *22*, 369–377. [CrossRef] [PubMed]
247. Admiraal, S.J.; Walsh, C.T.; Khosla, C. The Loading Module of Rifamycin Synthetase Is an Adenylation–Thiolation Didomain with Substrate Tolerance for Substituted Benzoates. *Biochemistry* **2001**, *40*, 6116–6123. [CrossRef] [PubMed]
248. Yu, T.W.; Müller, R.; Müller, M.; Zhang, X.; Draeger, G.; Kim, C.G.; Leistner, E.; Floss, H.G. Mutational analysis and reconstituted expression of the biosynthetic genes involved in the formation of 3-amino-5-hydroxybenzoic acid, the starter unit of rifamycin biosynthesis in *Amycolatopsis mediterranei* S699. *J. Biol. Chem.* **2001**, *276*, 12546–12555. [CrossRef]
249. Yu, T.W.; Shen, Y.; Doi-Katayama, Y.; Tang, L.; Park, C.; Moore, B.S.; Hutchinson, C.R.; Floss, H.G. Direct evidence that the rifamycin polyketide synthase assembles polyketide chains processively. *Proc. Natl. Acad. Sci. USA* **1999**, *96*, 9051–9056. [CrossRef] [PubMed]
250. Doi-Katayama, Y.; Yoon, Y.J.; Choi, C.Y.; Yu, T.W.; Floss, H.G.; Hutchinson, C.R. Thioesterases and the premature termination of polyketide chain elongation in rifamycin B biosynthesis by *Amycolatopsis mediterranei* S699. *J. Antibiot. (Tokyo)* **2000**, *53*, 484–495. [CrossRef]
251. Floss, H.G.; Yu, T.W. Lessons from the rifamycin biosynthetic gene cluster. *Curr. Opin. Chem. Biol.* **1999**, *3*, 592–597. [CrossRef]
252. Xu, J.; Wan, E.; Kim, C.J.; Floss, H.G.; Mahmud, T. Identification of tailoring genes involved in the modification of the polyketide backbone of rifamycin B by *Amycolatopsis mediterranei* S699. *Microbiology* **2005**, *151*, 2515–2528. [CrossRef]
253. White, R.J.; Martinelli, E.; Lancini, G. Ansamycin biogenesis: Studies on a novel rifamycin isolated from a mutant strain of *Nocardia mediterranei*. *Proc. Natl. Acad. Sci. USA* **1974**, *71*, 3260–3264. [CrossRef]
254. Qi, F.; Lei, C.; Li, F.; Zhang, X.; Wang, J.; Zhang, W.; Fan, Z.; Li, W.; Tang, G.; Xiao, Y.; et al. Deciphering the late steps of rifamycin biosynthesis. *Nat. Commun.* **2018**, *9*, 2342. [CrossRef] [PubMed]
255. Li, C.; Liu, X.; Lei, C.; Yan, H.; Shao, Z.; Wang, Y.; Zhao, G.; Wang, J.; Ding, X. RifZ (AMED_0655) is a pathway-specific regulator for rifamycin biosynthesis in *Amycolatopsis mediterranei*. *Appl. Environ. Microbiol.* **2017**, *83*, e03201-16. [CrossRef] [PubMed]
256. Lei, C.; Wang, J.; Liu, Y.; Liu, X.; Zhao, G.; Wang, J. A feedback regulatory model for RifQ-mediated repression of rifamycin export in *Amycolatopsis mediterranei*. *Microb. Cell Fact.* **2018**, *17*, 14. [CrossRef] [PubMed]
257. Absalon, A.E.; Fernández, F.J.; Olivares, P.X.; Barrios-González, J.; Campos, C.; Mejía, A. RifP; a membrane protein involved in rifamycin export in *Amycolatopsis mediterranei*. *Biotechnol. Lett.* **2007**, *29*, 951–958. [CrossRef] [PubMed]
258. Wehrli, W. Rifampin: Mechanisms of action and resistance. *Rev. Infect. Dis.* **1983**, *5*, S407–S411. [CrossRef] [PubMed]

259. Boucher, H.W.; Talbot, G.H.; Benjamin, D.K., Jr.; Bradley, J.; Guidos, R.J.; Jones, R.N.; Murray, B.E.; Bonomo, R.A.; Gilbert, D.; The Infectious Diseases Society of America. 10×'20 progress—Development of new drugs active against gram-negative bacilli: An update from the Infectious Diseases Society of America. *Clin. Infect. Dis.* **2013**, *56*, 1685–1694. [CrossRef] [PubMed]
260. Ponziani, F.R.; Scaldaferri, F.; Petito, V.; Paroni Sterbini, F.; Pecere, S.; Lopetuso, L.R.; Palladini, A.; Gerardi, V.; Masucci, L.; Pompili, M.; et al. The role of antibiotics in gut microbiota modulation: The eubiotic effects of rifaximin. *Dig. Dis.* **2016**, *34*, 269–278. [CrossRef]
261. Weber, D.; Oefner, P.J.; Dettmer, K.; Hiergeist, A.; Koestler, J.; Gessner, A.; Weber, M.; Stämmler, F.; Hahn, J.; Wolff, D.; et al. Rifaximin preserves intestinal microbiota balance in patients undergoing allogeneic stem cell transplantation. *Bone Marrow Transplant.* **2016**, *51*, 1087. [CrossRef] [PubMed]
262. Aristoff, P.A.; Garcia, G.A.; Kirchhoff, P.D.; Showalter, H.D. Rifamycins-obstacles and opportunities. *Tuberculosis (Edinb.)* **2010**, *90*, 94–118. [CrossRef]
263. Conover, L.H.; Moreland, W.T.; English, A.R.; Stephens, C.R.; Pilgrim, F.J.; Terramycin, X.I. Tetracycline. *J. Am. Chem. Soc.* **1953**, *75*, 4622–4623. [CrossRef]
264. Nelson, M.L.; Levy, S.B. The history of the tetracyclines. *Ann. N. Y. Acad. Sci.* **2011**, *1241*, 17–32. [CrossRef] [PubMed]
265. Zhang, W.; Ames, B.D.; Tsai, S.C.; Tang, Y. Engineered biosynthesis of a novel amidated polyketide, using the malonamyl-specific initiation module from the oxytetracycline polyketide synthase. *Appl. Environ. Microbiol.* **2006**, *72*, 2573–2580. [CrossRef] [PubMed]
266. Wang, P.; Gao, X.; Chooi, Y.H.; Deng, Z.; Tang, Y. Genetic characterization of enzymes involved in the priming steps of oxytetracycline biosynthesis in *Streptomyces rimosus*. *Microbiology* **2011**, *157*, 2401–2409. [CrossRef] [PubMed]
267. Zhang, W.; Watanabe, K.; Wang, C.C.C.; Tang, Y. Heterologous biosynthesis of amidated polyketides with novel cyclization regioselectivity from oxytetracycline polyketide synthase. *J. Nat. Prod.* **2006**, *69*, 1633–1636. [CrossRef] [PubMed]
268. Pickens, L.B.; Tang, Y. Oxytetracycline biosynthesis. *J. Biol. Chem.* **2010**, *285*, 27509–27515. [CrossRef] [PubMed]
269. Petković, H.; Lukežič, T.; Šušković, J. Biosynthesis of oxytetracycline by *Streptomyces rimosus*: Past, present and future directions in the development of tetracycline antibiotics. *Food Technol. Biotechnol.* **2017**, *55*, 3–13. [CrossRef]
270. Wang, P.; Bashiri, G.; Gao, X.; Sawaya, M.R.; Tang, Y. Uncovering the enzymes that catalyze the final steps in oxytetracycline biosynthesis. *J. Am. Chem. Soc.* **2013**, *135*, 7138–7141. [CrossRef]
271. Ohnuki, T.; Katoh, T.; Imanaka, T.; Aiba, S. Molecular cloning of tetracycline resistance genes from *Streptomyces rimosus* in *Streptomyces griseus* and characterization of the cloned genes. *J. Bacteriol.* **1985**, *161*, 1010–1016.
272. Lešnik, U.; Gormand, A.; Magdevska, V.; Fujs, Š.; Raspor, P.; Hunter, I.; Petković, H. Regulatory elements in tetracycline-encoding gene clusters: The *otcG* gene positively regulates the production of oxytetracycline in *Streptomyces rimosus*. *Food Technol. Biotechnol.* **2009**, *47*, 323–330.
273. Yin, S.; Wang, W.; Wang, X.; Zhu, Y.; Jia, X.; Li, S.; Yuan, F.; Zhang, Y.; Yang, K. Identification of a cluster-situated activator of oxytetracycline biosynthesis and manipulation of its expression for improved oxytetracycline production in *Streptomyces rimosus*. *Microb. Cell Fact.* **2015**, *14*, 46. [CrossRef]
274. Jenner, L.; Starosta, A.L.; Terry, D.S.; Mikolajka, A.; Filonava, L.; Yusupov, M.; Blanchard, S.C.; Wilson, D.N.; Yusupova, G. Structural basis for potent inhibitory activity of the antibiotic tigecycline during protein synthesis. *Proc. Natl. Acad. Sci. USA* **2013**, *110*, 3812–3816. [CrossRef] [PubMed]
275. Nelson, M.L.; Park, B.H.; Levy, S.B. Molecular requirements for the inhibition of the tetracycline antiport protein and the effect of potent inhibitors on the growth of tetracycline-resistant bacteria. *J. Med. Chem.* **1994**, *37*, 1355–1361. [CrossRef] [PubMed]
276. Villano, S.; Steenbergen, J.; Loh, E. Omadacycline: Development of a novel aminomethylcycline antibiotic for treating drug-resistant bacterial infections. *Future Microbiol.* **2016**, *11*, 1421–1434. [CrossRef] [PubMed]
277. Barriere, J.C.; Berthaud, N.; Beyer, D.; Dutka-Malen, S.; Paris, J.M.; Desnottes, J.F. Recent developments in streptogramin research. *Curr. Pharm. Des.* **1998**, *4*, 155. [PubMed]
278. Mast, Y.; Wohlleben, W. Streptogramins—Two are better than one! *Int. J. Med. Microbiol.* **2014**, *304*, 44–50. [CrossRef] [PubMed]

279. Charney, J.; Fisher, W.P.; Curran, C.; Machlowitz, R.A.; Tytell, A.A. Streptogramin, a new antibiotic. *Antibiot. Chemother. (Northfield, Ill.)* **1953**, *3*, 1283–1286.
280. Arai, M.; Karasawa, K.; Nakamura, S.; Yonehara, H.; Umezawa, H. Studies on mikamycin. I. *J. Antibiot. (Tokyo)* **1958**, *11*, 14–20.
281. Watanabe, K. Studies on mikamycin. VII. Structure of mikamycin B. *J. Antibiot. Ser. A* **1961**, *14*, 14–17.
282. Bartz, Q.R.; Standiford, J.; Mold, J.D.; Johannessen, D.W.; Ryder, A.; Maretski, A.; Haskell, T.H. *Antibiotics Annual (1954–1955)*; Medical Encyclopedia Inc.: New York, NY, USA, 1954; pp. 777–783.
283. De Somer, P.; Van Dijck, P. A preliminary report on antibiotic number 899, a streptogramin-like substance. *Antibiot. Chemother. (Northfield, Ill.)* **1955**, *5*, 632–639.
284. Casewell, M.; Friis, C.; Marco, E.; McMullin, P.; Phillips, I. The European ban on growth-promoting antibiotics and emerging consequences for human and animal health. *J. Antimicrob. Chemother.* **2003**, *52*, 159–161. [CrossRef]
285. Musiol, E.M.; Greule, A.; Härtner, T.; Kulik, A.; Wohlleben, W.; Weber, T. The AT2 domain of KirCI loads malonyl extender units to the ACPs of the kirromycin PKS. *ChemBioChem* **2013**, *14*, 1343–1352. [CrossRef]
286. Weber, T.; Laiple, K.J.; Pross, E.K.; Textor, A.; Grond, S.; Welzel, K.; Pelzer, S.; Vente, A.; Wohlleben, W. Molecular analysis of the kirromycin biosynthetic gene cluster revealed β-alanine as precursor of the pyridone moiety. *Chem. Biol.* **2008**, *15*, 175–188. [CrossRef] [PubMed]
287. Mast, Y.; Guezguez, J.; Handel, F.; Schinko, E. A complex signaling cascade governs pristinamycin biosynthesis in *Streptomyces pristinaespiralis*. *Appl. Environ. Microbiol.* **2015**, *81*, 6621–6636. [CrossRef] [PubMed]
288. Wang, W.; Tian, J.; Li, L.; Ge, M.; Zhu, H.; Zheng, G.; Huang, H.; Ruan, L.; Jiang, W.; Lu, Y. Identification of two novel regulatory genes involved in pristinamycin biosynthesis and elucidation of the mechanism for AtrA-p-mediated regulation in *Streptomyces pristinaespiralis*. *Appl. Microbiol. Biotechnol.* **2015**, *99*, 7151–7164. [CrossRef] [PubMed]
289. Meng, J.; Feng, R.; Zheng, G.; Ge, M.; Mast, Y.; Wohlleben, W.; Gao, J.; Jiang, W.; Lu, Y. Improvement of pristinamycin I (PI) production in *Streptomyces pristinaespiralis* by metabolic engineering approaches. *Synth. Syst. Biotechnol.* **2017**, *2*, 130–136. [CrossRef] [PubMed]
290. Li, L.; Zhao, Y.; Ruan, L.; Yang, S.; Ge, M.; Jiang, W.; Lu, Y. A stepwise increase in pristinamycin II biosynthesis by *Streptomyces pristinaespiralis* through combinatorial metabolic engineering. *Metab. Eng.* **2015**, *29*, 12–25. [CrossRef]
291. Nyssen, E.; Di Giambattista, M.; Cocito, C. Analysis of the reversible binding of virginiamycin M to ribosome and particle functions after removal of the antibiotic. *Biochim. Biophys. Acta Gene Struct. Expr.* **1989**, *1009*, 39–46. [CrossRef]
292. Johnston, N.J.; Mukhtar, T.A.; Wright, G.D. Streptogramin antibiotics: Mode of action and resistance. *Curr. Drug Targets* **2002**, *3*, 335–344. [CrossRef] [PubMed]
293. Roberts, M.C. Environmental macrolide–lincosamide–streptogramin and tetracycline resistant bacteria. *Front. Microbiol.* **2011**, *2*, 40. [CrossRef] [PubMed]
294. Roberts, M.C. Resistance to macrolide, lincosamide, streptogramin, ketolide, and oxazolidinone antibiotics. *Mol. Biotechnol.* **2004**, *28*, 47. [CrossRef]
295. Poehlsgaard, J.; Douthwaite, S. The bacterial ribosome as a target for antibiotics. *Nat. Rev. Microbiol.* **2005**, *3*, 870. [CrossRef] [PubMed]
296. Allignet, J.; Loncle, V.; Mazodier, P.; El Solh, N. Nucleotide sequence of a staphylococcal plasmid gene, *vgb*, encoding a hydrolase inactivating the B components of virginiamycin-like antibiotics. *Plasmid* **1988**, *20*, 271–275. [CrossRef]
297. Allignet, J.; Loncle, V.; El Solh, N. Sequence of a staphylococcal plasmid gene, *vga*, encoding a putative ATP-binding protein involved in resistance to virginiamycin A-like antibiotics. *Gene* **1992**, *117*, 45–51. [CrossRef]
298. Aparicio, J.F.; Caffrey, P.; Gil, J.A.; Zotchev, S.B. Polyene antibiotic biosynthesis gene clusters. *Appl. Microbiol. Biotechnol.* **2003**, *61*, 179–188. [CrossRef] [PubMed]
299. Fjærvik, E.; Zotchev, S.B. Biosynthesis of the polyene macrolide antibiotic nystatin in *Streptomyces noursei*. *Appl. Microbiol. Biotechnol.* **2005**, *67*, 436–443. [CrossRef] [PubMed]
300. Hazen, E.L.; Brown, R. Two antifungal agents produced by a soil actinomycete. *Science* **1950**, *112*, 423. [PubMed]

301. Mechlinski, W.; Schaffner, C.P. Separation of polyene antifungal antibiotics by high-speed liquid chromatography. *J. Chromatogr. A* **1974**, *99*, 619–633. [CrossRef]
302. Matsuoka, M. Biological studies on antifungal substances produced by *Streptomyces fungicidicus*. *J. Antibiot. (Tokyo)* **1960**, *13*, 121–124.
303. Veiga, M.; Fabregas, J. Tetrafungin, a new polyene macrolide antibiotic. I. Fermentation, isolation, characterization, and biological properties. *J. Antibiot. (Tokyo)* **1983**, *36*, 770–775. [CrossRef]
304. Chong, C.N.; Rickards, R.W. Macrolide antibiotic studies. XVI. The structure of nystatin. *Tetrahedron Lett.* **1970**, *11*, 5145–5148. [CrossRef]
305. Sletta, H.; Borgos, S.E.F.; Bruheim, P.; Sekurova, O.N.; Grasdalen, H.; Aune, R.; Ellingsen, T.E.; Zotchev, S.B. Nystatin biosynthesis and transport: *nysH* and *nysG* genes encoding a putative ABC transporter system in *Streptomyces noursei* ATCC 11455 are required for efficient conversion of 10-deoxynystatin to nystatin. *Antimicrob. Agents Chemother.* **2005**, *49*, 4576–4583. [CrossRef] [PubMed]
306. Sekurova, O.N.; Brautaset, T.; Sletta, H.; Borgos, S.E.F.; Jakobsen, Ø.M.; Ellingsen, T.E.; Strøm, A.R.; Valla, S.; Zotchev, S.B. In vivo analysis of the regulatory genes in the nystatin biosynthetic gene cluster of *Streptomyces noursei* ATCC 11455 reveals their differential control over antibiotic biosynthesis. *J. Bacteriol.* **2004**, *186*, 1345–1354. [CrossRef] [PubMed]
307. Gupte, M.; Kulkarni, P.; Ganguli, B. Antifungal antibiotics. *Appl. Microbiol. Biotechnol.* **2002**, *58*, 46–57. [CrossRef] [PubMed]
308. Hamilton-Miller, J.M. Chemistry and biology of the polyene macrolide antibiotics. *Bacteriol. Rev.* **1973**, *37*, 166. [PubMed]
309. Lee, M.Y.; Myeong, J.S.; Park, H.J.; Han, K.; Kim, E.S. Isolation and partial characterization of a cryptic polyene gene cluster in *Pseudonocardia autotrophica*. *J. Ind. Microbiol. Biotechnol.* **2006**, *33*, 84–87. [CrossRef] [PubMed]
310. Kim, B.G.; Lee, M.J.; Seo, J.; Hwang, Y.B.; Lee, M.Y.; Han, K.; Sherman, D.H.; Kim, E.S. Identification of functionally clustered nystatin-like biosynthetic genes in a rare actinomycetes, *Pseudonocardia autotrophica*. *J. Ind. Microbiol. Biotechnol.* **2009**, *36*, 1425. [CrossRef] [PubMed]
311. Lee, M.J.; Kong, D.; Han, K.; Sherman, D.H.; Bai, L.; Deng, Z.; Lin, S.; Kim, E.S. Structural analysis and biosynthetic engineering of a solubility-improved and less-hemolytic nystatin-like polyene in *Pseudonocardia autotrophica*. *Appl. Microbiol. Biotechnol.* **2012**, *95*, 157–168. [CrossRef] [PubMed]
312. Kim, H.J.; Han, C.Y.; Park, J.S.; Oh, S.H.; Kang, S.H.; Choi, S.S.; Kim, J.M.; Kwak, J.H.; Kim, E.S. Nystatin-like *Pseudonocardia* polyene B1, a novel disaccharide-containing antifungal heptaene antibiotic. *Sci. Rep.* **2018**, *8*, 13584. [CrossRef] [PubMed]
313. Caffrey, P.; Lynch, S.; Flood, E.; Finnan, S.; Oliynyk, M. Amphotericin biosynthesis in *Streptomyces nodosus*: Deductions from analysis of polyketide synthase and late genes. *Chem. Biol.* **2001**, *8*, 713–723. [CrossRef]
314. Carmody, M.; Murphy, B.; Byrne, B.; Power, P.; Rai, D.; Rawlings, B.; Caffrey, P. Biosynthesis of amphotericin derivatives lacking exocyclic carboxyl groups. *J. Biol. Chem.* **2005**, *280*, 34420–34426. [CrossRef]
315. Carmody, M.; Byrne, B.; Murphy, B.; Breen, C.; Lynch, S.; Flood, E.; Finnan, S.; Caffrey, P. Analysis and manipulation of amphotericin biosynthetic genes by means of modified phage KC515 transduction techniques. *Gene* **2004**, *343*, 107–115. [CrossRef] [PubMed]
316. Ellis, D. Amphotericin B: Spectrum and resistance. *J. Antimicrob. Chemother.* **2002**, *49*, 7–10. [CrossRef] [PubMed]
317. Goldman, C.; Akiyama, M.J.; Torres, J.; Louie, E.; Meehan, S.A. *Scedosporium apiospermum* infections and the role of combination antifungal therapy and GM-CSF: A case report and review of the literature. *Med. Mycol. Case Rep.* **2016**, *11*, 40–43. [CrossRef] [PubMed]
318. Volmer, A.A.; Szpilman, A.M.; Carreira, E.M. Synthesis and biological evaluation of amphotericin B derivatives. *Nat. Prod. Rep.* **2010**, *27*, 1329–1349. [CrossRef] [PubMed]
319. Zhang, B.; Zhang, H.; Zhou, Y.; Huang, K.; Liu, Z.; Zheng, Y. Improvement of amphotericin B production by a newly isolated *Streptomyces nodosus* mutant. *Biotechnol. Appl. Biochem.* **2018**, *65*, 188–194. [CrossRef] [PubMed]
320. Aparicio, J.F.; Barreales, E.G.; Payero, T.D.; Vicente, C.M.; de Pedro, A.; Santos-Aberturas, J. Biotechnological production and application of the antibiotic pimaricin: Biosynthesis and its regulation. *Appl. Microbiol. Biotechnol.* **2016**, *100*, 61–78. [CrossRef]

321. Divekar, P.V.; Bloomer, J.L.; Eastham, J.F.; Holtman, D.F.; Shirley, D.A. The isolation of crystalline tennecetin and the comparison of this antibiotic with pimaricin. *Antibiot. Chemother. (Northfield, Ill.)* **1961**, *11*, 377.
322. Burns, J. Tennecetin: A new antifungal antibiotic. *Antibiot. Chemother.* **1959**, *9*, 398–405.
323. Sui, Q.; Liu, W.; Lu, C.; Liu, T.; Qiu, J.; Liu, X. Extraction and structural identification of the antifungal metabolite of *Streptomyces lydicus* A02. *Chin. J. Biotechnol.* **2009**, *25*, 840–846.
324. Wang, T.J.; Shan, Y.M.; Li, H.; Dou, W.W.; Jiang, X.H.; Mao, X.M.; Liu, S.P.; Guan, W.J.; Li, Y.Q. Multiple transporters are involved in natamycin efflux in *Streptomyces chattanoogensis* L10. *Mol. Microbiol.* **2017**, *103*, 713–728. [CrossRef]
325. Anton, N.; Santos-Aberturas, J.; Mendes, M.V.; Guerra, S.M.; Martin, J.F.; Aparicio, J.F. PimM, a PAS domain positive regulator of pimaricin biosynthesis in *Streptomyces natalensis*. *Microbiology* **2007**, *153*, 3174–3183. [CrossRef] [PubMed]
326. Anton, N.; Mendes, M.V.; Martin, J.F.; Aparicio, J.F. Identification of PimR as a positive regulator of pimaricin biosynthesis in *Streptomyces natalensis*. *J. Bacteriol.* **2004**, *186*, 2567–2575. [CrossRef] [PubMed]
327. Vicente, C.M.; Santos-Aberturas, J.; Guerra, S.M.; Payero, T.D.; Martin, J.F.; Aparicio, J.F. PimT, an amino acid exporter controls polyene production via secretion of the quorum sensing pimaricin-inducer PI-factor in *Streptomyces natalensis*. *Microb. Cell Fact.* **2009**, *8*, 33. [CrossRef] [PubMed]
328. Mendes, M.V.; Recio, E.; Antón, N.; Guerra, S.M.; Santos-Aberturas, J.; Martín, J.F.; Aparicio, J.F. Cholesterol oxidases act as signaling proteins for the biosynthesis of the polyene macrolide pimaricin. *Chem. Biol.* **2007**, *14*, 279–290. [CrossRef] [PubMed]
329. Aparicio, J.F.; Martín, J.F. Microbial cholesterol oxidases: Bioconversion enzymes or signal proteins? *Mol. Biosyst.* **2008**, *4*, 804–809. [CrossRef] [PubMed]
330. Du, Y.L.; Chen, S.F.; Cheng, L.Y.; Shen, X.L.; Tian, Y.; Li, Y.Q. Identification of a novel *Streptomyces chattanoogensis* L10 and enhancing its natamycin production by overexpressing positive regulator ScnRII. *J. Microbiol.* **2009**, *47*, 506–513. [CrossRef] [PubMed]
331. Wang, S.; Liu, F.; Hou, Z.; Zong, G.; Zhu, X.; Ling, P. Enhancement of natamycin production on *Streptomyces gilvosporeus* by chromosomal integration of the *Vitreoscilla* hemoglobin gene (vgb). *World J. Microbiol. Biotechnol.* **2014**, *30*, 1369–1376. [CrossRef]
332. Lee, K.M.; Lee, C.K.; Choi, S.U.; Park, H.R.; Kitani, S.; Nihira, T.; Hwang, Y.I. Cloning and in vivo functional analysis by disruption of a gene encoding the γ-butyrolactone autoregulator receptor from *Streptomyces natalensis*. *Arch. Microbiol.* **2005**, *184*, 249–257. [CrossRef]
333. Qi, Z.; Kang, Q.; Jiang, C.; Han, M.; Bai, L. Engineered biosynthesis of pimaricin derivatives with improved antifungal activity and reduced cytotoxicity. *Appl. Microbiol. Biotechnol.* **2015**, *99*, 6745–6752. [CrossRef]
334. Li, X.Z.; Plésiat, P.; Nikaido, H. The challenge of efflux-mediated antibiotic resistance in Gram-negative bacteria. *Clin. Microbiol. Rev.* **2015**, *28*, 337–418. [CrossRef]
335. Coates, A.R.M.; Halls, G.; Hu, Y. Novel classes of antibiotics or more of the same? *Br. J. Pharmacol.* **2011**, *163*, 184–194. [CrossRef] [PubMed]
336. Spellberg, B.; Bartlett, J.G.; Gilbert, D.N. The future of antibiotics and resistance. *N. Engl. J. Med.* **2013**, *368*, 299–302. [CrossRef] [PubMed]
337. Blunt, J.W.; Copp, B.R.; Munro, M.H.G.; Northcote, P.T.; Prinsep, M.R. Marine natural products. *Nat. Prod. Rep.* **2011**, *28*, 196–268. [CrossRef] [PubMed]
338. Katz, L.; Baltz, R.H. Natural product discovery: Past, present, and future. *J. Ind. Microbiol. Biotechnol.* **2016**, *43*, 155–176. [CrossRef] [PubMed]
339. Kealey, C.; Creaven, C.A.; Murphy, C.D.; Brady, C.B. New approaches to antibiotic discovery. *Biotechnol. Lett.* **2017**, *39*, 805–817. [CrossRef] [PubMed]
340. Iorio, M.; Tocchetti, A.; Cruz, J.; Del Gatto, G.; Brunati, C.; Maffioli, S.; Sosio, M.; Donadio, S. Novel Polyethers from Screening *Actinoallomurus* spp. *Antibiotics* **2018**, *7*, 47. [CrossRef] [PubMed]
341. Hug, J.; Bader, C.; Remškar, M.; Cirnski, K.; Müller, R. Concepts and methods to access novel antibiotics from actinomycetes. *Antibiotics* **2018**, *7*, 44. [CrossRef] [PubMed]
342. Genilloud, O. Mining actinomycetes for novel antibiotics in the omics era: Are we ready to exploit this new paradigm? *Antibiotics* **2018**, *7*, 85. [CrossRef]
343. Amoutzias, G.; Chaliotis, A.; Mossialos, D. Discovery strategies of bioactive compounds synthesized by nonribosomal peptide synthetases and type-I polyketide synthases derived from marine microbiomes. *Mar. Drugs* **2016**, *14*, 80. [CrossRef]

344. Adnani, N.; Chevrette, M.; Adibhatla, S.N.; Zhang, F.; Yu, Q.; Braun, D.R.; Nelson, J.; Simpkins, S.W.; McDonald, B.R.; Myers, C.L.; et al. Coculture of marine invertebrate-associated bacteria and interdisciplinary technologies enable biosynthesis and discovery of a new antibiotic, keyicin. *ACS Chem. Biol.* **2017**, *12*, 3093–3102. [CrossRef]
345. Goers, L.; Freemont, P.; Polizzi, K.M. Co-culture systems and technologies: Taking synthetic biology to the next level. *J. R. Soc. Interface* **2014**, *11*, 20140065. [CrossRef]
346. Dashti, Y.; Grkovic, T.; Abdelmohsen, U.; Hentschel, U.; Quinn, R. Production of induced secondary metabolites by a co-culture of sponge-associated actinomycetes, *Actinokineospora* sp. EG49 and *Nocardiopsis* sp. RV163. *Mar. Drugs* **2014**, *12*, 3046–3059. [CrossRef]
347. Piel, J. Metabolites from symbiotic bacteria. *Nat. Prod. Rep.* **2009**, *26*, 338–362. [CrossRef]
348. Ling, L.L.; Schneider, T.; Peoples, A.J.; Spoering, A.L.; Engels, I.; Conlon, B.P.; Mueller, A.; Schäberle, T.F.; Hughes, D.E.; Epstein, S.; et al. A new antibiotic kills pathogens without detectable resistance. *Nature* **2015**, *517*, 455. [CrossRef]
349. Nichols, D.; Cahoon, N.; Trakhtenberg, E.M.; Pham, L.; Mehta, A.; Belanger, A.; Kanigan, T.; Lewis, K.; Epstein, S.S. Use of ichip for high-throughput in situ cultivation of "uncultivable" microbial species. *Appl. Environ. Microbiol.* **2010**, *76*, 2445–2450. [CrossRef]
350. Piddock, L.J.V. Teixobactin, the first of a new class of antibiotics discovered by iChip technology? *J. Antimicrob. Chemother.* **2015**, *70*, 2679–2680. [CrossRef]
351. Sherpa, R.T.; Reese, C.J.; Aliabadi, H.M. Application of iChip to grow "uncultivable" microorganisms and its impact on antibiotic discovery. *J. Pharm. Pharm. Sci.* **2015**, *18*, 303–315. [CrossRef]
352. Alessi, A.M.; Redeker, K.R.; Chong, J.P.J. A practical introduction to microbial molecular ecology through the use of isolation chips. *Ecol. Evol.* **2018**, *8*, 12286–12298. [CrossRef]
353. Lodhi, A.F.; Zhang, Y.; Adil, M.; Deng, Y. Antibiotic discovery: Combining isolation chip (iChip) technology and co-culture technique. *Appl. Microbiol. Biotechnol.* **2018**, *102*, 7333–7341. [CrossRef]
354. Mohana, N.C.; Rao, H.C.Y.; Rakshith, D.; Mithun, P.R.; Nuthan, B.R.; Satish, S. Omics based approach for biodiscovery of microbial natural products in antibiotic resistance era. *J. Genet. Eng. Biotechnol.* **2018**, *16*, 1–8. [CrossRef]
355. Vijayakumar, S.; Conway, M.; Lió, P.; Angione, C. Optimization of multi-omic genome-scale models: Methodologies, hands-on tutorial, and perspectives. In *Metabolic Network Reconstruction and Modeling*; Springer: Berlin/Heidelberg, Germany, 2018; pp. 389–408.
356. Franzosa, E.A.; Hsu, T.; Sirota-Madi, A.; Shafquat, A.; Abu-Ali, G.; Morgan, X.C.; Huttenhower, C. Sequencing and beyond: Integrating molecular 'omics' for microbial community profiling. *Nat. Rev. Microbiol.* **2015**, *13*, 360. [CrossRef]
357. Palazzotto, E.; Weber, T. Omics and multi-omics approaches to study the biosynthesis of secondary metabolites in microorganisms. *Curr. Opin. Microbiol.* **2018**, *45*, 109–116. [CrossRef]
358. Nikolouli, K.; Mossialos, D. Bioactive compounds synthesized by non-ribosomal peptide synthetases and type-I polyketide synthases discovered through genome-mining and metagenomics. *Biotechnol. Lett.* **2012**, *34*, 1393–1403. [CrossRef]
359. Medema, M.H.; Fischbach, M.A. Computational approaches to natural product discovery. *Nat. Chem. Biol.* **2015**, *11*, 639. [CrossRef]
360. Carbonell, P.; Currin, A.; Jervis, A.J.; Rattray, N.J.W.; Swainston, N.; Yan, C.; Takano, E.; Breitling, R. Bioinformatics for the synthetic biology of natural products: Integrating across the Design-Build-Test cycle. *Nat. Prod. Rep.* **2016**, *33*, 925–932. [CrossRef]
361. Ito, T.; Masubuchi, M. Dereplication of microbial extracts and related analytical technologies. *J. Antibiot. (Tokyo)* **2014**, *67*, 353–360. [CrossRef]
362. Seger, C.; Sturm, S.; Stuppner, H. Mass spectrometry and NMR spectroscopy: Modern high-end detectors for high resolution separation techniques–state of the art in natural product HPLC-MS, HPLC-NMR, and CE-MS hyphenations. *Nat. Prod. Rep.* **2013**, *30*, 970–987. [CrossRef]
363. Perez-Victoria, I.; Martin, J.; Reyes, F. Combined LC/UV/MS and NMR Strategies for the Dereplication of Marine Natural Products. *Planta Med.* **2016**, *82*, 857–871. [CrossRef]
364. Spraker, J.E.; Luu, G.T.; Sanchez, L.M. Imaging mass spectrometry for natural products discovery: A review of ionization methods. *Nat. Prod. Rep.* **2019**. [CrossRef]

365. Zhu, H.; Sandiford, S.K.; van Wezel, G.P. Triggers and cues that activate antibiotic production by actinomycetes. *J. Ind. Microbiol. Biotechnol.* **2014**, *41*, 371–386. [CrossRef]
366. Rutledge, P.J.; Challis, G.L. Discovery of microbial natural products by activation of silent biosynthetic gene clusters. *Nat. Rev. Microbiol.* **2015**, *13*, 509–523. [CrossRef]
367. Seyedsayamdost, M.R. High-throughput platform for the discovery of elicitors of silent bacterial gene clusters. *Proc. Natl. Acad. Sci. USA* **2014**, *111*, 7266–7271. [CrossRef]
368. Rosen, P.C.; Seyedsayamdost, M.R. Though Much Is Taken, Much Abides: Finding New Antibiotics Using Old Ones. *Biochemistry* **2017**, *56*, 4925–4926. [CrossRef]
369. Okada, B.K.; Seyedsayamdost, M.R. Antibiotic dialogues: Induction of silent biosynthetic gene clusters by exogenous small molecules. *FEMS Microbiol. Rev.* **2017**, *41*, 19–33. [CrossRef]
370. Altaee, N.; Kadhim, M.J.; Hameed, I.H. Characterization of metabolites produced by *E. coli* and analysis of its chemical compounds using GC-MS. *Int. J. Curr. Pharm. Rev. Res.* **2017**, *7*, 13–19.
371. Wexler, M.; Johnston, A.W.B. Wide host-range cloning for functional metagenomics. *Methods Mol. Biol.* **2010**, *668*, 77–96.
372. Ongley, S.E.; Bian, X.; Neilan, B.A.; Muller, R. Recent advances in the heterologous expression of microbial natural product biosynthetic pathways. *Nat. Prod. Rep.* **2013**, *30*, 1121–1138. [CrossRef]
373. Kallifidas, D.; Jiang, G.; Ding, Y.; Luesch, H. Rational engineering of *Streptomyces albus* J1074 for the overexpression of secondary metabolite gene clusters. *Microb. Cell Fact.* **2018**, *17*, 25. [CrossRef]
374. Gomez-Escribano, J.P.; Bibb, M.J. Engineering *Streptomyces coelicolor* for heterologous expression of secondary metabolite gene clusters. *Microb. Biotechnol.* **2011**, *4*, 207–215. [CrossRef]
375. Bonet, B.; Teufel, R.; Crusemann, M.; Ziemert, N.; Moore, B.S. Direct capture and heterologous expression of *Salinispora* natural product genes for the biosynthesis of enterocin. *J. Nat. Prod.* **2015**, *78*, 539–542. [CrossRef]
376. Deng, Y.; Zhang, X.; Zhang, X. Recent advances in genetic modification systems for Actinobacteria. *Appl. Microbiol. Biotechnol.* **2017**, *101*, 2217–2226. [CrossRef]
377. Dhakal, D.; Sohng, J.K.; Pandey, R.P. Engineering actinomycetes for biosynthesis of macrolactone polyketides. *Microb. Cell Fact.* **2019**, *18*, 137. [CrossRef]
378. Baltz, R.H. Genetic manipulation of secondary metabolite biosynthesis for improved production in *Streptomyces* and other actinomycetes. *J. Ind. Microbiol. Biotechnol.* **2016**, *43*, 343–370. [CrossRef]
379. Lee, N.; Hwang, S.; Lee, Y.; Cho, S.; Palsson, B.; Cho, B.K. Synthetic Biology Tools for Novel Secondary Metabolite Discovery in *Streptomyces*. *J. Microbiol. Biotechnol.* **2019**, *29*, 667–686. [CrossRef]
380. Palazzotto, E.; Tong, Y.; Lee, S.Y.; Weber, T. Synthetic biology and metabolic engineering of actinomycetes for natural product discovery. *Biotechnol. Adv.* **2019**, *37*, 107366. [CrossRef]
381. Genilloud, O. Actinomycetes: Still a source of novel antibiotics. *Nat. Prod. Rep.* **2017**, *34*, 1203–1232. [CrossRef]
382. Mazzetti, C.; Ornaghi, M.; Gaspari, E.; Parapini, S.; Maffioli, S.; Sosio, M.; Donadio, S. Halogenated spirotetronates from *Actinoallomurus*. *J. Nat. Prod.* **2012**, *75*, 1044–1050. [CrossRef]

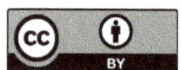

© 2019 by the authors. Licensee MDPI, Basel, Switzerland. This article is an open access article distributed under the terms and conditions of the Creative Commons Attribution (CC BY) license (http://creativecommons.org/licenses/by/4.0/).

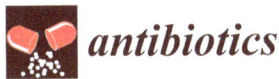

Review

Bacteriophages as Alternatives to Antibiotics in Clinical Care

Danitza Romero-Calle [1], Raquel Guimarães Benevides [1], Aristóteles Góes-Neto [1] and Craig Billington [2,*]

[1] Postgraduate Program in Biotechnology, State University of Feira de Santana (UEFS), Av. Transnordestina S/N, Feira de Santana-BA 44036-900, Brazil
[2] Health & Environment Group, Institute of Environmental Sciences and Research, PO Box 29-181, Christchurch 8540, New Zealand
* Correspondence: craig.billington@esr.cri.nz

Received: 2 August 2019; Accepted: 3 September 2019; Published: 4 September 2019

Abstract: Antimicrobial resistance is increasing despite new treatments being employed. With a decrease in the discovery rate of novel antibiotics, this threatens to take humankind back to a "pre-antibiotic era" of clinical care. Bacteriophages (phages) are one of the most promising alternatives to antibiotics for clinical use. Although more than a century of mostly ad-hoc phage therapy has involved substantial clinical experimentation, a lack of both regulatory guidance standards and effective execution of clinical trials has meant that therapy for infectious bacterial diseases has yet to be widely adopted. However, several recent case studies and clinical trials show promise in addressing these concerns. With the antibiotic resistance crisis and urgent search for alternative clinical treatments for bacterial infections, phage therapy may soon fulfill its long-held promise. This review reports on the applications of phage therapy for various infectious diseases, phage pharmacology, immunological responses to phages, legal concerns, and the potential benefits and disadvantages of this novel treatment.

Keywords: bacteriophages; clinical trials; antibiotic resistance; infectious disease; phage therapy

---

1. Introduction

There are approximately 10^{30-31} bacteriophages (phages) in the biosphere [1,2], which is estimated to be 10-fold higher than the total number of bacterial cells [3]. Phages are also an inherent part of the human microbiome, and so are usually well-tolerated when used in phage therapy [4–6]. Phages are one of the most promising alternatives to antibiotics, which can be used for medicine, agriculture, and related fields [7]. The evolution of multidrug-resistant and pan-drug-resistant bacteria poses a real threat to the control of infectious diseases globally, so it is urgent to have new therapeutic tools available. The United States National Institutes of Health have stated that phages are promising tools for combatting microbial resistance [8].

A post-antibiotic era in which minor injuries and common infections can kill because of the lack of drugs or their ineffectiveness is nowadays not an apocalyptic fantasy, but a real 21st-century threat. For example, ESKAPE organisms (*Enterococcus faecium*, *Staphylococcus aureus*, *Klebsiella pneumoniae*, *Acinetobacter baumannii*, *Pseudomonas aeruginosa*, and *Enterobacter* spp.) are extremely resistant to multiple antimicrobial agents [9] and are a serious challenge in medicine today. On the other hand, there historically has been no fit for purpose regulatory framework to deal with novel flexible and sustainable therapeutic approaches such as phages. For phages, this includes oversight of the setup and approval of adequate clinical trials, so as a result, there is no standard protocol for phage therapy.

In this review, we summarize the phage therapy clinical trials that have shown promising results in patients. We cover several diseases, immunological responses to phages, phage pharmacology, legal concerns about phage therapy, phage genetic modification, and a description of the advantages and disadvantages of phage therapy when compared to conventional treatments with antibiotics.

2. Phage Biology

Viruses that infect bacteria and *Achaea* are called phages, which have no machinery for generating energy and no ribosomes for making proteins. They are obligate bacterial parasites that carry all the genetic information required to undertake their reproduction in an appropriate host. The genome size of phages varies from a few thousand base pairs up to 498 kilobase pairs in phage G, which is the largest phage sequenced to date [10]. Most phages have a high level of host specificity (though some are broad in range), high durability in natural systems, and the inherent potential to reproduce rapidly in an appropriate host. They can be found associated with a great diversity of bacterial species in any natural ecosystem [11].

Phages can be characterized by their size and shape into three general groups: icosahedron, filamentous, and complex. Members of these groups may contain nucleic acid of various types including single-stranded DNA (ssDNA), double-stranded DNA (dsDNA), single-stranded RNA (ssRNA), or double-stranded RNA (dsRNA). Phages can be further classified with respect to their actions that follow infection of the bacterial cell. Virulent bacteriophages reproduce immediately and induce lysis of the cell to enable progeny release, whereas temperate phages insert their genetic material into the host genome or accessory elements, where they reproduce with the host until triggered to enter the lytic pathway as observed for virulent phages [12].

Virulent tailed phages of the Caudovirales order have been the best described for phage therapeutic applications. Within this group, the Myoviridae have a large capsid head and contractile tail, the Siphoviridae have a relatively small capsid and a long flexible non-contractile tail, and the Podoviridae have a small capsid head and short tail [13]. The virulent tailed phages follow a lytic cycle that begins with the specific attachment of phage anti-receptors to host cell surface receptor molecules. This interaction is often two-step, with an initial reversible phase and then irreversible phase. Once irreversibly bound, enzymes degrade the cell wall and the genetic material is ejected into the cell with (usually) the assistance of processive host enzymes. Once transcribed, the phage genome begins to redirect the host cell metabolism including DNA replication and protein biosynthesis to the reproduction of viral nucleic acid and proteins. Often, the host genome is degraded during this process. Once complete daughter viral particles are assembled, cell lysis is initiated to release the particles. Bacterial lysis is triggered by late encoded phage proteins including holins (to permeabilize the inner cell membrane) and endolysins (to degrade the peptidoglycan) with the loss of cell wall integrity causing lysis due to osmotic differential [14].

Specificity

Host specificity (range) of phages is variable, with some phages infecting multiple species and others only growing on one known isolate. However, their specificity is much higher than that of antibiotics. The phage host cell surface receptors and antiviral defense mechanisms (genetic and physical) are the main properties that determine specificity. For some highly conserved species, a single phage can kill the majority of strains (e.g., phage P100 infects >90% *Listeria monocytogenes* isolates tested [15]). Phages that propagate on species with high clonal diversity (e.g., *Pseudomonas aeruginosa*) typically only kill a small cohort of strains [16].

Establishment of phage banks or training (in vitro evolution) of phages to become more active and to elicit less bacterial resistance against the infecting bacterial strain can be valid strategies to overcome limited host specificity for targeted phage therapy [16]. This strategy likely works best for chronic infections where the target bacterium is well characterized. In order to treat acute infections, phage cocktails including phages that together span the whole spectrum of potential strains are proposed. However, the research and resources needed for the production of suitable and stable multi-component cocktails are disadvantages of this approach. An alternative approach is to use phage lytic enzymes (endolysins), which show broader host specificity at the genus and species level. Endolysins have been the subject of a recent review by our group [17], so are not discussed further here.

Antibiotics typically kill a broad-spectrum of either Gram-positive and Gram-negative bacteria including benign flora, which is increasingly considered to be non-desirable due to their adverse effects on the whole microbiota and potential to spread antibiotic resistance [18,19]. Phage therapy meets these challenges by its superior specificity and ability to treat drug-resistant isolates.

3. Phage Pharmacology

The pharmacology of phages necessitates the study of interactions between phages and bacteria as well as interactions between phages and body tissues [14]. Successful and safe phage therapy involves the effective control of phage–host interactions involving two fundamental components: pharmacodynamics and pharmacokinetics [20].

3.1. Pharmacodynamics

Pharmacodynamics is the study of the interaction of drugs with their receptors, the transduction systems to which they are related, and the changes in cells, organs, and the whole organism. The drugs' impact on the body can either be positive, thus maintaining or restoring health, or negative such as causing toxic side effects [20].

Phages can be applied via active or passive therapeutic strategies. In active treatment regimes, phages are introduced at low concentrations relative to the bacteria concentration and therapy relies on the production and release of progeny phages to infect all bacteria. Active treatments with phages are considered to have features of automated dosing and to mimic the bodies' homeostatic mechanism better than standard pharmaceuticals through the targeted killing of bacteria and phage production at actual sites of infection rather than systemically [21]. In contrast, passive phage treatment relies on single, or multiple rounds of sufficient phage concentrations to infect all target bacteria.

Compared to antibiotics, only a single phage is required to kill a single bacterium and so fewer units are required per treatment. Phages also do not dissociate from bacterial targets once irreversibly adsorbed. However, multiple phages may adsorb to individual bacteria. For these reasons, it is important to understand the concepts of multiplicity of infection (MOI), which is the ratio of phage infections per bacteria, and MOI_{input}, which is the number of phages that are administered per cell. The killing titer is another concept that can be used to guide phage therapy and is the number of effective bactericidal phage particles delivered (c.f. the number of plaque-based phage counts) [14,20–23]. Failure to recognize the special requirements of phage pharmacodynamics could result in compromises to phage therapy efficacy [20].

The degradation of phages by antibodies and other aspects of the immune system do not lead to the production and accumulation of toxic by-products. The low toxicity of phages is a consequence of their composition which, for tailed phages, is entirely protein and nucleic acid. As a result, phage therapy can be considered comparatively physiologically benign when compared to standard antibiotic therapies.

3.2. Pharmacokinetics

Pharmacokinetics describes the absorption, distribution, metabolism, and excretion of a drug. Absorption and distribution of the drug require its movement throughout the body, at first to the blood and then beyond the blood into specific tissues or compartments where the drug may accumulate at different densities [20]. Phage pharmacokinetics are also influenced by decay and proliferation as a result of the self-replication of bacteriophages.

The route of administration for phages will also affect in situ pharmacokinetics. In clinical cases, phages are frequently delivered by parenteral administration with oral dosing, topical application, and aerosolization also common. Data on the relative effectiveness of these approaches is largely drawn from animal studies. For instance, intramuscular, intraperitoneal, and subcutaneous injection of a phage cocktail were compared for efficacy in treating a *P. aeruginosa* in a murine burn model where intraperitoneal injection was found to be the most effective, most likely due to the delivery of higher numbers of phages more quickly and for a greater sustained period than other routes [24]. When using oral phage dosing in mice, the addition of 0.025% CaCO$_3$ was found to effectively protect the phage from stomach acids and deliver the phage to the upper and lower gastrointestinal tract where they reduced numbers of the targeted *E. coli* O157:H7 [25]. When treating *Burkholderia* infections induced in mice, the aerosolization of phages was found to be superior to intraperitoneal injection [26]. Some advantages and disadvantages of the administration routes are shown in Table 1.

Table 1. Routes of administration for phage therapy.

Delivery Route	Advantages	Disadvantages	Mitigations to Hurdles
Intraperitoneal	Higher dosage volumes possible. Diffusion to other sites.	Extent of diffusion to other sites may be overestimated in humans (most data from small animals).	Multiple delivery sites.
Intramuscular	Phages delivered at infection site.	Slower diffusion of phages (possibly). Lower dosage volumes.	Multi-dose courses. Multi-dose courses.
Subcutaneous	Localized and systemic diffusion.	Lower dosage volumes.	Multi-dose courses.
Intravenous	Rapid systemic diffusion.	Rapid clearing of phages by the immune system.	In vivo selection of low-immunogenic phages may be possible.
Topical	High dose of phages delivered at infection site.	Run-off from target site if phages suspended in liquid.	Incorporate phages into gels and dressings.
Suppository	Slow, stable release of phages over long time.	Limited applications/sites. Risk of insufficient dosing. Technically challenging to manufacture.	Careful consideration of phage kinetics required.
Oral	Ease of delivery. Higher dosage volumes possible.	Stomach acid reduces phage titer. Non-specific adherence of phages to stomach contents and other microflora.	Add calcium carbonate to buffer pH. Microencapsulation to deliver phages to target area.
Aerosol	Relative ease of delivery. Can reach poorly perfused regions of infected lungs.	High proportion of phages lost. Delivery can be impaired by mucus and biofilms	Use of depolymerases to reduce mucus.

In vitro studies of phage pharmacokinetics using mathematical models do not necessarily reflect the in vivo phage kinetics observed. For instance, phage T4 was reported to not replicate in vitro at host concentrations below 10^4 per mL, but evidence suggests that this is possible in murine models [27]. Phage feeding experiments in animals and humans frequently report irregular shedding and the passage of high percentages (up to 90% administered) of phages in feces [27]. The failure of many phage therapy experiments has been related to a poor understanding of phage pharmacokinetics, for instance, when dosing relies too much on the self-replicating nature of phages [20].

Phage lytic enzymes (endolysins) can also be used for therapy, but their kinetics are more similar to conventional treatments. For example, Jun et al. [28] determined that a *Staphylococcus aureus* specific endolysin had a half-life between 0.04 and 0.38 h after intravenous administration in healthy volunteers. The decay kinetics of this endolysin is likely explained by the presence of plasma proteases. Other endolysins have demonstrated a longer half-life such as 11.3 h for CF-301 and 5.2–5.6 h (for 30 and 60 mg/kg, respectively) for P128 [29,30].

Toxin (e.g., endotoxin) release due to significant bacterial cell lysis could potentially trigger septic shock during phage therapy. However, antibiotics like amikacin, cefoxitin, and imipenem have been shown to induce higher amounts of released endotoxin than coliphages [31]. The increase in endotoxin produced after 180 min incubation of *E. coli* LM33 was 3.8-fold with phage LM33_P1, 5.5-fold with amikacin, 8.7-fold with cefoxitin, and 30-fold with imipenem. With *E. coli* strain 536, there was a 19.8-fold increase in endotoxin with amikacin, 29.9-fold with phage 536_P1, 53.7-fold with imipenem, and 125.1-fold with ceftriaxone [31].

So, whilst less of an issue than for most conventional antibiotics, high fragmentation of the cell wall must be minimized with either phage or phage endolysin therapies to prevent an increase in pro-inflammatory cytokines [19,32]. To address this potential issue, several groups have proposed genetically engineering phages to prevent or reduce cell lysis, whilst still causing cell death by mechanisms such as degrading the host genome (see Section 7 and [33]).

4. Role of the Immune Response in Phage Therapy

Phages can potentially trigger innate and adaptive immune cells that may influence the success of phage therapy. Three major fields of phage-immune interaction can be discerned. First, involving immune recognition via pattern recognition receptor (PRR), which is a means for the recruitment of phagocytes to the infection site [34]. Phages can mediate the activation of innate immune cells when PRR recognizes phage-derived DNA and RNA. The extent of immune activation will differ depending on the phage type, the phage dose, and in vivo nucleic acid synthetic activity.

Second, promoted phage-neutralizing antibodies can hamper therapeutic success and this effect can increase with repeated administration [35]. Antibody induction against phages is considered to be highly variable, thus immunogenicity should be considered during phage screening prior to phage therapy. There are several externally presenting proteins on phages such as Hoc, which can potentially induce such an immune response [36–38]. Strategies to avoid phage-induced neutralizing antibody formation include refining dose concentrations, the use of low-multi-dose regimes, or low-dose passive therapy approaches.

Third, the inhibitory effect of humoral (adaptive) immunity and anti-phage antibody production on phages in the mammalian system is broadly known. Effects seem dose-dependent, with only high doses for long periods inducing specific responses. For instance, Majewska [39] developed a long-term study of antibody induction (IgM, IgG, secretory IgA) in mice fed T4 phage orally at high doses (10^9 PFU/mL drinking water). No effect was noted in the first two weeks, then in weeks 3–5, there was an increase in blood serum IgG. IgM did not increase until IgG began increasing, while IgA did not increase until days 63–79, but when it reached its maximum, no phage was found in the mouse feces. Increased IgA concentrations antagonized the gut transit of active phage and phage resistant hosts dominated the gut flora by day 92. However, IgA was rapidly cleared after phage withdrawal [39]. A similar study determined the immunological response of *Pseudomonas* phage F8 and T4 treatment in a murine systemic inflammatory response syndrome (SIR) model. The primary (IgM) and the secondary (IgG) responses inhibited the phages, and phage concentration in the spleen was significantly decreased [40].

Human trials in 26 patients with immunodeficiency diseases were undertaken to evaluate immunologic responses to phage ϕX174. An intravenous dose of 10^9 PFU/kg body weight was given, and the phage titer measured in blood. No antibody response was detected in eight cases of infantile X-linked agammaglobulinemia with circulating phages present for up to 11 days. The other 18 patients produced antibodies and phages were cleared from circulation within four days. Ten of these patients showed the IgM antibody, and eight patients produced both IgM and IgG [41]. Other work using ϕX174 [42] has demonstrated that repeated (up to quaternary) dosing of phages does not lead to serious adverse reactions.

It is currently not well understood if anti-phage antibodies could prevent bacterial resistance development to phages and if the pre-existing immunity to natural phages could affect phage therapy. Furthermore, there is no clear information about the impact of phage-specific factors on phage clearance mechanisms. There are also gaps in our understanding of the clinical relevance of the phage immune interaction. Nevertheless, the immunogenicity of phages itself does not seem to represent a significant safety risk for patients. Reports about immune effects in clinical studies using virulent phages are limited. The introduction of validated in vitro and in vivo methods to determine the comparability of immune effects of different phages and phage combinations would be indispensable. This would allow for valid conclusions on the value of immune-based parameters for the selection of phages, identification of responsive patient populations, exchangeability of phages, and the importance of individualized phage cocktails [33]. The engineering of phages to make them less immunogenic is also an area of active research (see Section 7).

5. Resistance to Phages

An important consideration for phage therapy is the potential for bacterial resistance. Phage-resistant bacteria have been noted in up to 80% of studies targeting the intestines and 50% of studies using sepsis models, with phage-resistant variants also observed in human studies [43].

As with resistance to classical antibiotics, spontaneous resistance to phages may occur through a number of mechanisms. For example, the cell surface target receptor(s) may not be expressed or become mutated, thus causing a complete loss of adsorption or decreased adsorption. This is a limitation of both phage and conventional antibiotic therapy. For both approaches, knowing the receptor site(s), their stability, and conservation across strains will help with the mitigation of resistance.

Acquired resistance is another area that requires investigation for both therapeutic approaches. Accessory genetic elements such as plasmids, temperate phages, and mobile genetic islands can carry genes coding for resistance to antibiotics. For phages, acquired resistance can encompass CRISPR-Cas systems [33], immunity proteins produced by temperate phages (though rare) and the acquisition of DNA restriction-modification systems.

A key advantage of phage therapy over conventional treatments for the avoidance of resistance development is the deployment of phage cocktails. The use of several phages, each targeting different receptors and each of a diverse genetic clade will enhance the ability to mitigate against the loss of adsorption or host genetic protection mechanisms. Genetic engineering may also provide a means to improve the diversity and targeting efficiency of phages for the avoidance of resistance (see Section 7). Another consideration is that bacterial mutations that confer phage-resistance often result in fitness costs to the resistant bacterium. Therefore, understanding and exploiting the fitness costs to resistant pathogens during therapy is a potentially promising research avenue [43].

6. Phage Therapy Clinical Trials in Humans

To date, human phage therapy trials have largely been empirical, with routine use limited to Georgia, Poland, and Russia [44]. In particular, the George Eliava Institute in Georgia has longstanding experience with the selection, isolation, and preparation of monophage and phage cocktails against a variety of bacterial pathogens for phage therapy. The therapeutic application of phages has also been undertaken for several decades at the Institute of Immunology and Experimental Therapy in Poland [45]. However, the experimental clinical data published in Russian and Polish journals are difficult to access due to security and language barriers.

Although the reporting and assessment of phage therapy need to improve, particularly with regard to efficacy and tolerability and the use of adequate patient numbers, several successful case reports have been published. The reports do provide some evidence that the development of phage therapy is a promising alternative to combat bacterial resistance to antibiotics.

In France, the national health regulator has authorized the first treatment of patients with extremely drug-resistant and difficult to treat infections using phage therapy. Since then, six cases with various bacterial infections have been successfully treated [44]. Even though several treatments were not conducted using clinical standards suitable for drug approval in the Western world, they showed therapeutic potential for phages and how phages can be applied [45].

New therapeutic products must usually go through a long and comprehensive process involving preclinical and clinical trials to gain regulatory approval for market access. In the US, the average time for the approval of a new drug from preclinical testing is 12 years and the costs run into millions of dollars due to the length, size, and complexity of human clinical trials. For these reasons, the number of formal phage therapy clinical trials (as listed on www.ClinicalTrials.gov or https://globalclinicaltrialdata.com/) is very limited [45]. However, some of the human phage therapy clinical trials underway are summarized in Figure 1 and are described in the following case studies.

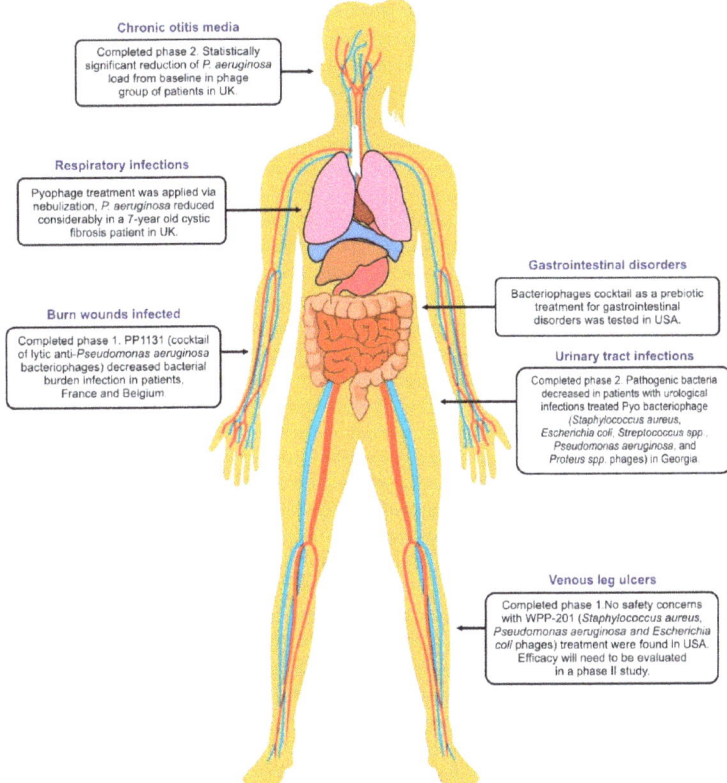

Figure 1. Human phage therapy trials and the range of target sites/infections. Image adapted from Furfaro et al. [46].

6.1. Phage Treatment of Burns

Phage therapy was applied in wound infections in 27 patients from hospitals in France and Belgium using a cocktail of virulent anti-*Pseudomonas aeruginosa* bacteriophages. Participants were randomly assigned (1:1) to a cocktail of 12 natural virulent anti-*P. aeruginosa* bacteriophages (10^6 plaque-forming units [PFU] per mL) or standard of care (1% sulfadiazine silver emulsion cream), and the route of administration was topical for seven days, with 14 days of follow-up [44].

The median of the primary endpoint was 144 h in the phage treatment group and 47 h in the standard of care group. Three (23%) of the 13 analyzable participants showed adverse events in the phage treatment group when compared with seven (54%) out of 13 in the standard care group. Bacteria isolated from patients of the failed phage treatment were resistant to low phage doses [44].

This study showed that phage treatment decreased bacterial burden in burn wounds in more time than the standard treatment. In this regard, studies increasing the phage concentration and the use of "phagograms" (as used for antibiograms) with more patients are warranted.

6.2. Treatment of A Septicemia Patient with Acute Kidney Damage

A man in his sixties was hospitalized for *Enterobacter cloacae* peritonitis and severe abdominal sepsis, dispersed intravascular coagulation, herniation, and bowel strangulation. Following prolonged treatment for these ailments, the patient developed gangrene and pressure sores colonized by drug-resistant *P. aeruginosa*. The infection developed to septicemia and colistin treatment (the only drug sensitivity) was carried out, however, acute kidney damage was detected, and the treatment was suspended. Subsequently, phage therapy against *P. aeruginosa* was conducted using a mixture of two phages active against the isolate in vitro, under the umbrella of Article 37 (Unproven Interventions in Clinical Practice) of the Declaration of Helsinki [46]. Following phage therapy, the patient showed improved kidney function, which returned to normal function after a few days, and blood cultures were negative.

However, the patient's pressure sores remained infected with *P. aeruginosa* and other species and four months later, the patient developed a refractory cardiac arrest due to blood culture-confirmed *Klebsiella pneumoniae* sepsis and the patient died. In vivo studies revealed that a *K. pneumoniae* strain isolated from the patient was sensitive to the antibiotics. According to historical reports, the use of phages by intravenous route in typhoid fever and *Staphylococcus aureus* [47] bacteremia were efficacious, nevertheless, this is the first contemporary report using phage monotherapy against *P. aeruginosa* septicemia in humans through the intravenous route [48].

6.3. Engineered Phages for Treatment of Mycobacteria in A Cystic Fibrosis Patient

Therapeutic phage treatment for mycobacteria has been explored in several animal models [49,50], but until recently had not been successfully used for mycobacterial infections in humans. A 15-year-old patient with cystic fibrosis and extensive comorbidities was referred for lung transplant with a disseminated infection of *Mycobacterium abscessus*. Following bilateral lung transplantation and persistent *M. abscessus* infections, phage genome engineering and forward genetics were used to engineer phages to target and kill the infectious *M. abscessus* strain. Therapy was conducted using an intravenous three-phage cocktail of 10^9 PFU of each phage every 12 h for 32 weeks [51].

Intravenous phage treatment was well tolerated, clinical improvement including sternal wound closure, improved liver and lung function, and substantial resolution of infected skin nodules were detected in the six months following therapy. No evidence of phage neutralization was detected in sera, although weak antibody responses to phage proteins were identified. Weak cytokine responses were reported for interferon-γ, interleukin-6, interleukin-10, and tumor necrosis factor-α [51]. Some evidence was presented that indicated active in vivo phage replication was taking place. Despite the apparent success of this therapy, the authors did caution that there was significant variation in *M. abscessus* phage susceptibility, so the treatment of similar patients will require more work to be undertaken to understand the science underlying this observation.

6.4. Phage Therapy for Respiratory Infections

There have been several pre-clinical studies describing the use of phage therapy against chronic bacterial lung infections using murine models. Pabary et. al. [52] determined that phage treatment reduced the infective burden and inflammatory response in the murine lung. All phage-treated mice cleared *P. aeruginosa* infection at 24 h, whereas infection persisted in all of the control mice. Phage also reduced infection and inflammation in bronchoalveolar lavage fluid when administered prophylactically. Another study showed that intranasal treatment with phage rescued mice from *Acinetobacter baumannii*-mediated pneumonia. Microcomputed tomography also indicated a reduction in lung inflammation in mice given phage [53]. In a study using a biofilm-associated murine model of chronic lung infection, phage therapy was effective seven days post-infection. Additionally, these studies established the potential for phage therapy in established and recalcitrant chronic respiratory tract infections [54].

Notwithstanding the reported treatment of *Mycobacterium* described in Section 6.3, reports of phage therapy of human bacterial respiratory infections are rare. In a 2011 case study from Georgia, a seven-year-old cystic fibrosis (CF) patient presented with chronic colonization of *P. aeruginosa* and *S. aureus* with antibiotic treatments having limited effect. Phage therapy was undertaken using a "Pyo phage" phage cocktail produced by the Eliava Institute, which reportedly contains phages active against *S. aureus*, *Streptococcus*, *Proteus*, *P. aeruginosa*, and *E. coli* [55]. The Pyo phage cocktail was delivered to the patient via nebulization at four-to-six week intervals for nine rounds of treatment. The *P. aeruginosa* numbers reduced considerably, however, the treatment was not effective against *S. aureus*. Consequently, Sb-1 phage (a phage targeting *S. aureus*) was added to the Pyo phage cocktail and administered five times with a nebulizer. This treatment reduced the concentration of *S. aureus* significantly. No adverse effects were detected in the patient upon Sb-1 phage treatment [55].

Recent advances in the spray drying of phages that have achieve increased numbers of phages delivered to the lungs (up to 10^8 PFU/aspiration) may considerably improve clinical outcomes for respiratory infections such as these [56]. Work has also shown that a cocktail of ten phages significantly decreased *P. aeruginosa* numbers in sputum samples from 58 CF patients collected from hospitals in Paris [45,57]. Forty-eight of 58 samples were positive for *P. aeruginosa* and the addition of phages significantly decreased the concentrations of *P. aeruginosa* in the sputum. An increase in the number of bacteriophages in 45.8% of these samples was also detected, demonstrating the potential for active phage therapy of respiratory infections in vivo.

6.5. Phage Therapy for Urinary Tract Infections

Therapy for treating urinary tract infections (UTIs) is one of the most promising applications for phages and one of the few that have been studied in a multi-stage clinical trial. In the first stage of the trial, 130 patients planned for transurethral resection of the prostate were screened for UTIs and 118 patients enrolled [58]. Criteria for inclusion in the trial were having $\geq 10^4$ cfu/mL of the pathogens *S. aureus*, *E. coli*, *Streptococcus*, *P. aeruginosa*, or *Proteus mirabilis* in their urine culture. Initial in vitro screening of these cultures against the Pyo phage cocktail, a commercial product produced by the Eliava Institute, revealed that the sensitivity was 41% (48/118). Directed evolution experiments were applied to the cocktail to select for expanded host range phages, and the sensitivity was improved to 75% (88/118).

In the second stage, nine patients who had infections caused by bacteria sensitive to the Pyo cocktail underwent non-blinded phage therapy. Administration of 20 mL 10^7–10^9 PFU/mL phages was via a suprapubic catheter twice every 24 h for seven days, starting the first day after surgery. Urine from the patients was subsequently cultured seven days after surgery or at the time of adverse indications. Prior to therapy, the patients' urine screening revealed the presence of *E. coli* in four cases, *Enterococcus* in two cases, *Streptococcus* in two cases, and *P. aeruginosa* in one case. Following therapy, titers of the pathogens decreased by 1–5 log cfu/mL in six out of nine patients. One of the four *E. coli* cases had no detectable pathogen, one of two *Streptococcus* cases had no detectable pathogen, one of the *Enterococcus* cases had no pathogens, but the other case detected *E. coli*. The patient with the *P. aeruginosa* infection required antibiotic therapy following a spike in fever and became asymptomatic; however, *P. aeruginosa* was detected in his urine. No adverse effects of phage therapy were detected. The study authors hope to further progress this work to full randomized and blinded control studies in the future.

6.6. Phage Therapy for Diarrhea

Whilst no longer an active partnership, the Nestlé Research Centre in Switzerland and the International Centre for Diarrhoeal Diseases Research in Bangladesh have undertaken joint research projects over a number of years that have explored the efficacy of phage therapy for the treatment of diarrheal diseases. In one of the studies, 120 Bangladeshi male children (6–24 months) presenting with acute bacterial diarrhea were given either 3.6×10^8 PFU of a T4-like coliphage cocktail (39 children), 1.4×10^9 PFU of a commercial coliphage preparation (Coliproteus from Microgen, 40 children), or a placebo (0.9% NaCl, 41 children) suspended in oral rehydration solution.

Results of this randomized blind trial indicated no adverse effects of oral phage treatment of the children. The phage survived the gastric passage, but there was no strong evidence of intestinal replication occurring in patients. Neither the T4-like nor the Microgen coliphage cocktail showed a significant clinical effect when compared to the control group for stool output or frequency, or rehydration. Likely reasons for the lack of significant effects were the lower than expected incidence of *E. coli* (60%) and the incidence of mixed species infections, the presence of non-susceptible coliforms (phage cocktail was not optimized for local isolates), and insufficient phage titer [59,60].

6.7. Treatment of Peri-Prosthetic Joint Infection

In this case study [61], an 80-year-old female patient with obesity and a history of relapsing prosthetic joint infection of the right hip presented with a *S. aureus* postoperative infection and was treated with debridement, antibiotics, and implant retention (DAIR). Four years later, another DAIR was performed for fluoroquinolone-resistant *E. coli*, following reimplantation surgery in the prior year. Then, due to a relapse including positive *E. coli* cultures, another DAIR was performed three weeks later. Antibacterial therapy with ceftriaxone was started; however, there were further signs of relapse and antibiotic treatment was stopped. Multidrug-resistant *P. aeruginosa* and penicillin-resistant *S. aureus* were identified in swabs of the wound discharge.

To undertake phage therapy, three phages targeted against the *P. aeruginosa* isolate were first prepared by Pherecydes Pharma (France). The *S. aureus* isolate was lost, so three phages from the Pherecydes Pharma phage bank were used. Phages were produced in a research environment with the manufacture overseen by The French National Agency for Medicines and Health Products Safety (ANSM). The final formulation of the *P. aeruginosa* and *S. aureus* phages were undertaken by the hospital pharmacy by mixing equal volumes of 10^{10} PFU/mL phage stocks. During the following DAIR, 20 mL of the phage cocktail was injected into the joint region. Co-therapy with antibiotics (daptomycin, amoxicillin, and clindamycin) was followed for the next six months without signs of *P. aeruginosa* or *S. aureus* infection. The patient later had a *Citrobacter* infection, which required DAIR, but once this was treated with Ciprofloxacin, no further infection was found in the joint (18 months post-phage therapy).

The bespoke use of phage and antibiotic combinations to treat a patient's infection has the potential to be utilized to create personalized therapy for deep and persistent tissue infections such as those found associated with peri-prosthetic joints (Figure 2).

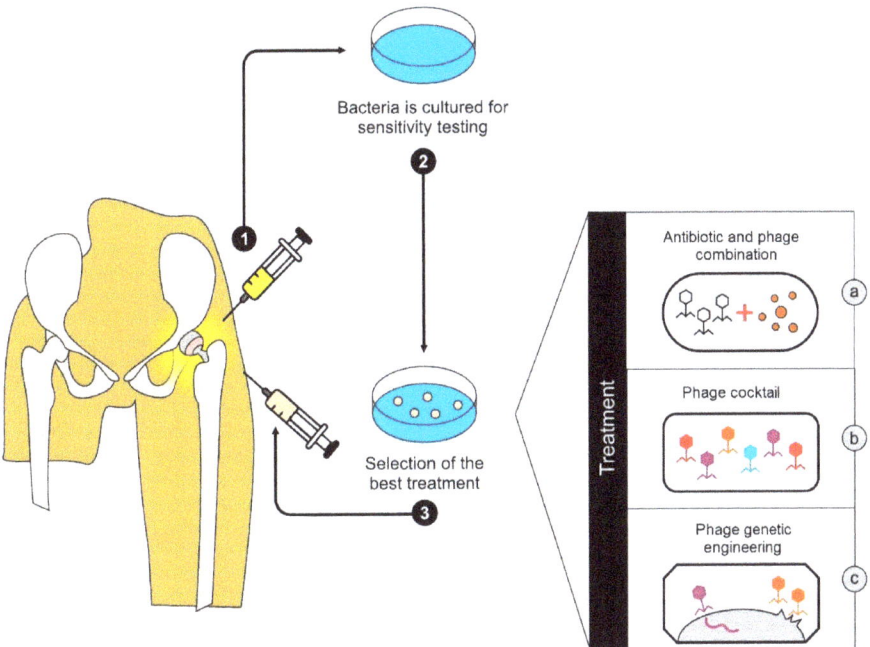

Figure 2. Personalized combinatorial phage therapy. Image adapted from Akanda et al. [62].

6.8. Treatment of Leg Ulcers

A Phase I trial of phage therapy with 42 patients with chronic venous leg ulcers has been undertaken [63]. Ulcers were treated for 12 weeks with a phage cocktail (WPP-201; 8×10^7 PFU/mL) or a control (saline). The phage cocktail targeted *P. aeruginosa, S. aureus,* and *E. coli*. Patient follow-up continued until week 24 and no adverse events were attributed to the phage treatment. There was no significant difference between the phage therapy group and the control group for the rate or frequency of ulcer healing. Efficacy of the preparation will need to be evaluated in a phase II efficacy study.

6.9. Therapy of Drug-Resistant Craniectomy Infection

A previously healthy 77-year-old male who suffered assault, subdural hematoma, and traumatic brain injury underwent a craniectomy, which was complicated by postoperative intracranial infection with multidrug-resistant *A. baumannii*. The isolate was resistant to all antibiotics; however, some isolates were sensitive to colistin [64]. An emergency investigational new drug application to use phage therapy on the patient was approved by the US Food and Drug Administration. Phages from the Naval Medical Research Center-Frederick were screened against the isolate and the most active phage prepared.

The phage (2.1×10^7 PFU/mL) was administered intravenously through a central catheter line every 2 h for eight days, with 98 total doses given. Following phage treatment, the patient initially seemed more alert, but continued to be unresponsive. The craniotomy site and skin flap healed well, though fevers and leukocytosis continued. There were no further signs of infection at the craniotomy site after surgical debridement. However, bacterial cultures obtained prior to phage administration were negative, therefore it was not possible to directly measure phage efficacy. Before the receipt of a second phage cocktail, the patient's family decided to withdraw care and the patient died.

The authors concluded that administration of phages through the surgical drain would likely have had more benefit than parenteral administration, less targeted phages with broader activity may have been more efficacious, and a better outcome might have been possible if personalized phage therapy had been developed more quickly and administered earlier in the course of infection.

6.10. Therapy of Ear Infections

A Phase I/II research trial was conducted in the UK to test the efficacy and safety of phages for the treatment of chronic ear infections (otitis media), where the infection is known to harbor antibiotic-resistant *P. aeruginosa* [65]. In this randomized double-blinded study, a cocktail of six phages produced by Biocontrol Limited (BiophagePA, 6×10^5 PFU), or placebo (glycerol-PBS solution) were administered to the ear canal of 24 patients. The follow-up to treatment was at 7, 21, and 43 days and revealed a statistically significant improvement in both clinical condition and patient-reported indicators for the phage treated group when compared to the control. No adverse reactions were noted in the phage-treated group.

In vivo replication of phages in the patients was evident for up to 23 days, with the mean recovery of phages during the trial sampling points being 200 times the input concentration. Clearance of phages was noted when the *P. aeruginosa* infection was resolved in patients. Reductions in overall *P. aeruginosa* numbers in the phage treatment group, whilst statistically significant, were generally modest, but measurement was likely to be compromised by the lack of access to deep parts of the ear canal. When *P. aeruginosa* was not completely cleared by phage therapy, there was an increase in clinical scores for some patients. The study authors suggest that repeated phage therapy after three to four weeks may be beneficial to these types of patients in any future work.

7. Engineering and Other Genetic Technologies for Phage Therapy

The advent of whole-genome sequencing and metagenomics have rapidly increased the number of phage genomes sequenced and is unlocking new insights into phage genetics. The use of this new knowledge for phage engineering holds great potential to increase the utility of phages for therapy, however, there are additional considerations such as ethical, safety, and regulatory, which need to be accounted for above that of 'natural' phage therapy. Engineering can be used to produce new variants of phages with expanded host range, decreasing the number of phage strains needed to cover bacterial diversity, and generating patentable phage variants [66–68]. For example, the host specificity of the *E. coli* K12-specific phage T2 was able to be changed by swapping gene products expressed at the tip of the long tail fiber with those of the PP01 phage, which is an *E. coli* O157: H7-specific phage [66]. The recombinant phage was able to infect *E. coli* O157: H7 and related strains, but could not infect *E. coli* K12 or its derivatives. Similarly, homologous recombination was used to replace the long tail fiber genes (genes 37 and 38) from the genome of T2 with those of the IP008 phage. The recombinant T2 phage had a host range identical to that of IP008 [67]. Lin et. al. [68] were also able to modify the *E. coli* female-specific T7 phage to overcome male exclusion by recombination with phage T3. The recombinant phages of T3 and T7 carried altered tail fibers and had better adsorption efficiency than T3.

Genetic engineering of phage permits the addition of novel functionality such as bacteriocins, enzybiotics, quorum sensing inhibitors, CRISPRs, and biofilm degrading enzymes that can enhance their killing potential [69–73]. Phages can be modified using the RNA-guided nuclease Cas9 to create sequence-specific antimicrobials. Cas9 was reprogrammed to target virulence genes and killed virulent, but not avirulent, strains of *S. aureus* in a mouse skin colonization model [65]. Another study used CRISPR-Cas technology to create RNA-guided nucleases delivered by phages to target specific DNA sequences in carbapenem-resistant *Enterobacteriaceae* and enterohemorrhagic *E. coli* [70]. Delivery of the nucleases improved the survival in a *Galleria mellonella* infection model. Phage-borne CRISPR-Cas systems can also be used to enable site-specific cleavage to induce cytotoxicity, activate toxin-antitoxin systems, re-sensitize bacterial populations to antibiotics, and modulate bacterial consortia [70].

Biofilms are the major cause of persistent infections in clinical settings, thus phage treatment to lyse bacteria in biofilms has attracted growing interest. An engineered T7 phage was constructed to encode a lactonase enzyme with broad-range activity for the quenching of quorum sensing molecules necessary for biofilm formation. The T7 phage incorporating the AHL lactonase *aiiA* gene from *Bacillus anthracis* degraded AHLs from diverse bacteria and caused the inhibition of a mixed-species biofilm composed of *P. aeruginosa* and *E. coli* [71]. In another approach using the T7 phage, a biofilm-degrading enzyme, DspB, produced by *Actinobacillus actinomycetemcomitans*, was inserted into the T7 genome and the resultant phage reduced *E. coli* biofilm cell counts by an additional 2 log when compared to the unmodified T7 [72].

As described in Section 4, components of the innate immune system can remove a significant proportion of administered phage. Studies have shown that long-circulating phage mutants can be isolated to address this issue. Vitiello et. al. [73] determined that a single specific substitution in the major phage capsid (E) protein of the lambda Argo phage was enough to confer a long-circulating phenotype that enhanced phage survival in the mouse circulatory system by more than a 1000-fold. Merril et. al. [74] used a serial passage selection method to isolate phage mutants with a greater capacity to remain in the circulatory system of the mouse. Lambda phage mutants with 13,000–16,000-fold better capacity to stay in the mouse circulatory system for 24 h after intraperitoneal injection were isolated.

Many antibiotics, as well as phage therapy, can present side effects due to endotoxin release from Gram-negative bacteria. To address this, genetic engineering was used to generate non-replicating non-lytic phage targeting *P. aeruginosa*. An export protein gene of the *P. aeruginosa* filamentous phage Pf3 was replaced with a restriction endonuclease gene and the variant (Pf3R) was non-replicative and prevented the release of phage from the target cell. Endotoxin release was kept to a minimum and the Pf3R phage efficiently killed a wild-type host in vitro. Phage therapy using Pf3R showed comparable or increased survival rates (depending on dose) when compared to Pf3 upon challenge in the mice model. Higher survival rates were correlated with a reduced inflammatory response when using Pf3R treatment [75]. Matsuda et. al. [76] also produced lysis-deficient T4 phages for this purpose. Mutant t amber A3 T4 phages were compared to wild-type T4 in mouse bacterial peritonitis model. Survival was significantly higher in mice treated with the lysis deficient phage when compared to the wild-type, and enterotoxin levels were significantly lower in the t A3 T4-treated mice at 12 hours after infection [76].

8. The Medicinal Regulatory Status of Phages

Phages are not specifically classified as living or chemical agents in any national medicinal legislation (as far as we are aware). This considerably complicates the regulation of human phage therapy clinical trials and commercialization of phage products as well-established safety, good manufacturing practice, and efficacy benchmarks are lacking [77]. Another barrier is that in order to prove the efficiency of phage preparations, their effectiveness and host range toward currently circulating pathogenic strains must be constantly monitored. This is most likely why the Russian Federation and Georgia approved phage preparations are continuously updated to target newly emerging pathogenic strains [78]. Therefore, any specific legislation regarding phage products would ideally permit these formulation updates as required to avoid repeated registration procedures.

A breakthrough for the regulation of phage therapy occurred in 2016, when the Belgian Minister of Social Affairs and Public Health defined the status of therapeutic phage preparations as industrially-prepared medicinal products (subjected to constraints related to marketing authorization) or as magistral (compounded) preparations prepared in the pharmacies' officinal [79]. Natural phages and their products can be processed by a pharmacist as raw materials (active ingredients) in magistral preparations, providing there is compliance with several provisions of the European Directive requirements for medicinal products for human use [78].

Several jurisdictions also permit the use of phages on compassionate grounds, where all other therapies have failed, and the condition is immediately life-threatening. These include the US FDA Expanded Access Program (www.fda.gov/news-events/public-health-focus/expanded-access) and Investigational Drug Program (https://www.fda.gov/drugs/types-applications/investigational-new-drug-ind-application) and the European Medicines Agency (https://www.ema.europa.eu/en/human-regulatory/research-development/compassionate-use).

9. Advantages and Disadvantages of Phage Therapy

Compared to conventional antibiotic therapy for bacterial infections, phage therapy has both a number of great advantages, but also some disadvantages. Some of these have been summarized in Table 2 and some aspects are discussed in more detail in the following subsections.

Table 2. Advantages and disadvantages of phage vs. antibiotic therapy for the treatment of bacterial infections.

Consideration	Antibiotic Therapy	Phage Therapy
Specificity	Low	High
Development costs	High	Low-moderate
Side effects	Moderate-high	Usually low, but yet to be fully established
Resistance	Increasing incidence of multi-drug resistant isolates.	Can treat multi-drug-resistant isolates. Phage resistant isolates generally lack fitness.
Delivery to target	Moderate	Moderate to good. Can penetrate the blood-brain barrier.
Formulation	Fixed	Fixed or variable
Regulation	Well established	Underdeveloped
Kinetics	Single hit	Single hit or self-amplifying
Immunogenicity	Variable	Likely low, but not well established
Clinical validation	Many trial studies	Relatively few trial studies

9.1. Key Advantages

Phage therapy has several key advantages that make it an attractive alternative to antibiotics. First, phages have high specificity to their hosts and unlike antibiotics, which have a much wider spectrum, are unlikely to cause dysbiosis and secondary infections (e.g., fungal infections). To date, phages have also not shown any significant side effects or risks of toxicity on mammalian cells [80]. Moreover, the process of isolation and selection of new phages is less expensive, in terms of time and costs, than the development process required for antibiotics: it typically takes millions of dollars and numerous years to develop an effective antibiotic drug [81].

The development of the resistance of bacteria to phage therapy is likely less significant than for antibiotics because of the ability to adapt phage cocktails by the substitution of phages, applying in vitro evolutionary pressure, or by genetic engineering. The variant resistant mutants are also generally of lower fitness. Phages are also able to successfully treat multi-drug-resistant bacteria as they use different mechanisms for targeting cells.

The ability of phages to widely spread through the body when applied by systemic administration, along with self-replication in the presence of the host, are qualities that most antibiotics do not have. Unlike most antibiotics, phages can also pass through the blood–brain barrier [82]. Some phages can also infiltrate and disrupt the biofilms that many pathogens naturally inhabit [82,83].

For patients with allergies to antibiotics, their treatment options can be restricted. About 1% of hospitalized patients have an allergy to penicillin-group drugs, the most common antibiotic allergy, followed by sulfonamides and tetracyclines [84]. Cross-reaction of penicillin allergies to next-generation cephalosporins and carbapenems has also been reported, but this remains controversial [85]. Phage therapy may be a valuable option for patients with antibiotic allergies, but reports are rare. For example, 12 patients with inflammatory soft tissue shotgun wounds and allergy to antibiotics (not specified) were reported to have been treated by polyvalent phage therapy (*Staphylococcus, Streptococcus, Proteus vulgaris, Proteus mirabilis, P. aeruginosa, E. coli,* and *K. pneumoniae*) for 15 days [86]. The concentrations of bacteria and the areas of wound healing were similar in the phage treatment group when compared to a control group of 35 patients receiving antibiotics. The authors concluded that phages were a reliable method for reducing microbial infection and that treatment led to a rapid epithelialization of the wound site [86].

9.2. Key Disadvantages

There are currently some key disadvantages of using phages as alternatives for antibiotics. However, these are predominantly due to gaps in knowledge and regulations, which may be resolved in the future. Critically, there is a lack of depth of information about the clinical application of phages for controlling bacterial infections. Much experimental clinical data published in Russian and Polish journals are difficult to access due to security and language barriers. There are also many more challenges for scientists in obtaining regulatory approval for phage-based therapeutic applications when compared to conventional therapies [80].

There is a lack of common established and validated protocols for the routes of administration, dose, frequency, and duration of phage treatment, which hampers inter-study comparison [87]. Often, the purity and stability of phage preparations used for clinical trials are also uncertain, with insufficient quality control data presented.

The concentration of phages may be reduced significantly during therapy by the reticuloendothelial system or be neutralized by antibodies, thus inhibiting their antimicrobial activity [39,88]. However, the effect of phage-neutralizing antibodies can be mitigated by refining dosing regimens and breeding phages to evade the immune system.

The genetic biosafety of phages is complex to assess. Phages used for therapy must not contain toxin or virulence genes, antibiotic resistance genes, or be able to horizontally transfer genes in the human microflora. Whilst whole-genome sequencing is a powerful tool to assist with these analyses, there is still an incomplete understanding of the functions of all encoded phage genes. Genetic engineering of phages will also likely invite greater scrutiny of safety which practitioners will need to address before application.

10. Conclusions

Antimicrobial resistance is increasing globally, and new treatments are urgently needed to meet this challenge in medical care. Whilst phage therapy for bacterial infections has been around for more than a century, the antibiotic-resistance crisis is providing renewed impetus for phage therapy to deliver on its long-held promise as a clinical treatment. As described here, there is an increasing number of well-executed Phase I/II clinical trials describing the safety and efficacy of phage therapy. There is an improved understanding of the pharmacology, immunology, safety, and potential for bacterial resistance. Technologies such as genetic engineering, whole-genome sequencing, and metagenomics also provide new tools to optimize phage therapeutic strategies. However, there are still data gaps on its efficacy and a lack of standardization and suitable regulatory frameworks that need to be resolved before phage therapy can take its place in mainstream medicine. Given the renewed interest and impetus in the field of phage therapy, there are reasons to be optimistic that these challenges can be met in the coming years.

Author Contributions: Conceptualization, D.R.-C. and C.B.; methodology, D.R.-C.; writing—original draft preparation, D.R.-C. and C.B.; writing—review and editing, D.R.-C., R.G.-B., A.G.-N. and C.B.; visualization, D.R.-C.; supervision, R.G.-B., A.G.-N. and C.B.; project administration, C.B.; funding acquisition, C.B.

Funding: This research was funded by an ESR Strategic Science Investment Fund grant to CB.

Conflicts of Interest: The authors declare no conflict of interest. The funders had no role in the design of the study; in the collection, analyses, or interpretation of data; in the writing of the manuscript, or in the decision to publish the results.

References

1. Hendrix, R.W.; Smith, M.C.M.; Burns, R.N.; Ford, M.E.; Hatfull, G.F. Evolutionary relationships among diverse bacteriophages and prophages: All the world's a phage. *Proc. Natl. Acad. Sci. USA* **1999**, *96*, 2192–2197. [CrossRef] [PubMed]
2. Hendrix, R.W. Bacteriophages: Evolution of the Majority. Theoretical Population Biology. *Popul. Biol.* **2002**, *61*, 471–480. [CrossRef]
3. Abedon, S.T.; Kuhl, S.J.; Blasdel, B.G.; Kutter, E.M. Phage treatment of human infections. *Bacteriophage* **2011**, *1*, 66–85. [CrossRef] [PubMed]
4. Międzybrodzki, R.; Borysowski, J.; Weber-Dabrowska, B.; Fortuna, W.; Letkiewicz, S.; Szufnarowski, K.; Pawełczyk, Z.; Rogóż, P.; Kłak, M.; Wojtasik, E.; et al. Clinical aspects of phage therapy. *Adv. Virus Res.* **2012**, *83*, 73–121. [PubMed]
5. Reyes, A.; Semenkovich, N.P.; Whiteson, K.; Rohwer, F.; Gordon, J.I. Going viral: Next-generation sequencing applied to phage populations in the human gut. *Nat. Rev. Microbiol.* **2012**, *10*, 607–617. [CrossRef] [PubMed]
6. Weber-Dabrowska, B.; Jónczyk-Matysiak, E.; Zaczek, M.; Łobocka, M.; Łusiak-Szelachowska, M.; Górski, A. Bacteriophage Procurement for Therapeutic Purposes. *Front. Microbiol.* **2016**, *7*, 1177. [CrossRef] [PubMed]
7. Aminov, R.; Caplin, J.; Chanishvili, N.; Coffey, A.; Cooper, I.; De Vos, D.; Doškar, J.; Friman, V.; Kurtböke, I.; Pantucek, R.; et al. Application of bacteriophages. *Microbiol. Aust.* **2018**, *38*, 63–66.
8. NIH NIAID's Antibacterial Resistance Program: Current Status and Future Directions. 2014. Available online: http://www.niaid.nih.gov/topics/antimicrobialresistane/documents/arstrategicplan2014.pdf (accessed on 23 September 2015).
9. Moellering, R.C. NDM-1—A cause for worldwide concern. *N. Eng. J. Med.* **2010**, *363*, 2377–2379. [CrossRef] [PubMed]
10. Ceyssens, P.-J.; Lavigne, R. Introduction to Bacteriophages Biology and Diversity. In *Bacteriophages in Control of Food and Waterborne Pathogens*; Sabour, P.M., Griffiths, M.W., Eds.; American Society of Microbiology: Washington, DC, USA, 2010.
11. Guttman, B.; Raya, R.; Kutter, E. Basic Phage Biology. In *Bacteriophages: Biology and Applications*; Kutter, E., Sulakvelidze, A., Eds.; CRC Press Florida: Boca Raton, FL, USA, 2011; pp. 29–66.
12. Engelkirk, G.; Duben-Engelkirk, P. *Burton's Microbiology for the Health Sciences*, 9th ed.; Lippincott Williams and Wilkins: Philadelphia, PA, USA, 2011.
13. Drulis-Kawa, Z.; Majkowska-Skrobek, G.; Maciejewska, B.; Delattre, A.S.; Lavigne, R. Learning from bacteriophages—Advantages and limitations of phage and phage-encoded protein applications. *Curr. Protein Pept. Sci.* **2012**, *13*, 699–722. [CrossRef] [PubMed]
14. Abubakar, S.; Hauwa-Suleiman, B.; Ali Abbagana, B.; Alhaji-Mustafa, I.; Abbas-Musa, I. Novel Uses of Bacteriophages in the Treatment of Human Infections and Antibiotic Resistance. *Am. J. Biosci.* **2016**, *4*, 34–40. [CrossRef]
15. Available online: https://en.wikipedia.org/wiki/Listeria_phage_P100 (accessed on 1 August 2019).
16. Friman, V.P.; Soanes-Brown, D.; Sierocinski, P.; Molin, S.; Johansen, H.K.; Merabishvili, M.; Pirnay, J.P.; De Vos, D.; Buckling, A. Pre-adapting parasitic phages to a pathogen leads to increased pathogen clearance and lowered resistance evolution with *Pseudomonas aeruginosa* cystic fibrosis bacterial isolates. *J. Evol. Biol.* **2016**, *29*, 188–198. [CrossRef] [PubMed]
17. Love, M.; Bhandari, D.; Dobson, R.; Billington, C. Potential for Bacteriophage Endolysins to Supplement or Replace Antibiotics in Food Production and Clinical Care. *Antibiotics* **2018**, *7*, 17. [CrossRef] [PubMed]
18. Rafii, F.; Sutherland, J.B.; Cerniglia, C.E. Effects of treatment with antimicrobial agents on the human colonic microflora. *Clin. Risk Manag.* **2008**, *4*, 1343. [CrossRef] [PubMed]
19. Abdelkader, K.; Gerstmans, H.; Saafan, H.; Dishisha, T.; Briers, Y. The Preclinical and Clinical Progress of Bacteriophages and Their Lytic Enzymes: The Parts are Easier than the Whole. *Viruses* **2019**, *24*, 11.
20. Abedon, S.T.; Thomas-Abedon, C. Phage therapy Pharmacology. *Cur. Pharm. Biotechnol.* **2010**, *11*, 28–47. [CrossRef]
21. Payne, R.J.H.; Phil, D.; Jansen, V.A. Phage therapy: The peculiar Kinetics of self-replicating pharmaceuticals. *Clin. Pharm. Ther.* **2000**, *68*, 225–230. [CrossRef]
22. Loc-Carrillo, C.; Abedon, S.T. Pros and Cons of phage therapy. *Bacteriophage* **2011**, *2*, 111–114. [CrossRef] [PubMed]

23. Bull, J.J.; Regoes, R.R. Pharmacodynamics of non-replicating viruses, bacteriocins and lysins. *Proc. Biol. Sci.* **2006**, *273*, 2703–2712. [CrossRef] [PubMed]
24. McVay, C.S.; Velasquez, M.; Fralick, J.A. Phage therapy of *Pseudomonas aeruginosa* infection in a mouse burn wound model. *Antimicrob. Agents Chemother.* **2007**, *51*, 1934–1938. [CrossRef]
25. Tanji, Y.; Shimada, T.; Fukudomi, H.; Miyanaga, K.; Nakai, Y.; Unno, H. Therapeutic use of phage cocktail for controlling *Escherichia coli* O157:H7 in gastrointestinal tract of mice. *J. Biosci. Bioeng.* **2005**, *100*, 280–287. [CrossRef]
26. Semler, D.D.; Goudie, A.D.; Finlay, W.H.; Dennis, J.J. Aerosol phage therapy efficacy in *Burkholderia cepacia* complex respiratory infections. *Antimicrob. Agents Chemother.* **2014**, *58*, 4005–4013. [CrossRef]
27. Brüssow, H. Phage therapy: The *Escherichia coli* experience. *Microbiology* **2005**, *151*, 2133–2140. [CrossRef] [PubMed]
28. Jun, S.Y.; Jang, I.J.; Yoon, S.; Jang, K.; Yu, K.-S.; Cho, J.Y.; Seong, M.-W.; Jung, G.M.; Yoon, S.J.; Kang, S.H. Pharmacokinetics and tolerance of the phage endolysin-based candidate drug SAL200 after a single intravenous administration among healthy volunteers. *Antimicrob. Agents Chemother.* **2017**, *24*, 61. [CrossRef] [PubMed]
29. Cassino, C.; Murphy, M.; Boyle, J.; Rotolo, J.; Wittekind, M. Results of the first in human study of lysin CF-301 evaluating the safety, tolerability and pharmacokinetic profile in healthy volunteers. In Proceedings of the 26th European Congress of Clinical Microbiology and Infectious Diseases, Amsterdam, The Netherlands, 9–12 April 2016.
30. Sriram, B.; Chikkamadaiah, S.C.R.; Durgaiah, M.; Hariharan, S.; Jayaraman, R.; Kumar, S.; Maheshwari, U.; Nandish, P. Pharmacokinetics and efficacy of ectolysin P128 in a mouse model of systemic Methicillin resistant *Staphylococcus aureus* (MRSA) infection. In Proceedings of the ASM Microbe 2017, New Orleans, LA, USA, 1–5 June 2017.
31. Dufour, N.; Delattre, R.; Ricard, J.D.; Debarbieux, L. The lysis of pathogenic *Escherichia coli* by bacteriophages releases less endotoxin than betalactams. *Clin. Infect. Dis.* **2017**, *64*, 1582–1588. [CrossRef]
32. Fischetti, V.A. Bacteriophage endolysins: A novel anti-infective to control Gram-positive pathogens. *Int. J. Med. Microbiol.* **2010**, *300*, 357–362. [CrossRef]
33. Pires, D.P.; Cleto, S.; Sillankorva, S.; Azeredo, J.; Lu, T.K. Genetically engineered phages: A review of advances over the last decade. *Microbiol. Mol. Biol. Rev.* **2016**, *80*, 523–543. [CrossRef] [PubMed]
34. Roach, D.R.; Leung, C.Y.; Henry, M.; Morello, E.; Singh, D.; Di Santo, J.P.; Weitz, J.S.; Debarbieux, L. Synergy between the host immune system and bacteriophage is essential for successful phage therapy against an acute respiratory pathogen. *Cell Host Microbe* **2017**, *22*, 38–47.e4. [CrossRef] [PubMed]
35. Biswas, B.; Adhya, S.; Washart, P.; Paul, B.; Trostel, A.N.; Powell, B.; Carlton, R.; Merril, C.R. Bacteriophage therapy rescues mice bacteremic from a clinical isolate of vancomycin-resistant *Enterococcus faecium*. *Infect. Immun.* **2002**, *70*, 204–210. [CrossRef]
36. Fishman, M. Antibody formation in vitro. *J. Exp. Med.* **1961**, *114*, 837–856. [CrossRef] [PubMed]
37. Dabrowska, K.; Switala-Jelen, K.; Opolski, A.; Górski, A. Possible association between phages, Hoc protein, and the immune system. *Arch. Virol.* **2006**, *151*, 209–215. [CrossRef]
38. Belleghem, J.D.; Clement, F.; Merabishvili, M.; Lavigne, R.; Vaneechoutte, M. Pro- and anti-inflammatory responses of peripheral blood mononuclear cells induced by *Staphylococcus aureus* and *Pseudomonas aeruginosa* phages. *Sci. Rep.* **2017**, *7*, 8004. [CrossRef] [PubMed]
39. Majewska, J.; Beta, W.; Lecion, D.; Hodyra-Stefaniak, K.; Kłopot, A.; Kaźmierczak, Z.; Miernikiewicz, P.; Piotrowicz, A.; Ciekot, J.; Owczarek, B.; et al. Oral application of T4 phage induces weak antibody production in the gut and in the blood. *Viruses* **2015**, *7*, 4783–4799. [CrossRef] [PubMed]
40. Hodyra-Stefaniak, K.; Miernikiewicz, P.; Drapa, J.; Drab, M.; Jonczyk-Matysiak, E.; Lecion, D.; Kazmierczak, Z.; Beta, M.; Harhala, J.M.; Bubak, B.; et al. Mammalian host-versus-phage immune response determines phage fate in vivo. *Sci. Rep.* **2015**, *5*, 14802. [CrossRef] [PubMed]
41. Ochs, H.D.; Davis, S.D.; Wedgwood, R.J. Immunologic responses to bacteriophage phi-X 174 in immunodeficiency diseases. *J. Clin. Investig.* **1971**, *50*, 2559–2568. [CrossRef] [PubMed]
42. Smith, L.L.; Buckley, R.; Lugar, P. Diagnostic Immunization with Bacteriophage ΦX 174 in Patients with Common Variable Immunodeficiency/Hypogammaglobulinemia. *Front. Immunol.* **2014**, *5*, 410. [CrossRef] [PubMed]

43. Oechslin, F. Resistance development to bacteriophages occurring during bacteriophage therapy. *Viruses* **2018**, *10*, 351. [CrossRef]
44. Jault, P.; Leclerc, T.; Jennes, S.; Pirnay, J.; Que, Y.A.; Resch, G.; Rousseau, A.F.; Ravat, F.; Carsin, H.; Floch, R.L.; et al. Efficacy and tolerability of a cocktail of bacteriophages to treat burn wounds infected by *Pseudomonas aeruginosa* (PhagoBurn): A randomised, controlled, double-blind phase 1/2 trial. *Lancet Infect. Dis.* **2019**, *19*, 35–45. [CrossRef]
45. Chang, R.Y.K.; Wallin, M.; Lin, Y.; Leung, S.S.Y.; Wang, H.; Morales, S.; Chan, H.K. Phage therapy for respiratory infections. *Adv. Drug Deliv. Rev.* **2018**, *133*, 76–86. [CrossRef]
46. Furfaro, L.L.; Payne, M.S.; Chang, B.J. Bacteriophage therapy: Clinical trials and regulatory hurdles. *Front. Cell. Infect. Microbiol.* **2018**, *8*, 376. [CrossRef]
47. Speck, P.; Smithyman, A. Safety and efficacy of phage therapy via the intravenous route. *FEMS Microbiol. Lett.* **2016**, *363*, 242. [CrossRef]
48. Jennes, S.; Merabishvili, M.; Soentjens, P.; Pang, K.W.; Rose, T.; Keersebilck, E.; Soete, O.; François, P.M.; Teodorescu, S.; Verween, G.; et al. Use of bacteriophages in the treatment of colistin-only-sensitive *Pseudomonas aeruginosa* septicaemia in a patient with acute kidney injury—A case report. *Crit. Care* **2017**, *21*, 129. [CrossRef] [PubMed]
49. Sula, L.; Sulova, J.; Stolcpartova, M. Therapy of experimental tuberculosis in guinea pigs with mycobacterial phages DS-6A, GR-21 T, My-327. *Czech. Med.* **1981**, *4*, 209–214. [PubMed]
50. Trigo, G.; Martins, T.G.; Fraga, A.G.; Longatto-Filho, A.; Castro, A.G.; Azeredo, J.; Pedrosa, J. Phage Therapy Is Effective against Infection by Mycobacterium ulcerans in a Murine Footpad Model. *PLoS Negl. Trop. Dis.* **2013**, *7*, 2183. [CrossRef] [PubMed]
51. Dedrick, R.M.; Guerrero-Bustamante, C.A.; Garlena, R.A.; Russell, D.A.; Ford, K.; Harris, K.; Gilmour, K.C.; Soothill, J.; Jacobs-Sera, D.; Schooley, R.T.; et al. Engineered bacteriophages for treatment of a patient with a disseminated drug-resistant Mycobacterium abscessus. *Nat. Med.* **2019**, *25*, 730–733. [CrossRef] [PubMed]
52. Pabary, R.; Singh, C.; Morales, S.; Bush, A.; Alshafi, K.; Bilton, D.; Alton, E.; Smithyman, A.; Davies, J. Anti pseudomonal bacteriophage reduces infective burden and inflammatory response in the murine lung. *Antimicrob. Agents Chemother.* **2016**, *60*, 744–751. [CrossRef] [PubMed]
53. Wang, Y.; Mi, Z.; Niu, W.; An, X.; Yuan, X.; Liu, H.; Li, L.; Liu, Y.; Feng, Y.; Huang, Y.; et al. Intranasal treatment with bacteriophage rescues mice from *Acinetobacter baumannii*-mediated pneumonia. *Future Microbiol.* **2016**, *11*, 631–641. [CrossRef]
54. Waters, E.M.; Neill, D.R.; Kaman, B.; Sahota, J.S.; Clokie, M.R.J.; Winstanley, C.; Kadioglu, A. Phage therapy is highly effective against chronic lung infections with *Pseudomonas aeruginosa*. *Thorax* **2017**, *72*, 666–667. [CrossRef]
55. Kutateladze, M.; Adamia, R. Phage therapy experience at the Eliava Institute. *Médecine et Maladies Infectieuses* **2008**, *38*, 426–430. [CrossRef]
56. Matinkhoo, S.; Lynch, K.; Dennis, J.; Finlay, W.; Vehring, R. Spray-dried respirable powders containing bacteriophages for the treatment of pulmonary infections. *J. Pharm. Sci.* **2011**, *100*, 5197–5205. [CrossRef]
57. Saussereau, E.; Vachier, I.; Chiron, R.; Godbert, B.; Sermet, I.; Dufour, N.; Pirnay, J.D.; De Vos, F.; Carrié, N.; Debarbieux, L. Effectiveness of bacteriophages in the sputum of cystic fibrosis patients. *Clin. Microbiol. Infect.* **2014**, *20*, 983–990. [CrossRef]
58. Ujmajuridze, A.; Chanishvili, N.; Goderdzishvili, M.; Leitner, L.; Mehnert, U.; Chkhotua, A.; Kessler, K.; Sybesma, W. Adapted Bacteriophages for Treating Urinary Tract Infections. *Front. Microbiol.* **2018**, *9*, 1832. [CrossRef] [PubMed]
59. Sarker, S.A.; Berger, B.; Deng, Y.; Kieser, S.; Foata, F.; Moine, D.; Descombes, P.; Sultana, S.; Huq, S.; Kumar-Bardhan, P.; et al. Oral application of *Escherichia coli* bacteriophage: Safety tests in healthy and diarrheal children from Bangladesh. *Environ. Microbiol.* **2016**, *19*, 237–250. [CrossRef] [PubMed]
60. Sarker, S.A.; Brüssow, H. From bench to bed and back again: Phage therapy of childhood *Escherichia coli* diarrhea. *Ann. N. Y. Acad. Sci.* **2016**, *1372*, 42–52. [CrossRef] [PubMed]
61. Ferry, T.; Leboucher, G.; Fevre, C.; Herry, Y.; Conrad, A.; Josse, J.; Batailler, C.; Chidiac, C.; Medina, M.; Lustig, S.; et al. Salvage Debridement, Antibiotics and Implant Retention ("DAIR") with local injection of a selected cocktail of bacteriophages: Is it an option for an elderly patient with relapsing *Staphylococcus aureus* prosthetic-joint infection? *Open Forum Infect. Dis.* **2018**, *24*, 5. [CrossRef] [PubMed]

62. Akanda, Z.Z.; Taha, M.; Abdelbary, H. Current review-The rise of bacteriophage as a unique therapeutic platform in treating peri-prosthetic joint infections. *J. Orthop. Res.* **2017**, *36*, 1051–1060. [CrossRef] [PubMed]
63. Rhoads, D.D.; Wolcott, R.D.; Kuskowski, M.A.; Wolcott, B.M.; Ward, L.S.; Sulakvelidze, A. Bacteriophage therapy of venous leg ulcers in humans: Results of a phase I safety trial. *J. Wound Care* **2009**, *238*, 240–243. [CrossRef]
64. Rose, T.; Verbeken, G.; De Vos, D.; Merabishvili, M.; Vaneechoutte, M.; Lavigne, R.; Jennes, S.; Zizi, M.; Pirnay, J.P. Experimental phage therapy of burn wound infection: difficult first steps. *Int. J. Burns Trauma* **2014**, *4*, 66–73. [PubMed]
65. Wright, A.; Hawkins, C.H.; Anggard, E.E.; Harper, D.R. A controlled clinical trial of a therapeutic phage preparation in chronic otitis due to antibiotic-resistant Pseudomonas aeruginosa; a preliminary report of efficacy. *Clin. Otolaryngol.* **2009**, *34*, 349–357. [CrossRef]
66. Yoichi, M.; Abe, M.; Miyanaga, K.; Unno, H.; Tanji, Y. Alteration of tail fiber protein gp38 enables T2 phage to infect *Escherichia coli* O157: H7. *J. Biotechnol.* **2005**, *115*, 101–107. [CrossRef]
67. Mahichi, F.; Synnott, A.J.; Yamamichi, K.; Osada, T.; Tanji, Y. Site-specific recombination of T2 phage using IP008 long tail fiber genes provides a targeted method for expanding host range while retaining lytic activity. *FEMS Microbiol. Lett.* **2009**, *295*, 211–217. [CrossRef]
68. Lin, T.-Y.; Lo, Y.-H.; Tseng, P.-W.; Chang, S.-F.; Lin, Y.-T.; Chen, T.-S. A T3 and T7 recombinant phage acquires efficient adsorption and a broader host range. *PLoS ONE* **2012**, *7*, e30954. [CrossRef] [PubMed]
69. Bikard, D.; Euler, C.W.; Jiang, W.; Nussenzweig, P.M.; Goldberg, G.W.; Duportet, X.; Fischetti, V.A.; Marraffini, L.A. Exploiting CRISPR-Cas nucleases to produce sequence-specific antimicrobials. *Nature Biotechnol.* **2014**, *32*, 1146. [CrossRef]
70. Citorik, R.J.; Mimee, M.; Lu, T.K. Sequence-specific antimicrobials using efficiently delivered RNA-guided nucleases. *Nature Biotechnol.* **2014**, *32*, 1141. [CrossRef] [PubMed]
71. Pei, R.; Lamas-Samanamud, G.R. Inhibition of biofilm formation by T7 bacteriophages producing quorum quenching enzymes. *Appl. Environ. Microbiol.* **2014**, *80*, 5340–5348. [CrossRef] [PubMed]
72. Lu, T.K.; Collins, J.J. Dispersing biofilms with engineered enzymatic bacteriophage. *Proc. Natl. Acad. Sci. USA* **2007**, *104*, 11197–11202. [CrossRef] [PubMed]
73. Vitiello, C.L.; Merril, C.R.; Adhya, S. An amino acid substitution in a capsid protein enhances phage survival in the mouse circulatory system more than a 1000-fold. *Virus Res.* **2005**, *114*, 101–103. [CrossRef] [PubMed]
74. Merril, C.R.; Biswas, B.; Carlton, R.; Jensen, N.C.; Creed, G.J.; Zullo, S.; Adhya, S. Long-circulating bacteriophage as antibacterial agents. *Proc. Natl. Acad. Sci. USA* **1996**, *93*, 3188–3192. [CrossRef] [PubMed]
75. Hagens, S.; Habel, A.; Von Ahsen, U.; Von Gabain, A.; Bläsi, U. Therapy of experimental *Pseudomonas* infections with a nonreplicating genetically modified phage. *Antimicrob. Agents Chemother.* **2004**, *48*, 3817–3822. [CrossRef]
76. Matsuda, T.; Freeman, T.A.; Hilbert, D.W.; Duff, M.; Fuortes, M.; Stapleton, P.P.; Daly, J.M. Lysis-deficient bacteriophage therapy decreases endotoxin and inflammatory mediator release and improves survival in a murine peritonitis model. *Surgery* **2005**, *137*, 639–646. [CrossRef]
77. Fauconnier, A. Regulating phage therapy: The biological master file concept could help to overcome the regulatory challenge of personalized medicines. *EMBO Rep.* **2017**, *18*, 198–200. [CrossRef]
78. Kutter, E.; De Vos, D.; Gvasalia, G.; Alavidze, Z.; Gogokhia, L.; Kuhl, S.; Abedon, S.T. Bacteriophage therapy of venous leg ulcers in humans: Results of a phase I safety trial. *Curr. Pharm. Biotechnol.* **2010**, *11*, 69–86. [CrossRef] [PubMed]
79. Commission de la santé publique, de l'environnement et du renouveau de la société. Questions jointes de Mme Muriel Gerkenset, M. Philippe Blanchart àlaministredes Affaires sociales et de la Santé publiques ur'la phagothérapie' àla ministre des Affaires sociales et de la Santé publique' (N 11955 and N 12911). 2016. Available online: https://www.dekamer.be/doc/CCRA/pdf/54/ac464.pdf (accessed on 1 August 2019).
80. El-Shibiny, A.; El-Sahhar, S. Bacteriophages: The possible solution to treat infections caused by pathogenic bacteria. *Can. J. Microbiol.* **2017**, *63*, 865–879. [CrossRef] [PubMed]
81. Golkar, Z.; Bagasra, O.; Pace, D.G. Bacteriophage therapy: A potential solution for the antibiotic resistance crisis. *J. Infect. Dev. Ctries.* **2014**, *8*, 129–136. [CrossRef] [PubMed]
82. Wittebole, X.; De Roock, S.; Opal, S.M. A historical overview of bacteriophage therapy as an alternative to antibiotics for the treatment of bacterial pathogens. *Virulence* **2014**, *5*, 226–235. [CrossRef] [PubMed]

83. Azeredo, J.; Sutherland, I.W. The use of phages for the removal of infectious biofilms. *Cur. Pharm. Biotechnol.* **2008**, *9*, 261–266. [CrossRef]
84. Anon. When is an allergy to an antibiotic really an allergy? *Best Pract. J.* **2015**, *68*, 22.
85. Terico, A.T.; Gallagher, J.C. Beta-lactam hypersensitivity and cross-reactivity. *J. Pharm. Pract.* **2014**, *27*, 530–544. [CrossRef] [PubMed]
86. Ligonenko, O.V.; Borysenko, M.M.; Digtyar, I.I.; Ivashchenko, D.M.; Zubakha, A.B.; Chorna, I.O.; Shumeyko, I.A.; Storozhenko, O.V.; Gorb, L.I.; Ligonenko, O.O. Application of bacteriophages in complex of treatment of a shot-gun wounds of soft tissues in the patients, suffering multiple allergy for antibiotics. *Klin. Khir.* **2015**, *10*, 65–66.
87. Ghannad, M.S.; Mohammadi, A. Bacteriophage: Time to re-evaluate the potential of phage therapy as a promising agent to control multidrug-resistant bacteria. *Iran. J. Basic Med. Sci.* **2012**, *15*, 693–701.
88. Kucharewicz-Krukowsk, A.; Slopek, S. Immunogenic effect of bacteriophage in patients subjected to phage therapy. *Arch. Immunol. Ther. Exp. (Warsz.)* **1987**, *35*, 553–561.

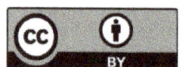
© 2019 by the authors. Licensee MDPI, Basel, Switzerland. This article is an open access article distributed under the terms and conditions of the Creative Commons Attribution (CC BY) license (http://creativecommons.org/licenses/by/4.0/).

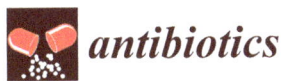

Review

Direct Measurement of Performance: A New Era in Antimicrobial Stewardship

Majdi N. Al-Hasan [1,2,*], Hana Rac Winders [3], P. Brandon Bookstaver [3,4] and Julie Ann Justo [3,4]

1. School of Medicine, University of South Carolina, Columbia, SC 29209, USA
2. Department of Medicine, Division of Infectious Diseases, Palmetto Health University of South Carolina Medical Group, Columbia, SC 29203, USA
3. Department of Clinical Pharmacy and Outcomes Sciences, University of South Carolina College of Pharmacy, Columbia, SC 29208, USA
4. Department of Pharmacy, Prisma Health Richland, Columbia, SC 29203, USA
* Correspondence: majdi.alhasan@uscmed.sc.edu; Tel.: +1-803-540-1062; Fax: +1-803-540-1079

Received: 18 July 2019; Accepted: 21 August 2019; Published: 24 August 2019

Abstract: For decades, the performance of antimicrobial stewardship programs (ASPs) has been measured by incidence rates of hospital-onset *Clostridioides difficile* and other infections due to multidrug-resistant bacteria. However, these represent indirect and nonspecific ASP metrics. They are often confounded by factors beyond an ASP's control, such as changes in diagnostic testing methods or algorithms and the potential of patient-to-patient transmission. Whereas these metrics remain useful for global assessment of healthcare systems, antimicrobial use represents a direct metric that separates the performance of an ASP from other safety and quality teams within an institution. The evolution of electronic medical records and healthcare informatics has made measurements of antimicrobial use a reality. The US Centers for Disease Control and Prevention's initiative for reporting antimicrobial use and standardized antimicrobial administration ratio in hospitals is highly welcomed. Ultimately, ASPs should be evaluated based on what they do best and what they can control, that is, antimicrobial use within their own institution. This narrative review critically appraises existing stewardship metrics and advocates for adopting antimicrobial use as the primary performance measure. It proposes novel formulas to adjust antimicrobial use based on quality of care and microbiological burden at each institution to allow for meaningful inter-network and inter-facility comparisons.

Keywords: Antibiotics; resistance; broad-spectrum agents; hospital epidemiology; antibiotic utilization; infection control; infection prevention; *Pseudomonas aeruginosa*; *Acinetobacter baumannii*; extended-spectrum beta-lactamases; carbapenem-resistant *Enterobacteriaceae*; methicillin-resistant *Staphylococcus aureus*

---

1. Introduction: Importance of Antimicrobial Stewardship Metrics

It is imperative for the success of any antimicrobial stewardship program (ASP) to have objective measures for performance evaluation. Direct measurement of ASP performance via process measures (e.g., antimicrobial use) and/or outcome measures (e.g., *Clostridioides difficile* infection [CDI]) is currently recommended by clinical guidelines to improve quality care and prevent antimicrobial resistance [1]. This process ensures that both hospital administration and ASP team members have consistent goals and expectations. It provides ASPs with the opportunity to periodically self-reflect on their performance and discuss long-term planning to achieve their aims. This also creates national and local standards to compare ASPs in different healthcare systems after adjustments for potential differences across institutions [1].

ASP metrics are often categorized by type into antimicrobial use (AU) measures, process measures, quality measures, costs and clinical outcome measures. Expert panels assembled among adult and pediatric stewards were challenged to develop a set of metrics perceived as both useful and logistically feasible for adoption by ASPs as performance metrics [2,3]. Variability in practice areas, institutions, resources and infrastructure all impede the utility of many proposed ASP metrics. The true impact of an ASP on quality and clinical outcome measures specifically is also debatable, given the patient complexities and confounders present. Do these metrics actually measure ASP "performance" or "value" or "efficiency", a combination of these factors, or none at all?

While several quantitative measures (e.g., antimicrobial use and costs) are often considered frontline metrics and central to ASP operations, noted expert stewards have proposed a shift in focus to quality and patient outcomes to demonstrate enhanced program value [4–6]. Many regulatory and quality improvement organizations (e.g., Agency for Healthcare Research and Quality) have established infectious diseases metrics designed to measure quality which are often tied to reimbursement [4]. The changing landscape of reimbursement in the US healthcare system and growing transparency of quality and safety measures through public reporting will likely impact ASPs and potentially influence key metrics tied to performance evaluation. Collaboration between ASPs, healthcare administration and quality divisions is imperative in order to maintain consistency in measured success. In this narrative review, we discuss the landscape of proposed ASP metrics and compare their value and utility as measures of ASP performance focusing on acute care hospitals.

2. Dynamics of Antimicrobial Stewardship and Infection Prevention and Control Programs

The re-emergence of CDI as a significant threat in the early 2000s was arguably the single most important factor increasing awareness of risks associated with antimicrobials at both the public and institutional level. The potential of patient-to-patient transmission of *C. difficile* spores make clusters or outbreaks of CDI an imminent threat to hospitals. CDI created a common target for both Infection Prevention and Control Programs and ASPs and facilitated a dynamic relationship between both teams. Contact isolation of hospitalized patients with CDI and hand hygiene of healthcare workers with soap and water have been the cornerstone of Infection Prevention and Control Program efforts to reduce transmission of *C. difficile* spores within the hospital. At the same time, reduction in unnecessary use of broad-spectrum antimicrobials may reduce the risk of hospital-onset CDI (HO-CDI). For this reason, many Infection Prevention and Control Programs started monitoring antimicrobial use in the hospital to enhance their CDI interventions, often utilizing the same team members. On other occasions, ASPs emerged under the Infection Prevention and Control Program umbrella. It was convenient to use the incidence rate of HO-CDI as a metric for both Infection Prevention and Control Programs and ASPs. The requirement for hospitals within the United States to publicly report the incidence rate of HO-CDI through National Healthcare Safety Network (NHSN) and paucity of other measures of ASP performance only emphasized this existing concept.

Similarly, institutional Infection Prevention and Control Programs have been monitoring and intervening to prevent patient-to-patient transmission of multidrug-resistant (MDR) bacteria: initially, extended-spectrum beta-lactamase-producing Enterobacteriaceae (ESBLE) and methicillin-resistant *Staphylococcus aureus* (MRSA), then carbapenem-resistant Enterobacteriaceae (CRE). Since antimicrobial use predisposes to colonization and infections with MDR bacteria [7,8], incidence rates of infections or colonization with MDR bacteria were often used as a quality measure of ASP performance. Mandatory reporting of these infections added another layer of convenience.

Over time, ASPs have evolved and have become more focused on quality of patient care, including optimization of antimicrobial management. At the same time, *C. difficile*, MRSA and ESBLE have emerged as community-onset pathogens rather than predominant causes of nosocomial infections [9–12]. Antimicrobial resistance of predominantly hospital-onset bacteria, such as *Pseudomonas aeruginosa* and *Acinetobacter baumannii*, has become the most imminent threat to hospitals in the US [13].

Moreover, with the emergence of community-acquired MRSA, intravenous vancomycin has become the most commonly used antimicrobial in US hospitals. The increasing use of vancomycin, by itself or in combination with piperacillin/tazobactam, has contributed to an increase in antimicrobial-associated nephrotoxicity in hospitalized patients [14,15]. Monitoring the use of nephrotoxic antimicrobial agents has been added to the daily duties of ASPs. This shifting focus has allowed a greater degree of independence from Infection Prevention and Control Programs and has made it difficult to use the same personnel for both Infection Prevention and Control Programs and ASPs.

3. Comparison of Various Antimicrobial Stewardship Metrics

3.1. Clostridioides difficile Infection

Prevention of CDI is one of the main benefits of antimicrobial stewardship. Current or prior antimicrobial use contributes to CDI due to changes in intestinal microbiota and decreased competition against *C. difficile* [16]. Therefore, it is intuitive to use CDI as a measure of ASP performance in hospitals [1,2]. However, the multifactorial nature of CDI, possibility of person-to-person transmission irrespective of antimicrobial use and site of acquisition, and changing incidence rate of CDI based on diagnostic testing methods or algorithms, argue against its use as the primary ASP metric.

3.1.1. CDI Diagnosis

CDI can only be diagnosed based on laboratory testing. Using a highly sensitive test, such as PCR, would increase the incidence of CDI compared to toxin A/B antibody–antigen assays [17]. An increase in the incidence rate of HO-CDI was observed when switching from toxin A/B antibody–antigen testing to PCR [18]. The use of diagnostic tests with varying sensitivities makes comparison of HO-CDI incidence rates across hospitals impractical. A recent study demonstrated that only 20% of in-hospital testing for CDI was appropriate [19]. Inappropriate testing for CDI resulted in overtreatment and inaccurate publicly reported metrics [19]. Even when the same laboratory diagnostic test is used, a change in institutional policy or algorithm for CDI testing influenced CDI incidence rates. An institutional requirement for testing all hospitalized patients with liquid stools was associated with higher incidence rate of HO-CDI in Scotland [20]. *C. difficile* PCR does not differentiate colonization from infection. Given the large proportion of inappropriate CDI testing in hospitals, a clinical decision-making tool to improve the appropriateness of testing likely has a much higher impact in reducing HO-CDI rates than any ASP intervention. This confounding makes it difficult to correlate incidence of HO-CDI with ASP activities aiming to optimize antimicrobial use. Instead, this argues for design of a diagnostic stewardship metric in collaboration with microbiology, central laboratory and Infection Prevention and Control Programs.

3.1.2. Relatively Low Incidence of CDI

Most clinical studies of CDI adopt a case-control design due to the relative infrequency of CDI in hospitalized patients. In two cohorts, only 2–4% of hospitalized patients with gram-negative bloodstream infections developed CDI, despite receipt of broad-spectrum antimicrobial therapy [21,22]. Although still considered a major risk, the relatively large number needed to harm constitutes a challenge for ASPs attempting to demonstrate effectiveness of their interventions. Based on such data, ASPs are required to streamline or discontinue 25–50 courses of broad-spectrum antimicrobials to potentially prevent one case of CDI. Discontinuation of antimicrobial therapy is one of the most impactful outcomes of any ASP intervention; however, it is a much less frequent intervention than de-escalation of antimicrobial therapy or reduction in proposed treatment duration [23]. Designing an ASP intervention to reduce the incidence rate of CDI requires a tremendous amount of time, resources and dedication. This is likely the reason for the relatively small number of published studies demonstrating successful reduction in CDI via ASP interventions, despite several decades of focus in this area. To our knowledge, only early de-escalation of broad-spectrum antimicrobial therapy (within 48 h) has been associated with a reduction in CDI risk [22]. Early de-escalation of antimicrobial therapy requires robust ASP, rapid diagnostics, timely electronic alerts, and experienced personnel to act on these alerts. Conventional de-escalation of antimicrobial therapy (after 4 days) has demonstrated non-inferiority to broad-spectrum therapy, but is yet to show a significant reduction in CDI [24].

3.1.3. Multifactorial Etiology of CDI

In addition to antimicrobials, many other independent risk factors have been associated with development of CDI, such as chemotherapy and proton-pump inhibitors [25]. Moreover, potential for person-to-person transmission of *C. difficile* spores makes Infection Prevention and Control Program efforts far more important than those of ASPs in reducing the incidence of HO-CDI. Given the large number of ASP interventions required to prevent CDI, a cluster of CDI in one unit of the hospital may cancel out an entire year's worth of ASP efforts. Another factor that has not been widely studied is the impact of antimicrobials used prior to hospital admission on the risk of HO-CDI. Hospital admissions secondary to community-onset CDI continue to rise and are not as intensely monitored by Infection Prevention and Control Programs or ASPs, but may also pose similar risk to institutional outbreaks. Most institutional ASPs have no control over antimicrobials received in ambulatory settings or other hospitals prior to referral.

3.1.4. Difficulty of Designing a Successful ASP Intervention for CDI

Although the association between antimicrobial use and CDI is strong, it remains controversial which antimicrobial agents/classes are more likely to contribute to CDI [26]. There is general agreement that the broader the spectrum of antimicrobials, the higher the risk of CDI; however, there are notable exceptions to this rule, such as clindamycin [27]. Interpretation of the literature is difficult, due to use of different definitions and inconsistent methodology. To increase sample size and power, community-onset and HO-CDI were merged despite vast differences in the spectrum of activity of oral and intravenous antimicrobials used in the two respective settings [28]. Moreover, all penicillins were classified in one category, despite the huge difference in the spectrum of activity of piperacillin-tazobactam and penicillin G, for example [29]. Even the well-designed interventions which have reported a reduction in the incidence rate of CDI after antimicrobial formulary changes did not assess the collateral damage of the intervention on antimicrobial resistance [20,30]. It is worrisome that some formulary restrictions designed for reducing CDI risk may encourage the use of antipseudomonal beta-lactams and carbapenems [30]. This contradicts recent large cohorts demonstrating the highest odds of CDI among hospitalized patients receiving antipseudomonal beta-lactams [22,31]. In addition, the linear increase in antimicrobial resistance of *E. coli* and other Enterobacteriaceae bloodstream isolates to aminopenicillins and first-generation cephalosporins limits de-escalation options from antipseudomonal beta-lactams to intravenous ceftriaxone or oral fluoroquinolones on many occasions [22,32,33]. The long-term consequences of increasing antimicrobial resistance rates to antipseudomonal beta-lactams and carbapenems secondary to excessive use may exceed any potential early benefits from this strategy [34,35]. A subtle decline in CDI at the expense of increasing antimicrobial resistance rates of already difficult to treat bacteria, such as *P. aeruginosa* and *A. baumannii*, constitutes one step forward and two steps back for the longevity of the ASP and the institution.

3.2. Incidence Rates of Infections or Colonization with MDR Bacteria

3.2.1. Extended-Spectrum Beta-Lactamase-Producing *Enterobacteriaceae* (ESBLE)

Controlling outbreaks and reducing transmission of ESBLE in the hospital setting have been common goals for both Infection Prevention and Control Programs and ASPs since this resistance mechanism was first described in 1983 [36]. This is conceivable since exposure to antimicrobials, particularly beta-lactams and fluoroquinolones, is a risk factor for infection or colonization with ESBLE [7,8]. Moreover, ESBLE may be transmitted from person-to-person within hospitals or other settings. At the turn of the century, ESBLE emerged as community-onset bacteria likely due to availability and widespread use of broad-spectrum oral antimicrobials in the community, such as extended-spectrum cephalosporins and fluoroquinolones [11,37]. The incidence rate of hospital-acquired ESBLE infections have remained relatively stable over the past decade, due to effective Infection Prevention and Control Programs and ASPs [12]. On the other hand, the lack of such programs in ambulatory settings and long-term care facilities has contributed to an increase in the incidence rate of community-onset ESBLE infections [12]. It is estimated that 80% of ESBLE infections in the US are acquired outside the hospital [8,12].

Another limitation of using ESBLE as a measure of ASP performance is the lag between ESBLE colonization and infection. Colonization with ESBLE within the past one year has been associated with increased risk of ESBLE infections [8,38]. Patients may be colonized with ESBLE due to antimicrobial use in the community. If a urinary culture is obtained on the fourth day of hospitalization for appropriate or inappropriate indications, the ESBLE isolate will be classified as nosocomial, even in the absence of any antimicrobial use during the index hospitalization [39]. This limits the utility of ESBLE as a measure of ASP performance.

3.2.2. Methicillin-Resistant *Staphylococcus aureus* (MRSA)

The emergence of MRSA as community-acquired bacteria by the end of last century makes the incidence of hospital-onset MRSA infections or colonization a less useful ASP metric. There is a suggestion that antimicrobial use may predispose to MRSA colonization or infection. A recent study demonstrated that the restriction of fluoroquinolone and macrolide use, among other antimicrobials, was associated with a reduction in MRSA infection rates [40]. However, this association was temporal, at best, and a decline in MRSA infection/colonization rates was demonstrated elsewhere without formulary changes [41–43]. In the era of increasing antimicrobial resistance rates, class restrictions of already limited antimicrobial treatment options for hospitalized patients with serious infections seem counterproductive. Given the high prevalence of community-acquired MRSA strains and widespread use of fluoroquinolones in the community, it is unrealistic to expect formulary restrictions of fluoroquinolones in hospitals to impact overall MRSA rates. Restricting fluoroquinolone use in the community to specific indications, such as acute pyelonephritis and community-onset pneumonia, seems more reasonable [44].

3.2.3. Carbapenem-Resistant *Enterobacteriaceae* (CRE)

Carbapenem exposure is a risk factor for CRE infections or colonization [45]. Since carbapenems are currently only available in intravenous form in the US, the incidence rate of CRE appears more relevant to institutional ASPs than that of ESBLE and MRSA. The potential for person-to-person transmission have made long-term care facilities reservoirs for CRE, likely due to lack of effective Infection Prevention and Control Programs and ASPs. The lag between CRE colonization and infection, as well as the potential for receiving carbapenems at other facilities, pose some limitations to using CRE incidence rates to evaluate ASP performance. The potential availability of oral carbapenems in the US in the near future may change the epidemiology of CRE infections, in an unfortunate repeat of the community-onset ESBLE phenomenon.

3.2.4. Antimicrobial-Resistant *P. aeruginosa* and *A. baumannii*

P. aeruginosa and *A. baumannii* are predominantly hospital-onset pathogens [46]. They are ubiquitous bacteria which are difficult to eliminate from hospital environments. Hospitalized patients may become colonized with these bacteria due to either heavy exposure from prolonged hospitalization or antimicrobial selection pressure [47,48]. The presence of open wounds, mechanical ventilation, and urinary or central venous catheters place hospitalized patients at higher risk of infections with these bacteria [46,49,50]. Resistance to antipseudomonal beta-lactams and carbapenems among these isolates poses serious challenges to hospitals due to the lack of safe and effective antimicrobial treatment options [35]. Outbreaks of infections due to MDR *P. aeruginosa* and *A. baumannii* are devastating to both patients and hospitals, associated with high mortality rates and high costs of treatment. The amount of time, resources and personnel dedicated to the containment of such outbreaks is enormous, occasionally requiring unit closures and massive financial burdens [51,52]. For this reason, *P. aeruginosa* and *A. baumannii* are at the top of the World Health Organization global list of critical priority [13].

Inpatient antimicrobial use is by far the most important factor influencing antimicrobial resistance rates of these hospital-onset isolates [53–57]. The recent increase in utilization of antipseudomonal beta-lactams and carbapenems in US hospitals has been temporally associated with an increase in antimicrobial resistance rates of *P. aeruginosa* [34,35]. Using antimicrobial resistance of *P. aeruginosa* and *A. baumannii* as an ASP metric is logical and reasonable, but has limitations. First, changes in referral patterns may impact antimicrobial resistance at tertiary care centers. Second, nearly one-half of *P. aeruginosa* bloodstream isolates are acquired outside the hospital [48]. Community-onset *P. aeruginosa* infections are particularly common among immune compromised hosts and patients who received recent beta-lactams [48–50]. Antimicrobial resistance rates of strictly hospital-onset *P. aeruginosa* and *A. baumannii* isolates are a more equitable measure of ASP performance. This requires stratification by site of acquisition. If such stratification is not automated by clinical informatics, then resistance rates of hospital-onset isolates will have to be done manually. This is unlikely to be feasible for many ASPs, based on current resources in time and personnel.

3.3. Quality of Care

Quality of patient care is the most important antimicrobial stewardship principle [2–5]. The ultimate goal of ASPs is to optimize both empirical and definitive antimicrobial therapy for hospitalized patients with serious infections.

3.3.1. Appropriate Definitive Antimicrobial Therapy

Many ASPs utilize available healthcare informatics resources to identify suboptimal antimicrobial use among individual patient cases. The objective is to ensure patients who have positive clinical cultures, particularly from sterile sites, receive the most effective antimicrobial therapy. Appropriate therapy is not only a matter of receiving an antimicrobial agent with in vitro susceptibility against the microbial isolate. Rather, it is based on effectiveness as derived from large clinical studies and involves receiving an appropriately dosed agent based on the primary source of infection, the patient's renal and hepatic function, and the minimal inhibitory concentration of the clinical isolate. The antimicrobial should also be administered via the appropriate route based on severity of infection, reliability of the enteral route, and bioavailability of the agent [58–60].

Since most currently available software for identification of bug–drug mismatches use in vitro susceptibility as a screening measure for appropriateness, many patients receiving inappropriate definitive therapy will not be identified. This includes patients receiving antimicrobial agents without activity at the site of the infection (e.g., daptomycin for MRSA pneumonia or nitrofurantoin for *E. coli* bloodstream infections). It would require a separate ASP intervention to review all cases of pneumonia or bloodstream infection to identify such cases. The variety of factors associated with the "appropriateness" of antimicrobial therapy makes it difficult to measure ASP performance based on this metric alone.

3.3.2. Appropriate Empirical Antimicrobial Therapy

Receipt of appropriate empirical antimicrobial therapy is independently associated with survival and shorter duration of hospitalization in patients with serious bacterial infections [58,59,61–63]. Despite the excessive use of broad-spectrum agents in hospitals, up to 30% of patients still receive inappropriate empirical therapy [64]. As the focus of ASPs has shifted to quality, many ASPs have invested in measuring and improving the appropriateness of empirical therapy. The art is designing institutional management guidelines which increase the appropriateness of empirical therapy while also reducing overall use of broad-spectrum agents [65]. Institutional management guidelines based on local evidence, coupled with rapid microbial identification and vigorous ASP monitoring, have been demonstrated to successfully achieve both goals [66]. The proportion of patients receiving appropriate empirical antimicrobial therapy for serious infections is the most important measure for the quality of ASP performance. Many host factors, including age, comorbidities and acute severity of illness, impact both survival and hospital length of stay in patients with serious bacterial infections [58,63,67,68]. In reality, the only variable an ASP can directly control and modify is the selection of empirical antimicrobial therapy. In order to use appropriateness of empirical therapy as a metric for ASP performance, it would require identification of every patient with a particular clinical syndrome (e.g., bloodstream infections, sepsis, or pneumonia) or a representative random sample. Although this may be time-consuming and labor-intensive, many ASPs are currently monitoring the appropriateness of empirical therapy, particularly in patients with bloodstream infections [66,69–72].

3.4. Cost of Healthcare

Antimicrobial cost was, for the most part, the only specific measure of ASP performance. Nonetheless, an institutional antimicrobial budget may be influenced by changes in acquisition price or renegotiation of institutional contracts, as dictated by supply and demand in the market.

Cost reduction has historically been used to justify the presence of an ASP, including both the establishment of a new program and maintenance of an existing program. ASPs have demonstrated significant reductions in hospitals' antimicrobial budgets, mostly by targeting and restricting unnecessary use of expensive antimicrobials (e.g., daptomycin, ceftaroline) [73–76]. However, cost savings generally plateau after few years. The cost of the acquisition of antimicrobials varies across institutions based on purchase volume and the ability of the healthcare system to negotiate a better deal. Occasional price hikes of commonly used agents make cost a less attractive metric. More importantly, the biggest cost savings institutional ASPs provide are hard to measure. These cost savings include reduction in length of hospital stay by improving the appropriateness of empirical antimicrobial therapy for serious infections [62,63]. Second, measurement of cost avoidance is also challenging. An ASP's efforts in reducing antimicrobial resistance rates of hospital-onset bacteria minimizes the need for new and often expensive antimicrobials used for treatment of infections due to MDR bacteria (e.g., ceftolozane/tazobactam, ceftazidime/avibactam).

3.5. Antimicrobial Use

3.5.1. Direct and Specific ASP Metric

Since ASPs manage antimicrobial therapy on a daily basis, harnessing antimicrobial use as the primary ASP metric is intuitive. Antimicrobial use represents the most direct measure of ASP performance. Most other metrics (e.g., CDI, MDR bacteria, and cost) provide indirect assessment of antimicrobial use. The assumption is that the higher the antimicrobial use within a hospital, the higher the HO-CDI and antimicrobial resistance. Contrary to incidence rates of HO-CDI and infections with MDR bacteria, institutional antimicrobial use is not affected by antimicrobials used outside the hospital. In addition, since the incidence of HO-CDI and infections with MDR bacteria may be reduced by Infection Prevention and Control Program efforts, antimicrobial use remains the only metric which differentiates the performance of ASPs from other patient safety and quality teams.

3.5.2. Antimicrobial Use of Broad-Spectrum Agents

ASP priority should be given for measuring antimicrobial use of broad-spectrum agents, such as antipseudomonal beta-lactams and carbapenems. For long-term monitoring, it would be useful to measure collective antimicrobial use of all antipseudomonal beta-lactams (e.g., piperacillin/tazobactam, cefepime, meropenem). This would avoid fluctuations associated with a temporary shortage of one agent. Monitoring intravenous vancomycin use is also important given the potential risk of nephrotoxicity [14,15]. Monitoring aminoglycosides use is equally important, particularly in institutions with frequent use of aminoglycoside combination regimens. Measurement of antimicrobial use of commonly used agents for treatment of community-onset infections, such as third-generation cephalosporins and fluoroquinolones, is also useful to ensure antipseudomonal beta-lactams and carbapenems are not completely replaced by agents which are still associated with a high risk of CDI. It would be reasonable to monitor institutional antimicrobial use of all agents, resources permitting, in order to ensure a decline of overall antimicrobial use in the hospital. However, most ASPs would not be bothered if the decline in antimicrobial use of broad-spectrum agents was accompanied by an increase in antimicrobial use of narrower-spectrum agents (e.g., penicillin G, nafcillin, ampicillin/sulbactam, cefazolin). After all, this is reflective of their hard work in de-escalation of broad-spectrum antimicrobial therapy.

3.5.3. Benefits of Reducing Antimicrobial Use

A reduction in antimicrobial use of antipseudomonal beta-lactams and other broad-spectrum agents is possible through syndrome-specific and other ASP interventions [72]. In addition, monitoring antimicrobial use is also rewarding for an ASP as a decline in antimicrobial use of broad-spectrum agents may be observed as early as 6 months following a successful intervention [72,77,78]. In the long-term, reduction in antimicrobial use of broad-spectrum agents will result in a decline in HO-CDI and antimicrobial resistance assuming there are no major changes in the healthcare system (e.g., referral patterns, outpatient antimicrobial prescription rates, clusters of HO-CDI or MDR bacteria).

3.5.4. Measurement of Antimicrobial Use

There are advantages and disadvantages of using days of therapy (DOT) or defined daily dose (DDD) as measures of antimicrobial use which are beyond the scope of this review. However, the goal of an ASP is to optimize, rather than minimize, antimicrobial therapy. Using DDD as a measure of antimicrobial use may punish ASPs for optimization of antimicrobial regimens in patients who truly need high doses of antimicrobials, such as patients with serious infections and augmented renal clearance. Conversely, institutions with relatively high rates of acute kidney injury due to heavy use of nephrotoxic agents may benefit from measuring DDD rather than DOT. Overall, DOT seems a fair indicator of performance for a local ASP.

An added benefit of antimicrobial use measurement is the frequent ability to stratify antimicrobial use by location and by time. This requires detailed knowledge of the denominator used in the generation of the antimicrobial use measurement, i.e., patient-days or the newer standard, days-present. Such data allows antimicrobial use to be locally compared across locations, such as hospital campus (in a multi-campus health system) or hospital unit, and by time, such as calendar month. This, in turn, helps ASPs identify areas within the institution where antimicrobial use appears excessive and helps design unit-specific or other targeted interventions.

4. Proposed Novel Antimicrobial Use (AU) Metrics

4.1. Adjustment of AU by Quality of Care

AU by itself is a measure of quantity, not quality of care. It would be valuable to provide reassurance that a reduction in AU of broad-spectrum agents is not achieved at the expense of appropriateness of therapy. Adjusting AU of broad-spectrum agents to the proportion of patients receiving appropriate empirical therapy incorporates quality of care and AU in one formula (Equation (1)):

$$AU_{adjustedQ} = \frac{AU_{local}}{P_{appropriate}} \qquad (1)$$

Equation (1): Antimicrobial use adjusted by quality of care as determined by appropriateness of empirical antimicrobial therapy.

Where $AU_{adjustedQ}$ is the adjusted AU by quality of care at an institution, AU_{local} is the raw AU at a particular local institution; $P_{appropriate}$ is the proportion of patients receiving appropriate empirical antimicrobial therapy at that facility.

For example, using 100 DOT/1000 patient-days of antipseudomonal beta-lactams to provide appropriate empirical therapy to 90% of patients with gram-negative bloodstream infections at hospital A is better than using the same amount to cover only 80% appropriately at hospital B (100/0.9 = 111 vs. 100/0.8 = 125). This formula implies it would have taken 111 and 125 DOT/1000 patient-days, respectively, to provide appropriate empirical therapy to virtually all patients with this clinical syndrome at hospitals A and B, respectively (Table 1). This provides an assessment of the quantitative (AU) and qualitative (appropriateness of empirical antimicrobial therapy) performance of ASPs. It should be noted that antimicrobial resistance rates at an institution may influence the proportion of patients receiving appropriate empirical therapy.

Table 1. Proposed novel metrics for adjustment of antimicrobial use by quality of care.

Adjusted AU	Formula
APBL	$\dfrac{AU_{APBL}}{\text{Proportion of patients with gram–negative BSI or sepsis receiving appropriate empirical antimicrobial therapy}}$
Carbapenems	$\dfrac{AU_{Carbapenems}}{\text{Proportion of patients with gram–negative BSI or sepsis receiving appropriate empirical antimicrobial therapy}}$
Anti-MRSA agents	$\dfrac{AU_{Anti-MRSA\ agents}}{\text{Proportion of patients with gram–positive BSI or sepsis receiving appropriate empirical antimicrobial therapy}}$
Anti-VRE agents	$\dfrac{AU_{Anti-VRE\ agents}}{\text{Proportion of patients with gram–positive BSI or sepsis receiving appropriate empirical antimicrobial therapy}}$

Note: AU: antimicrobial use; APBL: antipseudomonal beta-lactams; MRSA: methicillin-resistant *Staphylococcus aureus*; VRE: vancomycin-resistant *Enterococcus* species; BSI: bloodstream infections.

Many ASPs are currently involved in management of bloodstream infections in order to optimize empirical therapy. The proportion of patients with bloodstream infections receiving appropriate empirical therapy is already available at such institutions [66,69–71]. Moreover, as institutions adopt new bundles for improvement of survival in patients with sepsis, it would be useful to measure the appropriateness of empirical antimicrobial therapy as part of this bundle. These bloodstream infection and sepsis cohorts may be used as representative samples for the adjustment of AU by the quality of care received at each institution.

4.2. Adjustment of AU by Institutional Microbiological Burden

Similar to any other ASP metric, comparisons of AU across institutions are not valuable without taking into account the differences in patient populations and microbiological burden at these facilities. For example, there is a wide variation in the incidence of *P. aeruginosa* among gram-negative bacteria at various institutions with higher incidence at tertiary care referral centers than community hospitals [79]. Since broad-spectrum antimicrobial agents are used to treat infections due to certain bacteria (e.g., antipseudomonal beta-lactams for *P. aeruginosa*), it is reasonable to adjust for the incidence of such isolates at a particular institution. Equation (2) can be used to adjust AU by institutional microbiological burden:

$$AU_{adjustedM} = \dfrac{AU_{local}}{\left(\dfrac{I_{local}}{I_{overall}}\right)} \quad (2)$$

Equation (2): Antimicrobial use adjusted by microbiological burden at the institution.

Where $AU_{adjustedM}$ is the adjusted AU of antipseudomonal beta-lactams by microbiological burden at an institution, AU_{local} is the raw AU of antipseudomonal beta-lactams at a particular local institution, I_{local} is the incidence of the relevant organism(s) (i.e., *P. aeruginosa*) at that local institution, and $I_{overall}$ is its average incidence within the overall network or region.

As an example, AU_{local} of antipseudomonal beta-lactams at hospitals A (tertiary care medical center) and B (rural community hospital) are both reported as 100 DOT/1000 patient-days. The $I_{overall}$ is 0.12 (12% of all gram-negative isolates within this network or region are *P. aeruginosa*, for instance). I_{local} for hospitals A and B are 0.15 and 0.09, respectively. $AU_{adjustedM}$ of antipseudomonal beta-lactams at hospitals A and B could then be calculated as 100/(0.15/0.12) = 80 and 100/(0.09/0.12) = 133, respectively. The adjustments indicate that hospitals A and B would have utilized 80 and 133 DOT/1000 patient-days of antipseudomonal beta-lactams, respectively, if the proportion of *P. aeruginosa* isolates at both institutions were comparable to the overall network/regional average. Using 100 DOT/1000 patient-days of antipseudomonal beta-lactams may be justifiable in hospital A due to high microbiological burden, but seems excessive in hospital B.

Similar adjustments may be made for AU of anti-MRSA agents relative to the proportion of MRSA among all gram-positive isolates and AU of carbapenems based on proportion of ESBL-producing or ceftriaxone-resistant *E. coli*, *Klebsiella* species, and *Proteus mirabilis* (Table 2).

Table 2. Proposed novel metrics for adjustment of antimicrobial use by microbiological burden at each healthcare facility.

Adjusted AU	Formula
APBL	$\dfrac{AU_{APBL}}{\left(\dfrac{\text{Incidence of } P.\ aeruginosa \text{ at local institution}}{\text{Average overall incidence of } P.\ aeruginosa \text{ in network}}\right)}$
Carbapenems	$\dfrac{AU_{Carbapenems}}{\left(\dfrac{\text{Incidence of ESBLE at local institution}}{\text{Average overall incidence of ESBLE in network}}\right)}$ *
Anti-MRSA agents	$\dfrac{AU_{Anti-MRSA\ agents}}{\left(\dfrac{\text{Incidence of MRSA at local institution}}{\text{Average overall incidence of MRSA in network}}\right)}$
Anti-VRE agents	$\dfrac{AU_{Anti-VRE\ agents}}{\left(\dfrac{\text{Incidence of VRE at local institution}}{\text{Average overall incidence of VRE in network}}\right)}$

Note: AU: antimicrobial use; APBL: antipseudomonal beta-lactams; ESBLE: extended-spectrum beta-lactamase-producing *Enterobacteriaceae*; MRSA: methicillin-resistant *Staphylococcus aureus*; VRE: vancomycin-resistant *Enterococcus* species. * If microbiology laboratories in one or more hospitals in the network do not perform the ESBL screening test, then the incidence of ceftriaxone-resistant *Enterobacteriaceae* may be used alternatively to calculate adjusted carbapenem utilization in all hospitals in the network.

To our knowledge, these novel AU metrics in Section 4 have not been proposed in prior reviews of the literature. While their simple calculation is logical and represents a reasonable approach to AU interpretation, further research is warranted to validate these metrics in the clinical setting.

5. NHSN Antimicrobial Use and Resistance Module

The US Centers for Disease Control and Prevention (CDC) NHSN offers an antimicrobial use and resistance module with AU and AR options [80,81]. Facilities can participate in one or both options, but at this time, neither is required.

5.1. Antimicrobial Use (AU) Option

The AU option facilitates risk-adjusted inter- and intra-facility benchmarking of antimicrobial use [80]. Primarily, antimicrobial use is measured as antimicrobial DOT/1000 days-present. Antimicrobial use is aggregated by month for each patient care location and facility-wide. Antimicrobial use is also separated by the spectrum of the antimicrobials into 6 categories (Table 3). The data are then analyzed, and facilities receive a Standardized Antimicrobial Administration Ratio (SAAR) for each category and total antimicrobials in each patient care location and facility-wide. A SAAR of 1 indicates antimicrobial use is equivalent to referent populations. A SAAR greater than 1 that achieves statistical significance demonstrates excessive antimicrobial use, and a SAAR significantly lower than 1 may demonstrate underuse. SAAR still does not take into account quality of care (e.g., appropriateness of antimicrobial therapy). It does, however, attempt to control for institutional specifics, such as hospital size and complexity of patient population. The ability to look specifically at the different categories of antimicrobials is important, as ASPs are focused on decreasing broad-spectrum antimicrobials and increasing use of narrow-spectrum agents. This still constitutes a positive change for the institution, especially if SAAR for overall antimicrobials is equivalent to, or smaller than, 1, as it implies successful de-escalation from broad- to narrower-spectrum agents.

Table 3. Centers for Disease Control and Prevention National Healthcare and Safety Network antimicrobial use module categories.

Category	Commonly Used Antimicrobials
Broad-spectrum agents predominantly used for hospital-onset infections	Piperacillin/tazobactam, ceftazidime, cefepime, meropenem, imipenem/cilastatin, aztreonam, gentamicin, tobramycin
Broad-spectrum agents predominantly used for community-acquired infections	Ceftriaxone, cefotaxime, cefuroxime, cefdinir, ertapenem, ciprofloxacin, levofloxacin, moxifloxacin
Agents predominantly used for resistant gram-positive infections	Vancomycin, daptomycin, linezolid, ceftaroline
Narrow-spectrum beta-lactam agents	Penicillin G, ampicillin, amoxicillin, ampicillin/sulbactam, amoxicillin/clavulanate, nafcillin, dicloxacillin, cefazolin, cephalexin, cefoxitin
Agents posing the highest risk for *C. difficile* infection	Clindamycin, cefepime, ceftriaxone, cefdinir, ciprofloxacin, levofloxacin, moxifloxacin
Antifungal agents predominantly used for invasive candidiasis	Fluconazole, voriconazole, posaconazole, caspofungin, micafungin, anidulafungin

An example of such a comparison is provided in Figure 1. Such a line graph allows for a local ASP to evaluate their SAAR data over time. The monthly SAAR for all adult antibacterial agents facility-wide is in bold as an overall metric for antimicrobial use. Relevant subcategories are then superimposed on the same graph to allow for simple visual comparison and analysis by the ASP. Because subcategories for antibacterial agents are only available from NHSN for either adult intensive care units (ICUs) (Figure 1A) or adult wards (Figure 1B), the two line graphs are generated to assess antimicrobial use in each unit type. In this example, the adult facility-wide SAAR for overall antimicrobials remains below 1 for the entire time period. Broad-spectrum antimicrobials in adult ICUs are also consistently under 1, yet use of narrow-spectrum beta-lactams in adult ICUs is routinely above 1.0. This suggests that the observed use of agents such as penicillin G, ampicillin, nafcillin, and cefazolin was significantly greater than predicted by the NHSN model. Again, this antimicrobial use metric cannot assess quality of care. In order to distinguish whether this narrow spectrum beta-lactam use represents an appropriate de-escalation that an ASP can celebrate, versus an aggressive de-escalation which needs to be addressed by the ASP, this SAAR data would have to be coupled with quality of care data from the ICUs, e.g., appropriateness of therapy as previously discussed. In this way, SAAR data can reveal interesting nuances to guide local ASP assessments and subsequent initiatives.

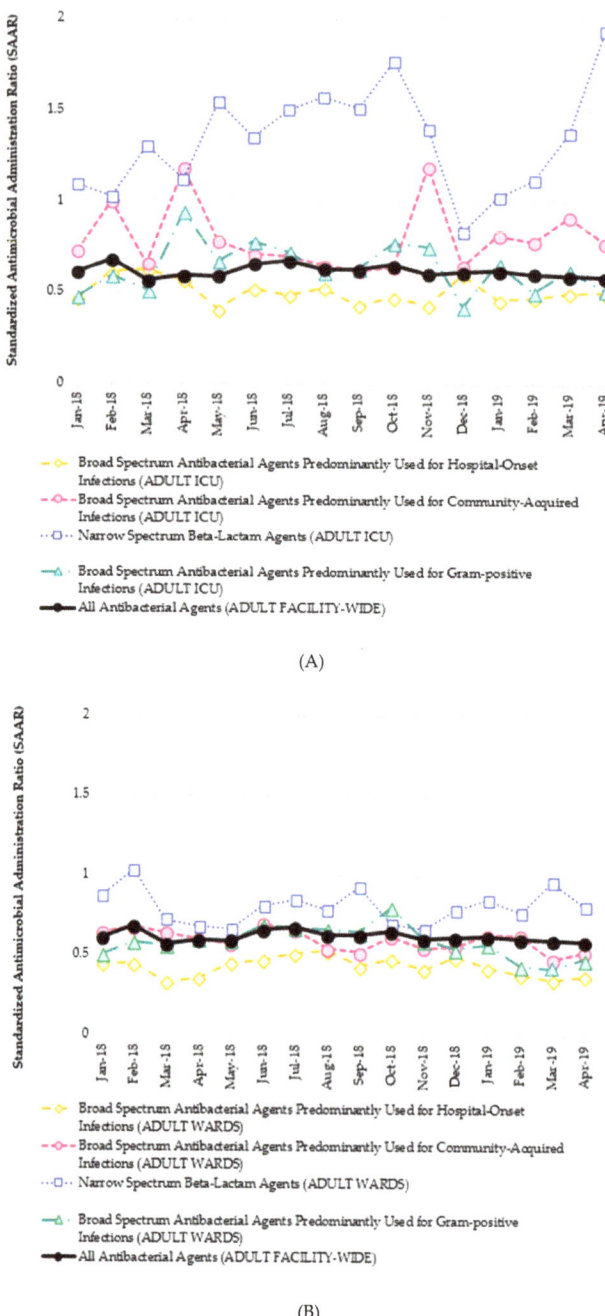

Figure 1. (**A**) Standardized Antimicrobial Administration Ratio (SAAR) report for all and select categories of antibacterial agents in adult intensive care units (ICUs) at a community-teaching hospital. (**B**) Standardized Antimicrobial Administration Ratio (SAAR) report for all and select categories of antibacterial agents at adult wards at a community-teaching hospital.

5.2. Antimicrobial Resistance (AR) Option

Facilities reporting to the AR option will receive a facility-wide antibiogram that can be stratified by source, time period, and specific antibiotics or organisms [80]. Participating facilities will also get a line list generated for all AR events including items such as date of birth, gender, specimen type, and organism. The benefits of this option for tracking the success of an ASP is similar to tracking MRSA, ESBLE, CRE, and resistance among *P. aeruginosa* and *A. baumannii* isolates. While short-term changes may be difficult to visualize, it may be possible to show long-term success. It also allows for benchmarking with other similar institutions. Both the AU and AR modules within the NHSN are promising ASP metrics with different potential uses.

6. Discussion

Historically, direct measurement of antimicrobial use was not feasible for most institutions; thus, surrogate metrics such as HO-CDI incidence and cost were derived. The assumption was that higher incidence rates of HO-CDI and infections due to MDR bacteria reflected excessive antimicrobial use of broad-spectrum agents at an institution. However, in the era of electronic medical records and progressive advancements of healthcare informatics, direct measurement of antimicrobial use has become a reality. CDC/NHSN module for reporting antimicrobial use and antimicrobial resistance provides the tools for direct measurements of ASP daily work and overall performance. Despite some initial hurdles, hospitals and ASPs are both determined to make this breakthrough advancement in the field of antimicrobial stewardship by improving ASP metrics. Adjustments of antimicrobial use by quality of care and institutional microbiological burden will evolve with time. Practical adjustment formulas, which demonstrate validity and generalizability across a broad mix of hospital types and geographical locations, will prove most useful.

ASP metrics may be classified into direct measures of ASP performance and global metrics for overall healthcare system evaluation. Antimicrobial use of broad-spectrum agents represents the primary direct ASP metric. Secondary direct metrics include incidence rate of CRE and antimicrobial resistance of predominantly hospital-onset pathogens, such as *P. aeruginosa* and *A. baumannii* (Table 4).

Table 4. Direct antimicrobial stewardship metrics.

ASP Metrics	Description
Antimicrobial use of broad-spectrum agents: Antipseudomonal beta-lactams Carbapenems Anti-MRSA agents Anti-VRE agents	• Most direct measure of ASP performance • Evaluates effectiveness of ASP interventions (e.g., syndrome-specific, prospective audit and feedback, de-escalation of therapy) • Measures both empirical and definitive therapy • Adjustments by quantity (facility size, patient population, or microbiological burden) and quality (appropriateness of therapy) at each healthcare facility are possible
Antimicrobial resistance of predominantly hospital-onset bacteria: *Pseudomonas aeruginosa* *Acinetobacter baumannii*	• Antimicrobial resistance of hospital-onset bacteria is associated with use of broad-spectrum antimicrobials at each institution • Antimicrobial resistance may also be influenced by referrals, especially at tertiary care centers • Patient-to-patient transmission of MDR bacteria may be reduced by effective infection prevention and control methods
Incidence rate of CRE	• Excessive use of carbapenems and other broad-spectrum antimicrobials increases risk of CRE infections or colonization • CRE rates may be influenced by transfers from other hospitals or skilled nursing facilities • Infection prevention and control programs are essential for reducing transmission of CRE in healthcare facilities

Note: ASP: antimicrobial stewardship programs; MRSA: methicillin-resistant *Staphylococcus aureus*; VRE: vancomycin-resistant *Enterococcus* species; MDR: multi-drug resistant; CRE: carbapenem-resistant *Enterobacteriaceae*.

In addition to these direct metrics, global metrics, including rates of CDI, MRSA, ESBLE, as well as cost of healthcare, should continue to be used in order to evaluate overall performance of healthcare systems (Table 5).

Table 5. Global metrics of overall healthcare system performance.

Global Metrics	Description
Incidence rate of hospital-onset *Clostridioides difficile* infection	• Indirect assessment of quantity and spectrum of AU in healthcare facilities • Tool for evaluation of IPCPs, clinical decision support programs, laboratory, and diagnostic stewardship
Incidence rate of ESBLE infections or colonization	• ESBLE predominantly cause community-onset infections in North America and Europe • Better metric for ambulatory ASPs and IPCPs than inpatient ASPs • Rates are influenced by prior colonization
Incidence rate of MRSA infections or colonization	• MRSA has emerged as community-onset bacteria as well • Association between MRSA and AU is not very clear • Measures performance of IPCPs more than ASPs
Sepsis or bloodstream infection case-fatality rate	• Evaluates clinical, diagnostic, and interventional critical care skills; clinical decision support programs; and laboratory diagnostics, including microbiology • ASPs may influence only one of many variables that determine outcome, that is, empirical antimicrobial therapy through institutional management guidelines and other interventions
Cost of healthcare	• Antimicrobial cost is a fraction of total healthcare cost • ASPs may indirectly contribute to reduction in healthcare cost by reducing length of hospital stay through selection of appropriate empirical antimicrobial therapy and reducing risk of antimicrobial adverse events such as acute kidney injury and *C. difficile* infection

Note: ASP: antimicrobial stewardship programs; AU: antimicrobial utilization; ESBLE: extended-spectrum beta-lactamase-producing *Enterobacteriaceae*; IPCP: infection prevention and control program.

7. Conclusions

In this new era of antimicrobial stewardship, direct measurement of ASP performance is feasible and preferable. Antimicrobial use within an institution represents the most direct and specific antimicrobial stewardship metric for hospital-based ASPs. Antimicrobial resistance of predominantly hospital-onset bacteria, such as *P. aeruginosa* and *A. baumannii*, represents a secondary antimicrobial stewardship metric. Participation of US hospitals in currently available CDC/NHSN modules for antimicrobial use and resistance is highly encouraged and represents a valuable step to improve antimicrobial stewardship at the national level. Novel stewardship metrics presented in this review allow adjustment of antimicrobial use by microbiological burden and quality of care as measured by appropriateness of empirical antimicrobial therapy at each institution. This enhances the antimicrobial stewardship mission in improving both the quantity and quality of patient care.

Author Contributions: Conceptualization, M.N.A.-H., H.R.W., P.B.B., and J.J.; Methodology, M.N.A.-H., H.R.W., P.B.B., and J.A.J.; Writing—original draft preparation, M.N.A.-H. and H.R.W.; writing—review and editing, M.N.A.-H., H.R.W., P.B.B., and J.A.J.; Visualization, M.N.A.-H., H.R.W., P.B.B., and J.A.J.; Supervision, M.N.A.-H., P.B.B., and J.A.J.; Project administration, M.N.A.-H.

Funding: This research received no external funding.

Acknowledgments: The authors thank Joseph Kohn and Prisma Health-Midlands Antimicrobial Stewardship and Support Team in South Carolina, USA for providing antimicrobial use data for demonstration in figures and for their valuable input in this narrative review.

Conflicts of Interest: H.R.W.: Speaker, ALK Abello. P.B.B.: Advisory board member, Melinta Therapeutics; Program content developer and speaker, FreeCE.com; Grant support, ALK Abello. M.N.A.-H. and J.A.J.: No conflicts.

Abbreviations

ASP = antimicrobial stewardship program; AR = antimicrobial resistance; AU = antimicrobial use; CDC = Centers for Disease Control and Prevention; CDI = *Clostridioides difficile* infection; CRE = carbapenem-resistant Enterobacteriaceae; DDD = defined daily dose; DOT = days of therapy; ESBLE = extended-spectrum beta-lactamase-producing Enterobacteriaceae; HO-CDI = hospital-onset *Clostridioides difficile* infection; ICU = intensive care unit; MDR = multidrug-resistant; MRSA = methicillin-resistant *Staphylococcus aureus*; NHSN = National Healthcare Safety Network; SAAR=Standardized Antimicrobial Administration Ratio

References

1. Barlam, T.F.; Cosgrove, S.E.; Abbo, L.M.; MacDougall, C.; Schuetz, A.N.; Septimus, E.J.; Srinivasan, A.; Dellit, T.H.; Falck-Ytter, Y.T.; Fishman, N.O.; et al. Implementing an antibiotic stewardship program: Guidelines by the Infectious Diseases Society of America and the Society for Healthcare Epidemiology of America. *Clin. Infect. Dis.* **2016**, *62*, e51–e77. [CrossRef] [PubMed]
2. Moehring, R.W.; Anderson, D.J.; Cochran, R.L.; Hicks, L.A.; Srinivasan, A.; Dodds Ashley, E.S. Structured Taskforce of Experts Working at Reliable Standards for Stewardship (STEWARDS) Panel. Expert consensus on metrics to assess the impact of patient-level antimicrobial stewardship interventions in acute-care settings. *Clin. Infect. Dis.* **2017**, *64*, 377–383. [CrossRef] [PubMed]
3. Science, M.; Timberlake, K.; Morris, A.; Read, S.; Le Saux, N. *Groupe Antibiothérapie en Pédiatrie Canada Alliance for Stewardship of Antimicrobials in Pediatrics (GAP Can ASAP)*; Quality metrics for antimicrobial stewardship programs; Pediatrics: Elk Grove, IL, USA, 2019; p. 143.
4. Nagel, J.L.; Stevenson, J.G.; Eiland, E.H.; Kaye, K.S. Demonstrating the value of antimicrobial stewardship programs to hospital administrators. *Clin. Infect. Dis.* **2014**, *59* (Suppl. 3), S146–S153. [CrossRef] [PubMed]
5. Brotherton, A.L. Metrics of antimicrobial stewardship programs. *Med. Clin. N. Am.* **2018**, *102*, 965–976. [CrossRef] [PubMed]
6. Bennett, N.; Schulz, L.; Boyd, S.; Newland, J.G. Understanding inpatient antimicrobial stewardship metrics. *Am. J. Health Syst. Pharm.* **2018**, *75*, 230–238. [CrossRef] [PubMed]
7. Tumbarello, M.; Trecarichi, E.M.; Bassetti, M.; De Rosa, F.G.; Spanu, T.; Di Meco, E.; Losito, A.R.; Parisini, A.; Pagani, N.; Cauda, R. Identifying patients harboring extended-spectrum-beta-lactamase-producing Enterobacteriaceae on hospital admission: Derivation and validation of a scoring system. *Antimicrob. Agents Chemother.* **2011**, *55*, 3485–3490. [CrossRef] [PubMed]
8. Augustine, M.R.; Testerman, T.L.; Justo, J.A.; Bookstaver, P.B.; Kohn, J.; Albrecht, H.; Al-Hasan, M.N. Clinical risk score for prediction of extended-spectrum beta-lactamase-producing Enterobacteriaceae in bloodstream isolates. *Infect. Control Hosp. Epidemiol.* **2017**, *38*, 266–272. [CrossRef]
9. Khanna, S.; Pardi, D.S.; Aronson, S.L.; Kammer, P.P.; Orenstein, R.; St Sauver, J.L.; Zinsmeister, A.R. The epidemiology of community-acquired *Clostridium difficile* infection: A population-based study. *Am. J. Gastroenterol.* **2012**, *107*, 89–95. [CrossRef]
10. Lambert, P.J.; Dyck, M.; Thompson, L.H.; Hammond, G.W. Population-based surveillance of *Clostridium difficile* infection in Manitoba, Canada, by using interim surveillance definitions. *Infect. Control Hosp. Epidemiol.* **2009**, *30*, 945–951. [CrossRef]
11. Pitout, J.D.; Hanson, N.D.; Church, D.L.; Laupland, K.B. Population-based laboratory surveillance for *Escherichia coli*-producing extended-spectrum beta-lactamases: Importance of community isolates with blaCTX-M genes. *Clin. Infect. Dis.* **2004**, *38*, 1736–1741. [CrossRef]
12. Thaden, J.T.; Fowler, V.G.; Sexton, D.J.; Anderson, D.J. Increasing incidence of extended-spectrum beta-lactamase-producing *Escherichia coli* in community hospitals throughout the Southeastern United States. *Infect. Control Hosp. Epidemiol.* **2016**, *37*, 49–54. [CrossRef] [PubMed]
13. Global Priority List of Antibiotic-Resistant Bacteria to Guide Research, Discovery, and Development of New Antibiotics. World Health Organization, 2017. Available online: https://www.who.int/medicines/publications/global-priority-list-antibiotic-resistant-bacteria/en/ (accessed on 30 June 2019).

14. Karino, S.; Kaye, K.S.; Navalkele, B.; Nishan, B.; Salim, M.; Solanki, S.; Pervaiz, A.; Tashtoush, N.; Shaikh, H.; Koppula, S.; et al. Epidemiology of acute kidney injury among patients receiving concomitant vancomycin and piperacillin-tazobactam: Opportunities for antimicrobial stewardship. *Antimicrob. Agents Chemother.* **2016**, *60*, 3743–3750. [CrossRef] [PubMed]
15. Hammond, D.A.; Smith, M.N.; Li, C.; Hayes, S.M.; Lusardi, K.; Bookstaver, P.B. Systematic review and meta-analysis of acute kidney injury associated with concomitant vancomycin and piperacillin/tazobactam. *Clin. Infect. Dis.* **2017**, *64*, 666–674. [CrossRef] [PubMed]
16. Piacenti, F.J.; Leuthner, K.D. Antimicrobial stewardship and *Clostridium difficile*-associated diarrhea. *J. Pharm. Pract.* **2013**, *26*, 506–513. [CrossRef] [PubMed]
17. Longtin, Y.; Trottier, S.; Brochu, G.; Paquet-Bolduc, B.; Garenc, C.; Loungnarath, V.; Beaulieu, C.; Goulet, D.; Longtin, J. Impact of the type of diagnostic assay on *Clostridium difficile* infection and complication rates in a mandatory reporting program. *Clin. Infect. Dis.* **2013**, *56*, 67–73. [CrossRef] [PubMed]
18. Grein, J.D.; Ochner, M.; Hoang, H.; Jin, A.; Morgan, M.A.; Murthy, A.R. Comparison of testing approaches for *Clostridium difficile* infection at a large community hospital. *Clin. Microbiol. Infect.* **2014**, *20*, 65–69. [CrossRef] [PubMed]
19. Kelly, S.G.; Yarrington, M.; Zembower, T.R.; Sutton, S.H.; Silkaitis, C.; Postelnick, M.; Mikolajczak, A.; Bolon, M.K. Inappropriate *Clostridium difficile* testing and consequent overtreatment and inaccurate publicly reported metrics. *Infect. Control Hosp. Epidemiol.* **2016**, *37*, 1395–1400. [CrossRef]
20. Graber, C.J. *Clostridium difficile* infection: Stewardship's lowest hanging fruit? *Lancet Infect. Dis.* **2017**, *17*, 123–124. [CrossRef]
21. Al-Hasan, M.N.; Wilson, J.W.; Lahr, B.D.; Thomsen, K.M.; Eckel-Passow, J.E.; Vetter, E.A.; Tleyjeh, I.M.; Baddour, L.M. Beta-lactam and fluoroquinolone combination antibiotic therapy for bacteremia caused by gram-negative bacilli. *Antimicrob. Agents Chemother.* **2009**, *53*, 1386–1394. [CrossRef]
22. Seddon, M.M.; Bookstaver, P.B.; Justo, J.A.; Kohn, J.; Rac, H.; Haggard, E.; Mediwala, K.N.; Dash, S.; Al-Hasan, M.N. Role of early de-escalation of antimicrobial therapy on risk of *Clostridioides difficile* infection following Enterobacteriaceae bloodstream infections. *Clin. Infect. Dis.* **2019**, *69*, 414–420. [CrossRef]
23. Tucker, K.; Lashkova, L.; Flemming, T.; Justo, J.; Kohn, J.; Al-Hasan, M.N.; Sanasi, K.; Bookstaver, P.B. Impact of antimicrobial stewardship initiatives on carbapenem utilization and antimicrobial resistance. In Proceedings of the 55th Interscience Conference on Antimicrobial Agents and Chemotherapy, San Diego, CA, USA, 17–21 September 2015. Abstract #2243.
24. Palacios-Baena, Z.R.; Delgado-Valverde, M.; Valiente Méndez, A.; Almirante, B.; Gómez-Zorrilla, S.; Borrell, N.; Corzo, J.E.; Gurguí, M.; de la Calle, C.; García-Álvarez, L.; et al. Impact of de-escalation on prognosis of patients with bacteraemia due to Enterobacteriaceae: A post-hoc analysis from a multicenter prospective cohort. *Clin. Infect. Dis.* **2018**. [CrossRef] [PubMed]
25. Tariq, R.; Singh, S.; Gupta, A.; Pardi, D.S.; Khanna, S. Association of gastric acid suppression with recurrent *Clostridium difficile* infection: A systematic review and meta-analysis. *JAMA Intern. Med.* **2017**, *177*, 784–791. [CrossRef] [PubMed]
26. Thomas, C.; Stevenson, M.; Riley, T.V. Antibiotics and hospital-acquired *Clostridium difficile*-associated diarrhoea: A systematic review. *J. Antimicrob. Chemother.* **2003**, *51*, 1339–1350. [CrossRef] [PubMed]
27. Brown, K.A.; Khanafer, N.; Daneman, N.; Fisman, D.N. Meta-analysis of antibiotics and the risk of community-associated *Clostridium difficile* infection. *Antimicrob. Agents Chemother.* **2013**, *57*, 2326–2332. [CrossRef]
28. Pagels, C.M.; McCreary, E.K.; Rose, W.E.; Dodds Ashley, E.S.; Bookstaver, P.B.; Dilworth, T.J. Designing antimicrobial stewardship initiatives to enhance scientific dissemination. *J. Am. Coll. Clin. Pharm.* **2019**, 1–7. [CrossRef]
29. McFarland, L.V.; Surawicz, C.M.; Stamm, W.E. Risk factors for *Clostridium difficile* carriage and, *C. difficile*-associated diarrhea in a cohort of hospitalized patients. *J. Infect. Dis.* **1990**, *162*, 678–684. [CrossRef] [PubMed]
30. Lawes, T.; Lopez-Lozano, J.M.; Nebot, C.A.; Macartney, G.; Subbarao-Sharma, R.; Wares, K.D.; Sinclair, C.; Gould, I.M. Effect of a national 4C antibiotic stewardship intervention on the clinical and molecular epidemiology of *Clostridium difficile* infections in a region of Scotland: A non-linear time-series analysis. *Lancet Infect. Dis.* **2017**, *17*, 194–206. [CrossRef]
31. Harris, A.D.; Sbarra, A.N.; Leekha, S.; Jackson, S.S.; Johnson, J.K.; Pineles, L.; Thom, K.A. Electronically available comorbid conditions for risk prediction of healthcare-associated *Clostridium difficile* infection. *Infect. Control Hosp. Epidemiol.* **2018**, *39*, 297–301. [CrossRef]

32. Al-Hasan, M.N.; Lahr, B.D.; Eckel-Passow, J.E.; Baddour, L.M. Antimicrobial resistance trends of *Escherichia coli* bloodstream isolates: A population-based study, 1998–2007. *J. Antimicrob. Chemother.* **2009**, *64*, 169–174. [CrossRef]
33. Waltner-Toews, R.I.; Paterson, D.L.; Qureshi, Z.A.; Sidjabat, H.E.; Adams-Haduch, J.M.; Shutt, K.A.; Jones, M.; Tian, G.B.; Pasculle, A.W.; Doi, Y. Clinical characteristics of bloodstream infections due to ampicillin-sulbactam-resistant, non-extended-spectrum-beta-lactamase-producing *Escherichia coli* and the role of TEM-1 hyperproduction. *Antimicrob. Agents Chemother.* **2011**, *55*, 495–501. [CrossRef]
34. Baggs, J.; Fridkin, S.K.; Pollack, L.A.; Srinivasan, A.; Jernigan, J.A. Estimating National trends in inpatient antibiotic use among US hospitals from 2006 to 2012. *JAMA Intern. Med.* **2016**, *176*, 1639–1648. [CrossRef]
35. Logan, L.K.; Gandra, S.; Mandal, S.; Klein, E.Y.; Levinson, J.; Weinstein, R.A.; Laxminarayan, R. Prevention Epicenters Program, US Centers for Disease Control and Prevention. Multidrug- and carbapenem-resistant *Pseudomonas aeruginosa* in children, United States, 1999–2012. *J. Pediatr. Infect. Dis. Soc.* **2017**, *6*, 352–359.
36. Knothe, H.; Shah, P.; Krcmery, V.; Antal, M.; Mitsuhashi, S. Transferable resistance to cefotaxime, cefoxitin, cefamandole and cefuroxime in clinical isolates of *Klebsiella pneumoniae* and Serratia marcescens. *Infection* **1983**, *11*, 315–317. [CrossRef]
37. Rodriguez-Bano, J.; Navarro, M.D.; Romero, L.; Martínez-Martínez, L.; Muniain, M.A.; Perea, E.J.; Pérez-Cano, R.; Pascual, A. Epidemiology and clinical features of infections caused by extended-spectrum beta-lactamase-producing *Escherichia coli* in nonhospitalized patients. *J. Clin. Microbiol.* **2004**, *42*, 1089–1094. [CrossRef]
38. Rottier, W.C.; Bamberg, Y.R.; Dorigo-Zetsma, J.W.; van der Linden, P.D.; Ammerlaan, H.S.; Bonten, M.J. Predictive value of prior colonization and antibiotic use for third-generation cephalosporin-resistant enterobacteriaceae bacteremia in patients with sepsis. *Clin. Infect. Dis.* **2015**, *60*, 1622–1630. [CrossRef]
39. Morgan, D.J.; Meddings, J.; Saint, S.; Lautenbach, E.; Shardell, M.; Anderson, D.; Milstone, A.M.; Drees, M.; Pineles, L.; Safdar, N.; et al. SHEA Research Network. Does nonpayment for hospital-acquired catheter-associated urinary tract infections lead to overtesting and increased antimicrobial prescribing? *Clin. Infect. Dis.* **2012**, *55*, 923–929. [CrossRef]
40. Lawes, T.; Lopez-Lozano, J.M.; Nebot, C.A.; Macartney, G.; Subbarao-Sharma, R.; Dare, C.R.; Wares, K.D.; Gould, I.M. Effects of national antibiotic stewardship and infection control strategies on hospital-associated and community-associated meticillin-resistant *Staphylococcus aureus* infections across a region of Scotland: A non-linear time-series study. *Lancet Infect. Dis.* **2015**, *15*, 1438–1449. [CrossRef]
41. Jain, R.; Kralovic, S.M.; Evans, M.E.; Ambrose, M.; Simbartl, L.A.; Obrosky, D.S.; Render, M.L.; Freyberg, R.W.; Jernigan, J.A.; Muder, R.R.; et al. Veterans Affairs initiative to prevent methicillin-resistant *Staphylococcus aureus* infections. *N. Engl. J. Med.* **2011**, *364*, 1419–1430. [CrossRef]
42. Klein, E.Y.; Mojica, N.; Jiang, W.; Cosgrove, S.E.; Septimus, E.; Morgan, D.J.; Laxminarayan, R. Trends in methicillin-resistant *Staphylococcus aureus* hospitalizations in the United States, 2010–2014. *Clin. Infect. Dis.* **2017**, *65*, 1921–1923. [CrossRef]
43. Kourtis, A.P.; Hatfield, K.; Baggs, J.; Mu, Y.; See, I.; Epson, E.; Nadle, J.; Kainer, M.A.; Dumyati, G.; Petit, S.; et al. Vital signs: Epidemiology and recent trends in methicillin-resistant and in methicillin-susceptible *Staphylococcus aureus* bloodstream infections—United States. *MMWR Morb. Mortal. Wkly. Rep.* **2019**, *68*, 214–219. [CrossRef]
44. FDA Updates Warnings for Fluoroquinolone Antibiotics. Available online: http://www.fda.gov/NewsEvents/Newsroom/PressAnnouncements/ucm513183.htm (accessed on 4 June 2019).
45. Orsi, G.B.; Bencardino, A.; Vena, A.; Carattoli, A.; Venditti, C.; Falcone, M.; Giordano, A.; Venditti, M. Patient risk factors for outer membrane permeability and KPC-producing carbapenem-resistant *Klebsiella pneumoniae* isolation: Results of a double case-control study. *Infection* **2013**, *41*, 61–67. [CrossRef]
46. Al-Hasan, M.N.; Wilson, J.W.; Lahr, B.D.; Eckel-Passow, J.E.; Baddour, L.M. Incidence of *Pseudomonas aeruginosa* bacteremia: A population-based study. *Am. J. Med.* **2008**, *121*, 702–708. [CrossRef]
47. Gransden, W.R.; Leibovici, L.; Eykyn, S.J.; Pitlik, S.D.; Samra, Z.; Konisberger, H.; Drucker, M.; Phillips, I. Risk factors and a clinical index for diagnosis of *Pseudomonas aeruginosa* bacteremia. *Clin. Microbiol. Infect.* **1995**, *1*, 119–123. [CrossRef]
48. Hammer, K.L.; Justo, J.A.; Bookstaver, P.B.; Kohn, J.; Albrecht, H.; Al-Hasan, M.N. Differential effect of prior beta-lactams and fluoroquinolones on risk of bloodstream infections secondary to *Pseudomonas aeruginosa*. *Diagn. Microbiol. Infect. Dis.* **2017**, *87*, 87–91. [CrossRef]

49. Cheong, H.S.; Kang, C.I.; Wi, Y.M.; Kim, E.S.; Lee, J.S.; Ko, K.S.; Chung, D.R.; Lee, N.Y.; Song, J.H.; Peck, K.R. Clinical significance and predictors of community-onset *Pseudomonas aeruginosa* bacteremia. *Am. J. Med.* **2008**, *121*, 709–714. [CrossRef]
50. Schechner, V.; Nobre, V.; Kaye, K.S.; Leshno, M.; Giladi, M.; Rohner, P.; Harbarth, S.; Anderson, D.J.; Karchmer, A.W.; Schwaber, M.J.; et al. Gram-negative bacteremia upon hospital admission: When should *Pseudomonas aeruginosa* be suspected? *Clin. Infect. Dis.* **2009**, *48*, 580–586. [CrossRef]
51. Decraene, V.; Ghebrehewet, S.; Dardamissis, E.; Huyton, R.; Mortimer, K.; Wilkinson, D.; Shokrollahi, K.; Singleton, S.; Patel, B.; Turton, J.; et al. An outbreak of multidrug-resistant *Pseudomonas aeruginosa* in a burns service in the North of England: Challenges of infection prevention and control in a complex setting. *J. Hosp. Infect.* **2018**, *100*, e239–e245. [CrossRef]
52. Milan, A.; Furlanis, L.; Cian, F.; Bressan, R.; Luzzati, R.; Lagatolla, C.; Deiana, M.L.; Knezevich, A.; Tonin, E.; Dolzani, L. Epidemic dissemination of a carbapenem-resistant *Acinetobacter baumannii* clone carrying armA two years after its first isolation in an Italian hospital. *Microb. Drug Resist.* **2016**, *22*, 668–674. [CrossRef]
53. Paramythiotou, E.; Lucet, J.C.; Timsit, J.F.; Vanjak, D.; Paugam-Burtz, C.; Trouillet, J.L.; Belloc, S.; Kassis, N.; Karabinis, A.; Andremont, A. Acquisition of multidrug-resistant *Pseudomonas aeruginosa* in patients in intensive care units: Role of antibiotics with antipseudomonal activity. *Clin. Infect. Dis.* **2004**, *38*, 670–677. [CrossRef]
54. Montero, M.; Sala, M.; Riu, M.; Belvis, F.; Salvado, M.; Grau, S.; Horcajada, J.P.; Alvarez-Lerma, F.; Terradas, R.; Orozco-Levi, M.; et al. Risk factors for multidrug-resistant *Pseudomonas aeruginosa* acquisition. Impact of antibiotic use in a double case-control study. *Eur. J. Clin. Microbiol. Infect. Dis.* **2010**, *29*, 335–339. [CrossRef]
55. Nakamura, A.; Miyake, K.; Misawa, S.; Kuno, Y.; Horii, T.; Kondo, S.; Tabe, Y.; Ohsaka, A. Meropenem as predictive risk factor for isolation of multidrug-resistant *Pseudomonas aeruginosa*. *J. Hosp. Infect.* **2013**, *83*, 153–155. [CrossRef]
56. Cobos-Trigueros, N.; Sole, M.; Castro, P.; Torres, J.L.; Hernández, C.; Rinaudo, M.; Fernández, S.; Soriano, Á.; Nicolás, J.M.; Mensa, J.; et al. Acquisition of *Pseudomonas aeruginosa* and its resistance phenotypes in critically ill medical patients: Role of colonization pressure and antibiotic exposure. *Crit. Care* **2015**, *19*, 218. [CrossRef]
57. Al-Jaghbeer, M.J.; Justo, J.A.; Owens, W.; Kohn, J.; Bookstaver, P.B.; Hucks, J.; Al-Hasan, M.N. Risk factors for pneumonia due to beta-lactam-susceptible and beta-lactam-resistant *Pseudomonas aeruginosa*: A case-case-control study. *Infection* **2018**, *46*, 487–494. [CrossRef]
58. Cain, S.E.; Kohn, J.; Bookstaver, P.B.; Albrecht, H.; Al-Hasan, M.N. Stratification of the impact of inappropriate empirical antimicrobial therapy for Gram-negative bloodstream infections by predicted prognosis. *Antimicrob. Agents Chemother.* **2015**, *59*, 245–250. [CrossRef]
59. Retamar, P.; Portillo, M.M.; Lopez-Prieto, M.D.; Rodríguez-López, F.; de Cueto, M.; García, M.V.; Gómez, M.J.; Del Arco, A.; Muñoz, A.; Sánchez-Porto, A.; et al. SAEI/SAMPAC Bacteremia Group. Impact of inadequate empirical therapy on the mortality of patients with bloodstream infections: A propensity score-based analysis. *Antimicrob. Agents Chemother.* **2012**, *56*, 472–478. [CrossRef]
60. Al-Hasan, M.N.; Rac, H. Transition from intravenous to oral antimicrobial therapy in patients with uncomplicated and complicated bloodstream infections. *Clin. Microbiol. Infect.* **2019**. [CrossRef]
61. Paul, M.; Shani, V.; Muchtar, E.; Kariv, G.; Robenshtok, E.; Leibovici, L. Systematic review and meta-analysis of the efficacy of appropriate empiric antibiotic therapy for sepsis. *Antimicrob. Agents Chemother.* **2010**, *54*, 4851–4863. [CrossRef]
62. Shorr, A.F.; Micek, S.T.; Welch, E.C.; Doherty, J.A.; Reichley, R.M.; Kollef, M.H. Inappropriate antibiotic therapy in Gram-negative sepsis increases hospital length of stay. *Crit. Care Med.* **2011**, *39*, 46–51. [CrossRef]
63. Battle, S.E.; Bookstaver, P.B.; Justo, J.A.; Kohn, J.; Albrecht, H.; Al-Hasan, M.N. Association between inappropriate empirical antimicrobial therapy and hospital length of stay in Gram-negative bloodstream infections: Stratification by prognosis. *J. Antimicrob. Chemother.* **2017**, *72*, 299–304. [CrossRef]
64. Sogaard, M.; Norgaard, M.; Dethlefsen, C.; Schonheyder, H.C. Temporal changes in the incidence and 30-day mortality associated with bacteremia in hospitalized patients from 1992 through 2006: A population-based cohort study. *Clin. Infect. Dis.* **2011**, *52*, 61–69. [CrossRef]
65. Nimmich, E.B.; Bookstaver, P.B.; Kohn, J.; Justo, J.A.; Hammer, K.L.; Albrecht, H.; Al-Hasan, M.N. Development of Institutional Guidelines for Management of Gram-Negative Bloodstream Infections: Incorporating Local Evidence. *Hosp. Pharm.* **2017**, *52*, 691–697. [CrossRef]

66. Bookstaver, P.B.; Nimmich, E.B.; Smith, T.J.; Justo, J.A.; Kohn, J.; Hammer, K.L.; Troficanto, C.; Albrecht, H.A.; Al-Hasan, M.N. Cumulative effect of an antimicrobial stewardship and rapid diagnostic testing bundle on early streamlining of antimicrobial therapy in Gram-negative bloodstream infections. *Antimicrob. Agents Chemother.* **2017**, *61*, e00189-17. [CrossRef]
67. Al-Hasan, M.N.; Lahr, B.D.; Eckel-Passow, J.E.; Baddour, L.M. Predictive scoring model of mortality in Gram-negative bloodstream infection. *Clin. Microbiol. Infect.* **2013**, *19*, 948–954. [CrossRef]
68. Al-Hasan, M.N.; Juhn, Y.J.; Bang, D.W.; Yang, H.J.; Baddour, L.M. External validation of bloodstream infection mortality risk score in a population-based cohort. *Clin. Microbiol. Infect.* **2014**, *20*, 886–891. [CrossRef]
69. Huang, A.M.; Newton, D.; Kunapuli, A.; Gandhi, T.N.; Washer, L.L.; Isip, J.; Collins, C.D.; Nagel, J.L. Impact of rapid organism identification via matrix-assisted laser desorption/ionization time-of-flight combined with antimicrobial stewardship team intervention in adult patients with bacteremia and candidemia. *Clin. Infect. Dis.* **2013**, *57*, 1237–1245. [CrossRef]
70. MacVane, S.H.; Nolte, F.S. Benefits of adding a rapid PCR-based blood culture identification panel to an established antimicrobial stewardship program. *J. Clin. Microbiol.* **2016**, *54*, 2455–2463. [CrossRef]
71. Banerjee, R.; Teng, C.B.; Cunningham, S.A.; Ihde, S.M.; Steckelberg, J.M.; Moriarty, J.P.; Shah, N.D.; Mandrekar, J.N.; Patel, R. Randomized trial of rapid multiplex polymerase chain reaction-based blood culture identification and susceptibility testing. *Clin. Infect. Dis.* **2015**, *61*, 1071–1080. [CrossRef]
72. Mediwala, K.N.; Kohn, J.E.; Bookstaver, P.B.; Justo, J.A.; Rac, H.; Tucker, K.; Lashkova, L.; Dash, S.; Al-Hasan, M.N. Syndrome-specific versus prospective audit and feedback interventions for reducing use of broad-spectrum antimicrobial agents. *Am. J. Infect. Control* **2019**. [CrossRef]
73. Sick, A.C.; Lehmann, C.U.; Tamma, P.D.; Lee, C.K.; Agwu, A.L. Sustained savings from a longitudinal cost analysis of an internet-based preapproval antimicrobial stewardship program. *Infect. Control Hosp. Epidemiol.* **2013**, *34*, 573–580. [CrossRef]
74. Beardsley, J.R.; Williamson, J.C.; Johnson, J.W.; Luther, V.P.; Wrenn, R.H.; Ohl, C.C. Show me the money: Long-term financial impact of an antimicrobial stewardship program. *Infect. Control Hosp. Epidemiol.* **2012**, *33*, 398–400. [CrossRef]
75. Ozkurt, Z.; Erol, S.; Kadanali, A.; Ertek, M.; Ozden, K.; Tasyaran, M.A. Changes in antibiotic use, cost and consumption after an antibiotic restriction policy applied by infectious disease specialists. *Jpn. J. Infect. Dis.* **2005**, *58*, 338–343.
76. Akpan, M.R.; Ahmad, R.; Shebl, N.A.; Ashiru-Oredope, D. A review of quality measures for assessing the impact of antimicrobial stewardship programs in hospitals. *Antibiotics* **2016**, *5*, 5. [CrossRef]
77. Bartlett, J.M.; Siola, P.L. Implementation and first-year results of an antimicrobial stewardship program at a community hospital. *Am. J. Health Syst. Pharm.* **2014**, *71*, 943–949. [CrossRef]
78. Tamma, P.D.; Avdic, E.; Keenan, J.F.; Zhao, Y.; Anand, G.; Cooper, J.; Dezube, R.; Hsu, S.; Cosgrove, S.E. What is the more effective antibiotic stewardship intervention: Preprescription authorization or postprescription review with feedback? *Clin. Infect. Dis.* **2017**, *64*, 537–543.
79. Al-Hasan, M.N.; Eckel-Passow, J.E.; Baddour, L.M. Influence of referral bias on the clinical characteristics of patients with Gram-negative bloodstream Infection. *Epidemiol. Infect.* **2011**, *139*, 1750–1756. [CrossRef]
80. Antimicrobial Use and Resistance Module. 2019. Available online: https://www.cdc.gov/nhsn/PDFs/pscManual/11pscAURcurrent.pdf (accessed on 1 June 2019).
81. van Santen, K.L.; Edwards, J.R.; Webb, A.K.; Pollack, L.A.; O'Leary, E.; Neuhauser, M.M.; Srinivasan, A.; Pollock, D.A. The standardized antimicrobial administration ratio: A new metric for measuring and comparing antibiotic use. *Clin. Infect. Dis.* **2018**, *67*, 179–185. [CrossRef]

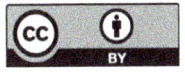

© 2019 by the authors. Licensee MDPI, Basel, Switzerland. This article is an open access article distributed under the terms and conditions of the Creative Commons Attribution (CC BY) license (http://creativecommons.org/licenses/by/4.0/).

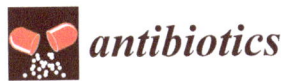

Review

The Perfect Bacteriophage for Therapeutic Applications—A Quick Guide

Lucía Fernández [1,2,*], Diana Gutiérrez [3], Pilar García [1,2] and Ana Rodríguez [1,2]

1. Instituto de Productos Lácteos de Asturias (IPLA-CSIC), (DairySafe Group), Paseo Río Linares s/n -Villaviciosa, 33300 Asturias, Spain
2. Instituto de Investigación Sanitaria del Principado de Asturias (ISPA), 33011 Oviedo, Spain
3. Laboratory of Applied Biotechnology, Department of Applied Biosciences, Faculty of Bioscience Engineering, Ghent University, 9000 Ghent, Belgium
* Correspondence: lucia.fernandez@ipla.csic.es; Tel.: +34-9858-92131

Received: 29 July 2019; Accepted: 21 August 2019; Published: 23 August 2019

Abstract: The alarming spread of multiresistant infections has kick-started the quest for alternative antimicrobials. In a way, given the steady increase in untreatable infectious diseases, success in this endeavor has become a matter of life and death. Perhaps we should stop searching for an antibacterial panacea and explore a multifaceted strategy in which a wide range of compounds are available on demand depending on the specific situation. In the context of this novel tailor-made approach to combating bacterial pathogens, the once forgotten phage therapy is undergoing a revival. Indeed, the compassionate use of bacteriophages against seemingly incurable infections has been attracting a lot of media attention lately. However, in order to take full advantage of this strategy, bacteria's natural predators must be taken from their environment and then carefully selected to suit our needs. In this review, we have explored the vast literature regarding phage isolation and characterization for therapeutic purposes, paying special attention to the most recent studies, in search of findings that hint at the most efficient strategies to identify suitable candidates. From this information, we will list and discuss the traits that, at the moment, are considered particularly valuable in phages destined for antimicrobial therapy applications. Due to the growing importance given to biofilms in the context of bacterial infections, we will dedicate a specific section to those characteristics that indicate the suitability of a bacteriophage as an antibiofilm agent. Overall, the objective is not just to have a large collection of phages, but to have the best possible candidates to guarantee elimination of the target pathogens.

Keywords: bacteriophages; biofilms; novel antimicrobials

1. Phage Therapy: A Major Comeback with Minor Setbacks

The existence of viruses that can infect and kill bacterial cells, known as bacteriophages (or phages), was discovered almost simultaneously by Frederick Twort and Félix d'Herelle about one century ago, but it is the latter who has been credited with introducing the concept of using these entities as antimicrobial agents [1,2]. Indeed, the French-Canadian microbiologist pioneered the so-called phage therapy and used phages to treat patients with various infectious diseases [3]. Since that time, the utilization of phages for therapeutic applications has remained common practice in Eastern Europe, saving countless human lives [4]. Conversely, in other parts of the world, the introduction of antibiotics pushed this anti-infective strategy out of center stage for many decades. After all, antibiotics were cheaper to manufacture and exhibited a broader spectrum of activity, thereby eliminating the need to identify the etiological agent prior to treatment prescription. However, with time, overuse and misuse of antibiotics became widespread in different fields, such as human and veterinary medicine or agriculture. In this context, antibiotics exerted the selective pressure that resulted in the spread of resistance markers and led up to the current antimicrobial resistance crisis [5]. Alarmingly, the number of deaths associated with bacterial infections is rising and threatens to reach levels not seen since the preantibiotic era. The reason for this is that more and more bacterial strains are acquiring multiresistance and are, consequently, able to survive treatment with most, if not all, antibiotics commonly used in the clinic. Given the severity of such a scenario, besides curtailing unnecessary antibiotic use, the scientific community has started a race to find as many alternatives to conventional antibiotics as possible [6]. Among the many options being explored, the revival of phage therapy presents itself as an attractive strategy to substitute or complement other therapies [7]. This is especially the case because phages, due to their unique mechanism of action, exhibit some notable differences compared to other types of antimicrobials, some of which are particularly advantageous. These positive attributes include their natural origin, lack of toxicity for humans or nontarget microbes (being harmless to the normal microbiota), and their effectiveness against antibiotic-resistant bacteria, amongst others. On the downside, phage therapy generally requires identification of the target pathogen and phage resistance development remains a possibility, although it is not usually as easily transferable to other microorganisms as antibiotic resistance determinants. Moreover, resistance could be easily overcome by using combinations of different phages (phage cocktails) instead of a single phage for therapeutic applications [8].

Nonetheless, not everything is rosy on the way toward normalizing the use of bacteriophages against unwanted bacteria in the context of human medicine. Most notably, it will be paramount to convince both the general public and the competent authorities that these antimicrobials are safe for human health and the environment, as well as provide undeniable proof of their efficacy in clinical settings. Indeed, these are two key aspects in order to surmount the current regulatory constraints that limit the use of bacterial viruses for infection treatment in humans. Until relatively recently, most evidence regarding the effectiveness of phage therapy was the result of direct use in patients, but well-organized and reproducible data will be essential in order to comply with the requirements set out for the approval of medicinal products [9]. In this regard, the growing number of completed clinical trials will certainly be invaluable. On the other hand, the growing utilization of phages as biocontrol agents for the disinfection of inert surfaces may also help to pave the way toward regulatory approval [10]. As a matter of fact, the relevant authorities in different countries (USA, Israel, Canada, Switzerland, Australia, New Zealand, and the Netherlands) have already approved this type of applications against several pathogens in the context of the food industry [11,12]. For example, there are several commercially available products to be used against various food pathogens, such as *Listeria monocytogenes*, *Salmonella*, or *Escherichia coli*, as surface disinfectants or processing aids. Indeed, the FDA has recognized some phage-based formulations as "generally regarded as safe" (GRAS) as food additives. Regarding medicinal use, phage therapy is now under the scrutiny of government agencies, which are trying to determine the most adequate regulatory framework considering the special characteristics of phages. In the meantime, patients in many countries can have access to this treatment as compassionate use [13]. One of the major challenges of regulating phage approval is the diversity of phages that will be necessary to successfully implement this therapeutic strategy. Indeed, in order to harness the full potential of phage therapy and its adaptability to changes in pathogenic strains, there should be room for making changes to phage-based formulations without the need for a lengthy and costly approval process. In addition to regulatory hurdles, bringing phage therapy to the market also has the problem of not being very attractive for pharmaceutical companies. To some extent, this is a consequence of their natural origin, as phages cannot be patented. Also, their use is aimed to be used as an acute course of treatment rather than for chronic administration, which obviously means that they would not be as profitable as other medicines. However, the relevant authorities can help by designing an affordable and straightforward pathway for regulatory compliance that might perhaps encourage the participation of smaller specialized companies.

Overall, it is apparent that phages are getting closer and closer to becoming a mainstream antimicrobial treatment option, especially in the case of difficult-to-cure multiresistant infections.

However, in order to get the most out of phage therapy, we will need to have an arsenal of well-chosen effective and safe bacteriophages at our disposal. This will involve a number of steps that, if not carefully planned, may hinder the successful development and subsequent implementation of this strategy (Figure 1). In order to maximize speed and minimize costs, it is necessary to establish clear guidelines indicating where and how to look for suitable therapeutic phages, as well as define the most valuable traits in the identified candidates.

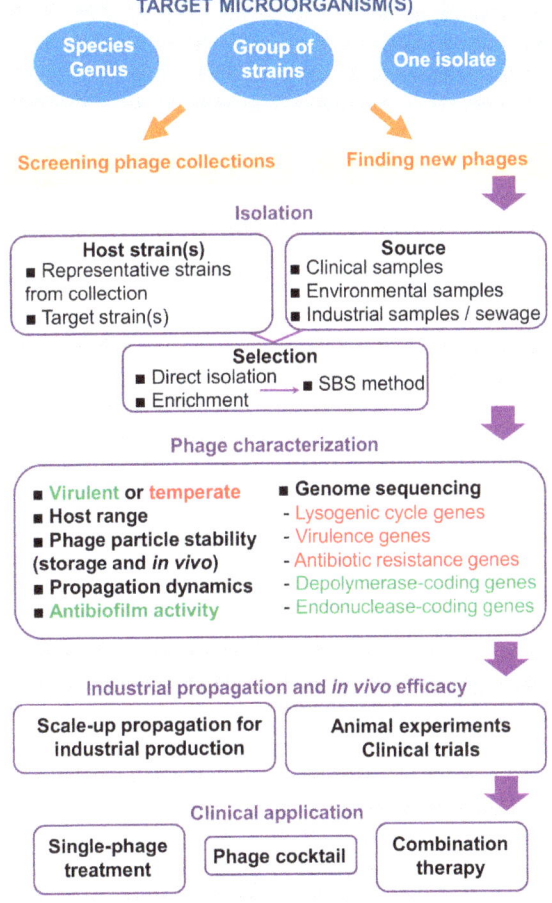

Figure 1. Steps involved in the development of phage therapy strategies. In the phage characterization step, text in green and red respectively correspond to desirable and undesirable characteristics in a phage for therapeutic applications. Abbreviations: SBS method, step-by-step method.

2. In Search of New Phages

One of the main advantages of using bacteriophages as antimicrobials is their sheer quantity and diversity. As a matter of fact, even without improvement by genetic engineering, nature represents an almost limitless source of new phage variants. It is well known that phages are the most abundant biological entities on earth (about 10^{31} phages in total) [14]. On top of that, bacterial viruses evolve at a dizzying rate and are, as a result, highly diverse. Indeed, there is evidence indicating that bacteriophages outpace their hosts in the coevolutionary race [15]. Now, this all sounds like good news from the perspective of the antimicrobial development pipeline until coming to the realization that finding the right phages for our purpose among this huge set of candidates is quite the gargantuan task. Nevertheless, it is also worth noting that vast phage collections are already available in different research centers and universities around the globe. As a result, this would be a good place to start once the target microbe is identified.

It is obviously impossible to screen for phages everywhere, so a major step consists in narrowing down the most probable reservoirs of viruses that infect and kill our target microbe. As is always the case with predators, these reservoirs are likely to coincide with the main habitats of their prey, that is, the target pathogen. In that sense, d'Hérelle suggested that the best source of bacterial viruses for antimicrobial applications are samples from patients who are recovering or who have just recovered from an infection [16]. Indeed, he first remarked the existence of "bacteria eaters" in stool samples of patients recovering from bacillary dysentery [1]. Similarly, phages against enterohemorrhagic *E. coli* (EHEC) O157:H7 were found in fecal samples from human patients and cattle [17]. Additionally, phages infecting *Cutibacterium acnes* (formerly *Propionibacterium acnes*) and *Actinobacillus* have respectively been isolated from human skin and dental plaque [18,19]. Given the prevalence of human pathogenic bacteria in infected patients, another good reservoir of phages infecting these microorganisms is wastewater from hospitals [20]. If clinical samples are not available, good results have also been obtained with sewage water, which has actually become a frequent starting point for phage hunts [21]. In the case of microbes with high prevalence in diverse ecological niches, different environmental sources like river or stream water have also been the place to isolate new bacteriophages [22,23]. Additionally, drinking water was the source of phages infecting *Enterococcus* and *Staphylococcus* [24], while silage from dairy farms proved a good source of listeriaphages [25].

In some cases, the phage titer in these reservoirs will be high enough to allow direct isolation of the virus after filtration of the sample; for example, by visualization of lysis plaques on plates containing the host (double layer assay). However, this is not always the case and enrichment steps are often required to detect the presence of the phage. Frequently, it is a good idea to collect large-volume samples in order to increase the chances of phage isolation, especially when dealing with samples taken from environmental sources. It must also be noted that some phages form very small plaques on a bacterial lawn, which would hinder their identification by the double layer method. For this reason, if no plaques are observed during the isolation step, it might be worth repeating the process but using techniques that increase plaque size, such as addition of subinhibitory concentrations of antibiotics [26,27] or other compounds like sodium thiosulfate, ferric ammonium citrate or 2,3,5-triphenyltetrazolium [28].

Another important aspect in the quest to find new phages with antimicrobial potential lies in the selection of the most appropriate host strain or strains. However, this choice will also depend on the specific goal of the search. Thus, if the objective is the identification of phages against as many strains of a given pathogen as possible, multihost selection protocols should be used. Additionally, the host strains should preferably be very varied in terms of their characteristics and origin so that they are representative of the species. In this sense, Casey et al. [29] recommend using bacteria reference collections for phage identification, as they offer a good representation of the intraspecies diversity, together with strains of clinical relevance. However, in some cases, there may be a specific target strain or group of strains that do not seem to be susceptible to the phages available in different collections. Then, it will be necessary to carry out screenings using these strains as selection hosts. Nonetheless, if finding a new virulent phage that infects our target strain proves to be very difficult, it is possible to carry out an adaptation strategy in which coevolution rounds may allow the selection of a phage variant that can effectively infect and kill the pathogenic strain. This protocol is called the step-by-step (SBS) method [30]. The phenomenon of local host adaptation also plays a role in the identification of new phages [31]. Indeed, phages are known to co-evolve very closely with their host strains. As a result, virulent phages from a given reservoir or geographic location are oftentimes more effective at targeting strains from that same milieu.

3. Desirable Traits in Phages with Antimicrobial Potential

3.1. Specific but Not Too Specific

One of the major advantages of bacteriophages as antimicrobials is their specificity. A consequence of this characteristic is that they are not only innocuous to eukaryotic cells, but also to all prokaryotic cells outside their host range. This would ensure that the normal microbiota remains intact during therapy, which in turn would be expected to help prevent secondary infections and probably accelerate recovery. Indeed, there is growing proof that the microorganisms inhabiting our bodies play very important roles in our overall health. Antibiotic treatment, by contrast, can severely affect our normal microbiota due to their more general, broad-range action, which often results in serious side effects [32]. Another benefit of this specific action is that we can technically try to identify viruses that only infect certain strains within a bacterial species, distinguishing, for example, between pathogenic and nonpathogenic isolates. Again, some microbes can potentially be helpful or harmful to their human hosts depending on the presence of sometimes only a few genes that turn them from friend to foe. As a result, it would be ideal to develop antimicrobials that can differentiate between commensal and pathogenic strains of the same species.

Notwithstanding the incredible target precision that can be achieved with phage therapy, it is generally preferable to isolate viruses able to attack a wide range of strains within a bacterial species. In some cases, it may also be desirable that a given phage can infect different pathogenic species within a genus. Staphylococcal phages are a good example of this, with some of them infecting the two opportunistic pathogens *Staphylococcus aureus* and *Staphylococcus epidermidis*, such as myophages phiIPLA-RODI and phiIPLA-C1C [33]. The polyvalent nature of staphylophages is also useful since it allows carrying out phage propagation on nonpathogenic species, such as *Staphylococcus xylosus* [34]. Remarkably, there are phages capable of infecting different genera within the *Enterobacteriaceae* family, including *E. coli* O157:H7, *Salmonella enterica* ser. Paratyphi, and *Shigella dysenteriae* [35].

At first glance, it would appear that having a broad host range would be a synonym of success for a bacteriophage, as it would increase its likelihood of encountering a susceptible bacterial cell, which is necessary for survival of the phage population [36]. However, this hypothesis is not supported by the available experimental data. Thus, the ability of a given phage to infect and multiply inside a host depends on factors from both prey and predator. As mentioned previously, some studies have observed a very well-tuned coevolution, leading to local specificity in phage–host interactions [31]. Indeed, there is evidence that greater specialization can be linked to increased infection efficacy and the other way around, which suggests that there is an evolutionary compromise between these two properties [37,38]. Therefore, while it is possible to broaden the host range of a given phage, this might lead to a "weaker virus" that cannot propagate as efficiently.

In any case, a bacteriophage used for therapeutic applications should at the very least be able to infect the different variations of the pathogen population inside the patient. As this is not always possible with single-phage preparations, the use of a phage cocktail, if available, is always a better option. Interestingly, study of the coexistence dynamics between the cyanobacterium *Prochlorococcus* and ten cyanophages revealed that acquisition of resistance to one phage sometimes resulted in enhanced infection by other phages [39]. In some cases, the authors could demonstrate that this was due to the increased adsorption of "the other phages" to the phage-resistant mutants than to the original bacterial strain. If this phenomenon is also observed in therapeutic phages, it would be useful in the context of phage cocktail administration, as it would manifest itself as a synergic rather than an additive effect between the different viruses. Identification of the potential phage receptors in the host is an important aspect of designing a phage cocktail. Evidently, it would be better to have experimental evidence of the nature of the receptor for a specific phage. However, if this information is not available, there are now resources to predict potential receptor molecules based on the phage genome data and information from literature or databases [40,41]. Indeed, it would help to avoid combining phages that can potentially exhibit cross-resistance. Moreover, it would be preferable to select phages whose target receptors are essential for bacterial fitness or virulence as the likelihood of phage resistance selection will be lower or, at the very least, might lead to lesser pathogenicity. Furthermore, if there is receptor modification, the probability of phage variants that can infect the altered receptor are much higher than they are in cases of receptor loss, a possibility with nonessential receptor molecules [42]. Indeed, infectivity evolution in phages during therapeutic applications should be studied more in depth. Especially, because it provides a unique opportunity of using an evolving antimicrobial that can potentially overcome by itself bacterial resistance mechanisms during therapy [42].

Another strategy for limiting phage resistance is the selection of phages harboring modified nucleotides, like archeosine or N6-(1-acetamido)-adenine, in their genomes. This would make the viral DNA resistant to the activity of many restriction endonucleases, one of bacteria's natural antiphage defense systems [43]. A hint of this trait can be found during genome sequencing through the identification of genes involved in the biosynthesis of these nucleotides. For instance, recent studies showed that siphophages Vid5 and BRET, which respectively infect the enterobacteria *Pantoea agglomerans* and *E. coli*, carry archeosine biosynthesis genes [44,45].

3.2. Virulent Phages Only, Please

In addition to the lytic cycle, which ends up with the death of the bacterial cell, some bacteriophages can also undergo the so-called lysogenic cycle. In this case, the viral genome integrates into and replicates with the bacterial chromosome. The viral genetic material, known as prophage, can stay in this state for generations until an environmental signal turns on the machinery leading to its excision from the bacterial genome and kick-starts the lytic cycle. This type of phage is called temperate and they are known to actively contribute to the phenomenon of horizontal gene transfer, one of the main mechanisms involved in the spread of antimicrobial resistance and virulence genes. As a result, temperate phages are not considered good candidates for phage therapy. In contrast, phages that can only undergo the lytic cycle, or virulent phages, are ideal for this purpose, as their multiplication is almost always followed by lysis of the infected cell. These phages are also sometimes called "professionally lytic" [46]. During the phage selection process, virulent and temperate phages can tentatively be differentiated as they respectively produce clear and turbid plaques on a bacterial lawn.

In some cases, phages that can infect and kill the target organism, especially if it is a specific strain, are scarce and utilization of virulent derivatives from temperate phages is required. This can be achieved by selecting or constructing mutant phage variants through different protocols. For example, phage deletion mutants can be easily isolated by exposing the phage particles to several rounds of a chelating agent such as ethylenediaminetetraacetic acid (EDTA), sodium citrate, or sodium pyrophosphate [47]. Chelating agents exert a destabilizing effect on the phage particles by binding the cations located on their surface, which results in conformational defects and, ultimately, in viability loss. However, viral particles carrying deletions in their genome are smaller and can retain their conformation and remain viable under these conditions. From the selected deletion mutants, it would be then possible to identify the virulent variants, as they would produce clear instead of turbid plaques. Alternatively, phages can be genetically manipulated to obtain a virulent variant by removing genes involved in lysogeny. Indeed, a cocktail containing engineered phages successfully eliminated an infection by a drug-resistant strain of *Mycobacterium abscessus* from a cystic fibrosis patient [48]. However, the use of genetically modified organisms is still shrouded in controversy and is not even a viable option in many countries.

Nevertheless, strictly virulent phages are not completely free from the danger of facilitating transfer of antibiotic resistance genes. For instance, Keen et al. [49] recently described the existence of "superspreader" virulent phages, which do not carry endonucleases in their genome and release the bacterial DNA to the environment. This would make it possible that this now extracellular DNA can enter other microorganisms by natural transformation and potentially spread resistance or virulence markers. In fact, this study reported that addition of the phage to cocultures of a kanamycin-sensitive *Bacillus* sp. and kanamycin-resistant *E. coli* strains led to a 1000-fold increase in transfer of the antibiotic resistance marker to *Bacillus*. This would not be a desirable situation so it would be important to ensure that a phage with therapeutic potential does degrade the bacterial chromosome prior to cell lysis.

Once confirmed that a candidate phage is strictly virulent and not a superspreader, the next step is to determine if it can propagate efficiently both in vitro and in vivo. First, it is necessary to study propagation under in vitro conditions, for example, by performing a one-step growth curve. This technique requires achieving the synchronous infection of all bacterial cells in a population in order to then monitor how the number of extracellular and intracellular viable phage particles changes throughout the lytic cycle. This data will allow calculation of valuable propagation parameters, such as burst size (average number of new phage particles released per infected cell) and latent period (part of the lytic cycle between virion attachment to the cell and start of new phage particle release). In some cases, a shorter latent period has been associated with the possession of DNA-dependent RNA polymerases in the phage genome [50]. Theoretically, this protein might shut down host transcription and increase the efficiency of the phage replication cycle, although this phenomenon has not been supported by experimental evidence yet. After confirming that the phage can propagate under in vitro conditions, which is essential for phage production, in vivo experiments should be performed to confirm that the virus can also multiply effectively at the infection site if the target host is present. This ability to self-propagate during treatment is undoubtedly a major advantage compared to other types of antimicrobials, whose concentration invariably decreases after administration to the patient.

3.3. Safe for Human Health and the Environment

Following the isolation of a phage with therapeutic potential, it is necessary to perform genome sequencing and analysis. Thanks to the advances made in this field, this has become an easy and affordable task that can actually save us a lot of time and money on additional experiments. On the one hand, examination of the phage genome can confirm that there are no genes involved in lysogeny, such as the lytic cycle repressor, integrases or site-specific recombinases. Identification of genes encoding potential endonucleases can also suggest that it is not a "superspreader". On top of that, genomic analysis is the single most reliable way to know whether the phage genome encodes toxins or antimicrobial resistance determinants. Indeed, if there are any such genes, the phage should never be considered for therapeutic applications. If possible, it is also preferable to choose a propagation host (a so-called surrogate strain) that does not carry prophages or virulence/antibiotic resistance markers [51].

Besides not being carriers of "bad genes", bacteriophages must be innocuous when administered to the patients. As mentioned above, one key aspect of phages as therapeutics is the fact that they do not infect nontarget bacteria, leaving the normal microbiota largely undisturbed after therapy. Regarding their safety for the patient, all clinical trials so far indicate that they do not exhibit significant toxicity. Nonetheless, it is worth noting that phages need to be well purified in order to remove toxic substances before administration. A clear example of this is endotoxin, which could lead to serious side-effects if not thoroughly removed from the phage suspension. The importance of endotoxin removal depends, however, on the type of application. For example, it is essential for intravenous administration, while purification does not need to be so strict for topical or oral administration to the patient [51,52]. In that sense, it is also important to consider the potential effect of widespread lysis of the target bacteria inside the patient. It is worth noting, however, that studies in which filtered lysates were administered directly to patients without further purification led to mild or, most frequently, no symptoms [53]. Overall, the available data suggests that the doses required for bacteriophages to trigger toxicity exceed the effective concentrations necessary for their application. This holds true not only for the administered doses but also considering the propagation inside the patient. As such, phages typically exhibit a high therapeutic index, a quantitative measurement of the relative safety of a drug, which is obtained as the ratio between the dose leading to toxicity and the amount that displays antimicrobial activity.

Due to the relative simplicity and lack of diversity of bacteriophages in terms of their chemical composition, basically consisting of proteins and nucleic acids, their potential interactions with the immune system are relatively easy to study and predict in stark contrast to other types of antimicrobials. Given that the outward structure of the viral particle consists basically of proteins, phages can be immunogenic. This issue would be especially problematic when intravenous (i.v.) administration is required, as it could potentially lead to an anaphylactic response. However, i.v. administration of phages has been performed repeatedly without observing major negative side effects [52].

Widespread phage application as an antimicrobial also poses questions regarding its potential impact on natural environments [54]. Indeed, it is very important to assess the risk of altering the composition of natural microbial communities due to the release of phages from clinical, veterinary or agricultural applications. These changes could be deleterious to ecosystems as they might alter nutrient cycling. Given the structure of these communities, an impact of phages on soil ecological dynamics (phage to bacteria ratios of 1:1) would be more expected than on aquatic communities (phage to bacteria ratios of 1:100). However, this disruptive effect would be expected to be much lower than that of antibiotics given the specificity of bacteriophage activity.

A key aspect to ensure the safety of phages aimed for therapeutic applications is the development of well-defined bacteriophage production and quality control protocols that allow manufacturing of pharmaceutical-grade phage products [55]. These methods should maximize phage yield in the production stage followed by highly effective purification steps [55,56]. Thus, while satisfying health and environmental concerns should be a priority, the economic viability of industrial phage production must also be taken into account. All of these steps are also very important in order to achieve regulatory approval of phage-based formulations [57].

3.4. Stability

As mentioned above, phage particles consist of a nucleic acid molecule inside a proteinaceous envelope. As such, they are much more complex and labile compounds than other antimicrobials. This fact makes them unstable outside a specific range of environmental conditions (temperature, pH, UV-light, salt concentrations, proteases). Thorough analysis of phage particle stability is, therefore, an integral part of the phage characterization process. For example, a very effective virulent phage that has a very narrow stability range may not be well suited for therapy. Indeed, the viral particles must be able to withstand the production, storage and administration stages in sufficient numbers to reach their target. However, the conditions that allow phage stability maintenance vary enormously depending on the specific phage [58]. In fact, it appears that neither family nor close structural similarity are good predictors of stability range, although tailed phages generally seem to be the most stable under adverse environmental conditions [59].

After propagation, the bacteriophage should remain viable and infective throughout storage. As mentioned above, specific storage conditions have to be tested for each phage, as they may vary depending on its characteristics. For example, different storage temperatures are better suited for different phages [59]. Thus, while some are more stable at temperatures around 4 °C, others must be kept at freezing temperatures of −20 °C or even −80 °C. In contrast, some phages exhibit very good stability at room temperature or even 37 °C. Another important factor is the format for storing the phage particles. For instance, some phages remain viable for longer periods of time when stored in a liquid (which can be growth medium or a buffer). An alternative possibility is storing the phage particles in a dry powder, which can be produced by different techniques such as lyophilization (freeze drying) or spray drying. In this case, it is necessary to consider that the drying process itself may be deleterious for the viral particles, which might lead to a considerable titer loss prior to storage [22,60]. Sometimes, preservation in both liquid and dry form can be improved by adding different stabilizing agents, such as skim milk, glycerol, trehalose, or sorbitol [61]. Alternatively, the phages can be kept as a nucleic acid inside infected cells, which can then be stored frozen at −80 °C [62]. The lytic cycle would continue as soon as bacterial growth is resumed. However, González-Menéndez et al. [60] showed that this technique does not always improve phage particle stability compared to storage of the naked phages. Some studies have also shown that phage encapsulation in nanovesicles can enhance stability by protecting the particles from environmental factors, although a study showed that this improvement was only noticeable during short-term but not during long-term storage [63].

In order to be a good candidate for phage therapy, the viral particles must be stable not only during the production and storage stages, but also during its application, that is, it has to remain infective from the moment of administration to the patient until it reaches the target pathogen. In that context, the characteristics of the phage and the type of formulation used will depend on the administration route and target organs. With regards to temperature, for example, the phage should be able to withstand the body temperature for long enough to reach its target host. Additionally, if application is to be carried out by topical administration, it would be desirable that the phage is not exceedingly sensitive to UV-light exposure, so that it is not inactivated before infecting the bacterial cells. If treatment is aimed at respiratory infections, the phage particles should be able to withstand techniques used for the preparation of aerosols, such as freeze- or spray-drying [64–66]. In turn, the ability to withstand an acidic pH will be very important if the phage is to be administered by the oral route.

As was the case with storage, encapsulation of the phage particles can also be helpful in order to improve stability during treatment. For example, by facilitating skin absorption of the product so that the phage can reach deeper layers of the epidermis, or by protecting the phage particles from the acid in the stomach or from bile salts [67]. Encapsulation can also be suitable for inhalation of a phage formulation that has to reach the lungs. For instance, a study by Singla et al. [68] showed that phages in liposomes were more effective than nonencapsulated phages for treating pneumonia caused by *Klebsiella pneumoniae*. Additionally, encapsulated phages displayed a greater ability to enter eukaryotic cells than their nonencapsulated counterparts [69]. This indicates that they have greater potential for reaching intracellular pathogens. Recent work by Nobrega et al. [70] demonstrated that improved phage stability during oral administration could be achieved by genetically engineering the phage particles of the *E. coli* phage T7 to display lipids on their surface. The authors proposed this strategy as a good alternative to encapsulation. This high stability is very important as otherwise, oral administration of phages requires very high phage titers ($\geq 10^{11}$ PFU/mL) so that at least a dose of 10^6 PFU can reach the intestine.

Topical application of phages is the preferred form of treatment for various skin infections, ranging from acne to serious burn wound infections. In these cases, the phage will typically be applied as a cream. Good results for phage stability in this format have been obtained so far. For example, phages against *C. acnes* remained viable for 90 days in a semisolid preparation if stored protected from light and at 4 °C [18]. In the case of the staphylococcal phage K, stability for several days could be achieved with a cream stored at room temperature, and the results were improved when using an oil-in-water nanoemulsion [71]. The authors hypothesized that this enhanced stability may be the result of electrostatic forces [72]. Additionally, the nanoemulsion may lead to decreased electrostatic repulsion between the negatively charged surfaces of the phage particle and the cell. In the case of products aimed at treating burn wound infections, Merabishvili et al. [73] examined the stability of phages against the main causative agents (*P. aeruginosa*, *A. baumanii*, *S. aureus*) in different antibiotic-containing formulations, including creams, ointments, and hydrogels. The results of this work indicate that the pH of the product is the most limiting factor for phage stability.

Finally, the bacteriophage must be able to resist the immune response of the patient. However, it seems that a very high dose of phage particles, much higher than that recommended for treatment, is necessary in order to elicit a significant immune response [74]. According to a study by Majewska et al. [74], this response is higher if the phage is applied by subcutaneous injection rather than by oral administration. This lack of a very intense response by the immune system is probably the result of continuous exposure to phages which are part of the human microbiome [75]. In any case, definitively showing that phages can remain viable and be effective will come from further studies in animal models and clinical trials. It is also important to make sure that the phage particles are not inactivated by neutralizing antibodies. However, a humoral immune response would be more of a problem when the phages are administered parenterally rather than after oral or topical application [76]. Moreover, antibody production dynamics would be expected to occur more slowly than pathogen elimination by the phage and, as a result, phage neutralization by the immune system should not constitute a problem during acute infection therapy. Additionally, PEGylation of the phage particles, that is, addition of monomethoxy-polyethylene glycol (mPEG), is known to reduce their immunogenicity and result in lesser levels of cytokine production in mice [77]. Nonetheless, these responses still must be studied in more depth.

3.5. Antibiofilm Potential

Biofilms are the most common lifestyle of bacteria in both natural and artificial environments, including inside the human body. As a result, it is now known that biofilms contribute to bacterial pathogenicity, especially in the case of chronic infections [78]. These multicellular structures allow the bacterial cells to survive under normally lethal conditions, resisting challenges by the immune system or antimicrobial compounds thanks to a combination of multiple mechanisms [79]. This makes biofilms very difficult to eliminate, and one of the major problems that need to be tackled in order to combat infections. In that sense, bacteriophages may, given their special characteristics, provide an interesting alternative to conventional disinfectants or antibiotics [80,81]. However, it is necessary to demonstrate that a given phage is a useful antibiofilm agent. Several studies have already shown that phage treatment of preformed biofilms can successfully reduce the amount of total attached biomass as well as the number of viable bacterial cells attached to the surface. For instance, phage phiIPLA-RODI, which infects different staphylococcal species, can successfully kill *S. aureus* cells from preformed single-species and multispecies biofilms [33,82]. A further example was provided by Khalifa et al. [83], who showed that an enterococcal phage could eliminate in vitro biofilms and prevent infection by *Enterococcus faecalis* in an ex vivo model of root canal infection. Likewise, phages have been used to kill biofilm cells from numerous important pathogens such as *P. aeruginosa* [84], *A. baumanii* [85], and uropathogenic *E. coli* [86], amongst others. Also, some studies have demonstrated that phages can move across these complex microbial populations (Figure 2A) and propagate if a suitable host is present (Figure 2B) [87,88]. Remarkably, phages also seem to be able to infect the infamous persister cells (Figure 2C) that are known to contribute to recalcitrant infections, even if they cannot proceed with the lytic cycle until bacterial growth is resumed [89].

An interesting feature of some phages is the possession of genes coding for exopolysaccharide depolymerases (Figure 2D) that can degrade the polysaccharidic component of the extracellular matrix of biofilms facilitating biofilm dispersion and access of the phage into the deeper layers of this structure [90,91]. It is clear that including at least one such phage in a therapeutic cocktail would be of help to all the different phages. Similarly, production by phage J8-65 of a colinidase, which targets polysaccharides in the cell envelope, was responsible for synergy between this phage and T7 in a temperature- and media-dependent manner [92]. Alternatively, a bacteriophage of interest could be genetically modified to encode a depolymerase in its genome, as Lu and Collins [93] demonstrated in their proof-of-principle work with phage T7. Although this strategy would be very controversial at the moment, if engineered phages become more widely accepted for therapy applications, this would open the door for modification with other types of genes that may control biofilm development. A very interesting example was provided by Pei et al. [94] who cloned a quorum-quenching enzyme in the genome of T7 bacteriophages. While phage degradation of the extracellular matrix is a very desirable outcome, phage inactivation by matrix components should be avoided (Figure 2E).

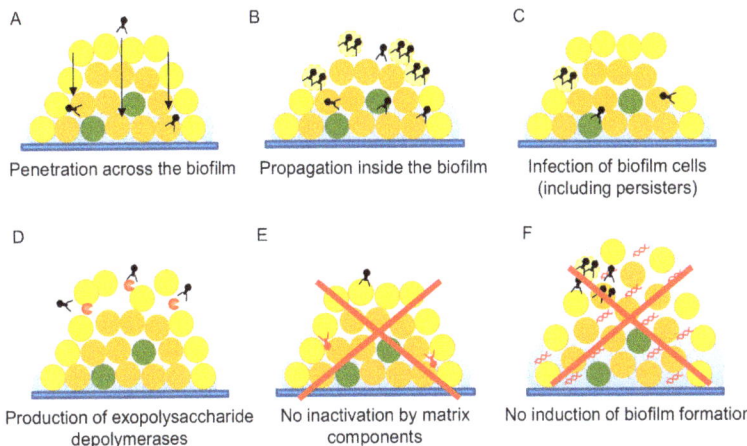

Figure 2. Analysis of the antibiofilm potential of a candidate bacteriophage.

Another important aspect to examine is whether a given phage can potentially promote biofilm formation of the target pathogen (Figure 2F). In this sense, there are examples showing that both biofilm enhancement and inhibition are possible depending on the phage–host pair, although studies concerning the impact of virulent phages have been so far outnumbered by those focusing on temperate viruses [95]. For example, different studies have shown that addition of some virulent phages leads to increased biofilm formation in strains of *S. aureus*, *P. aeruginosa*, *Salmonella*, and *Vibrio anguillarum* [96–98]. In some cases, such as *P. aeruginosa*, it is known that the phenotype is due to the selection of phage-resistant mutants with better biofilm-forming ability [97]. This could be solved by application of a phage cocktail, as selection of mutants against all phages in the cocktail would be less likely. In *V. anguillarum*, phage KVP40 promotes increased cell aggregation [98]. In contrast, accumulation of extracellular DNA was responsible for increased attached biomass upon low-level predation of *S. aureus* by phage phiIPLA-RODI [96]. Nonetheless, it is worth emphasizing the need to understand the specific mechanisms underlying biofilm increase by phages in order to take action to reduce or completely eliminate this undesirable phenomenon.

4. Conclusions

In the midst of a nearly apocalyptic scenario regarding our ability to cure infectious diseases, phage therapy seems like a saving grace. Perhaps not a perfect strategy by itself, it certainly is a good supplement to other therapies as part of a vast antimicrobial arsenal. Their specificity also fits very nicely within the tendency toward a more personalized approach to human medicine, especially when it comes to treatment strategies. However, it is paramount to have as much information as possible before phage therapy use in the clinic is generalized. This will hopefully prevent some of the errors made with antibiotics. Additionally, it is very important to have a crystal-clear view of the characteristics that make a bacteriophage a good candidate for therapeutic use. Once it is established where and how the search for new phages will be performed, careful analysis of the isolated phage should ensue. Perhaps the single most important trait is the selection of strictly lytic phages, while temperate phages should be either modified or discarded outright. In addition, phages should not carry virulence or antibiotic resistance genes in their genomes and preferably produce endonucleases that degrade the host chromosome prior to cell lysis, thereby preventing spread of bacterial genes to other microbes by natural transformation. Clearly, bacteriophages will never attain the spectrum of action of antibiotics, if only because of their particular multistep mechanism of bacterial killing, the lytic cycle, which involves several specific interactions at the molecular level. This may not necessarily be a drawback, as phage specificity also allows for tightly controlled killing of pathogenic targets without damaging eukaryotic cells or nontarget microbes. This feature is very important given the increasingly recognized role of the microbiota in human health. Another aspect that requires attention during phage selection is phage particle stability under different conditions, especially those occurring during storage and, above all, during treatment. Nonetheless, strategies that allow prolonged stability such as encapsulation should be also developed further. Last but not least, the interactions between phages and microbial biofilms should be analyzed in depth in order to maximize the potential use of bacterial viruses to reduce or eliminate these structures. Indeed, this might be a key step in the fight against chronic, recalcitrant infections that do not respond to other types of antimicrobial therapy. Overall, phage therapy seems like a viable, promising strategy that might play a major role in the antibacterial regimes of the future, perhaps even the near future. Nonetheless, further research is still necessary to fill in the gaps that will enable using this strategy while maximizing both efficacy and safety.

Author Contributions: L.F., D.G., P.G. and A.R. wrote the paper.

Funding: This study was funded by grants AGL2015-65673-R (Ministry of Science and Innovation, Spain), EU ANIWHA ERA-NET (BLAAT ID: 67)/PCIN-2017-001 (Ministry of Economy, Industry and Competitiveness, Spain), Proyecto Intramural CSIC201670E040, Proyecto Intramural CSIC 201770E016, GRUPIN14-139 (Program of Science, Technology and Innovation 2013-2017, Principado de Asturias), IDI/2018/000119 (iAsturias Innovation, Principado de Asturias) and FEDER EU funds.

Acknowledgments: P.G. and A.R. are members of the bacteriophage network FAGOMA II and the FWO Vlaanderen funded "Phagebiotics" research community (WO.016.14).

Conflicts of Interest: The authors declare no conflict of interest.

References

1. D'Hérelle, F. Sur un microbe invisible antagoniste des bacilles dysentériques. *C. R. Acad. Sci.* **1917**, *165*, 373–375.
2. Twort, F. An investigation on the nature of ultra-microscopic viruses. *Lancet* **1915**, *186*, 1241–1243. [CrossRef]
3. D'Hérelle, F.; Smith, G.H. *The Bacteriophage and Its Clinical Application*; Charles, C., Ed.; Thomas: Springfield, IL, USA, 1930.
4. Debarbieux, L.; Pirnay, J.P.; Verbeken, G.; de Vos, D.; Merabishvili, M.; Huys, I.; Patey, O.; Schoonjans, D.; Vaneechoutte, M.; Zizi, M.; et al. A bacteriophage journey at the European Medicines Agency. *FEMS Microbiol. Lett.* **2016**, *363*. [CrossRef] [PubMed]
5. Ventola, C.L. The antibiotic resistance crisis: Part 1: Causes and threats. *Pharm. Ther.* **2015**, *40*, 277–283.
6. World Health Organization. *Global Action Plan on Antimicrobial Resistance*; World Health Organization: Geneva, Switzerland, 2015.
7. Gordillo-Altamirano, F.L.; Barr, J.J. Phage therapy in the postantibiotic era. *Clin. Microbiol. Rev.* **2019**, *32*. [CrossRef] [PubMed]
8. Chan, B.K.; Abedon, S.T.; Loc-Carrillo, C. Phage cocktails and the future of phage therapy. *Future Microbiol.* **2013**, *8*, 769–783. [CrossRef] [PubMed]
9. Furfaro, L.L.; Payne, M.S.; Chang, B.J. Bacteriophage therapy: Clinical trials and regulatory hurdles. *Front. Cell Infect. Microbiol.* **2018**, *8*, 376. [CrossRef]
10. Moye, Z.D.; Woolston, J.; Sulakvelidze, A. Bacteriophage applications for food production and processing. *Viruses* **2018**, *10*, 205. [CrossRef]
11. Fernández, L.; Gutiérrez, D.; Rodríguez, A.; García, P. Application of bacteriophages in the agro-food sector: A long way toward approval. *Front. Cell Infect. Microbiol.* **2018**, *8*, 296. [CrossRef]
12. Endersen, L.; O'Mahony, J.; Hill, C.; Ross, R.P.; McAuliffe, O.; Coffey, A. Phage therapy in the food industry. *Annu. Rev. Food Sci. Technol.* **2014**, *5*, 327–349. [CrossRef]
13. McCallin, S.; Sacher, J.C.; Zheng, J.; Chan, B.K. Current state of compassionate phage therapy. *Viruses* **2019**, *11*, 343. [CrossRef] [PubMed]
14. Suttle, C.A. Viruses in the sea. *Nature* **2005**, *437*, 356–361. [CrossRef] [PubMed]
15. Vos, M.; Birkett, P.J.; Birch, E.; Griffiths, R.I.; Buckling, A. Local adaptation of bacteriophages to their bacterial hosts in soil. *Science* **2009**, *325*, 833. [CrossRef] [PubMed]

16. D'Herelle, F. *Le Phénomène de la Guérison des Maladies Infectieuses*; Masson: Paris, France, 1938.
17. O'Flynn, G.; Ross, R.P.; Fitzgerald, G.F.; Coffey, A. Evaluation of a cocktail of three bacteriophages for biocontrol of *Escherichia coli* O157:H7. *Appl. Environ. Microbiol.* **2004**, *70*, 3417–3424. [CrossRef] [PubMed]
18. Brown, T.L.; Petrovski, S.; Dyson, Z.A.; Seviour, R.; Tucci, J. The formulation of bacteriophage in a semi solid preparation for control of *Propionibacterium acnes* growth. *PLoS ONE* **2016**, *11*, e0151184. [CrossRef] [PubMed]
19. Tylenda, C.A.; Calvert, C.; Kolenbrander, P.E.; Tylenda, A. Isolation of *Actinomyces* bacteriophage from human dental plaque. *Infect. Immun.* **1985**, *49*, 1–6. [PubMed]
20. Latz, S.; Wahida, A.; Arif, A.; Häfner, H.; Hoß, M.; Ritter, K.; Horz, H.P. Preliminary survey of local bacteriophages with lytic activity against multi-drug resistant bacteria. *J. Basic Microbiol.* **2016**, *56*, 1117–1123. [CrossRef] [PubMed]
21. Weber-Dąbrowska, B.; JońCzyk-Matysiak, E.; Żaczek, M.; Łobocka, M.; Łusiak-Szelachowska, M.; Górski, A. Bacteriophage procurement for therapeutic purposes. *Front. Microbiol.* **2016**, *7*, 1177. [CrossRef] [PubMed]
22. Merabishvili, M.; Vervaet, C.; Pirnay, J.-P.; de Vos, D.; Verbeken, G.; Mast, J.; Chanishvili, N.; Vaneechoutte, M. Stability of *Staphylococcus aureus* phage ISP after freeze-drying (lyophilization). *PLoS ONE* **2013**, *8*, e68797. [CrossRef]
23. Ul Haq, I.; Chaudhry, W.N.; Andleeb, S.; Qadr, I.I. Isolation and partial characterization of a virulent bacteriophage IHQ1 specific for *Aeromonas punctata* from stream water. *Microb. Ecol.* **2011**, *63*, 954–963. [CrossRef]
24. Weber-Dąbrowska, B.; Żaczek, M.; Dziedzic, B.; Łusiak-Szelachowska, M.; Kiejzik, M.; Górski, A.; Gworek, B.; Wierzbicki, K.; Eymontt, A. Bacteriophages in green biotechnology—The utilization of drinking water. In *Industrial, Medical and Environmental Applications of Microorganisms: Current Status and Trends*; Wageningen Academic Publishers: Wageningen, The Netherlands, 2014; pp. 500–504.
25. Vongkamjan, K.; Switt, A.M.; den Bakker, H.C.; Fortes, E.D.; Wiedmann, M. Silage collected from dairy farms harbors an abundance of listeriaphages with considerable host range and genome size diversity. *Appl. Environ. Microbiol.* **2012**, *78*, 8666–8675. [CrossRef] [PubMed]
26. Loś, J.M.; Golec, P.; Wegrzyn, G.; Wegrzyn, A.; Loś, M. Simple method for plating *Escherichia coli* bacteriophages forming very small plaques or no plaques under standard conditions. *Appl. Environ. Microbiol.* **2008**, *74*, 5113–5120. [CrossRef] [PubMed]
27. Kaur, S.; Harjai, K.; Chhibber, S. Methicillin-resistant *Staphylococcus aureus* phage plaque size enhancement using sublethal concentrations of antibiotics. *Appl. Environ. Microbiol.* **2012**, *78*, 8227–8233. [CrossRef] [PubMed]
28. McLaughlin, M.R.; Balaa, M.F. Enhanced contrast of bacteriophage plaques in *Salmonella* with ferric ammonium citrate and sodium thiosulfate (FACST) and tetrazolium red (TZR). *J. Microbiol. Methods* **2006**, *65*, 318–323. [CrossRef] [PubMed]
29. Casey, E.; van Sinderen, D.; Mahony, J. In vitro characteristics of phages to guide 'real life' phage therapy suitability. *Viruses* **2018**, *10*, 163. [CrossRef] [PubMed]
30. Gu, J.; Liu, X.; Li, Y.; Han, W.; Lei, L.; Yang, Y.; Zhao, H.; Gao, Y.; Song, J.; Lu, R.; et al. A method for generation phage cocktail with great therapeutic potential. *PLoS ONE* **2012**, *7*, e31698. [CrossRef]
31. Kawecki, T.J.; Ebert, D. Conceptual issues of local adaptation. *Ecol. Lett.* **2004**, *7*, 1225–1241. [CrossRef]
32. Langdon, A.; Crook, N.; Dantas, G. The effects of antibiotics on the microbiome throughout development and alternative approaches for therapeutic modulation. *Genome Med.* **2016**, *8*, 39. [CrossRef]
33. Gutiérrez, D.; Vandenheuvel, D.; Martínez, B.; Rodríguez, A.; Lavigne, R.; García, P. Two phages, phiIPLA-RODI and phiIPLA-C1C, lyse mono- and dual-species staphylococcal biofilms. *Appl. Environ. Microbiol.* **2015**, *81*, 3336–3348. [CrossRef]
34. El Haddad, L.; Ben Abdallah, N.; Plante, P.L.; Dumaresq, J.; Katsarava, R.; Labrie, S.; Corbeil, J.; St-Gelais, D.; Moineau, S. Improving the safety of *Staphylococcus aureus* polyvalent phages by their production on a *Staphylococcus xylosus* strain. *PLoS ONE* **2014**, *9*, e102600. [CrossRef]
35. Hamdi, S.; Rousseau, G.M.; Labrie, S.J.; Tremblay, D.M.; Kourda, R.S.; Ben Slama, K.; Moineau, S. Characterization of two polyvalent phages infecting *Enterobacteriaceae*. *Sci. Rep.* **2017**, *7*, 40349. [CrossRef] [PubMed]
36. Koskella, B.; Meaden, S. Understanding bacteriophage specificity in natural microbial communities. *Viruses* **2013**, *5*, 806. [CrossRef] [PubMed]

37. Poullain, V.; Gandon, S.; Brockhurst, M.A.; Buckling, A.; Hochberg, M.E. The evolution of specificity in evolving and coevolving antagonistic interactions between a bacteria and its phage. *Evolution* **2008**, *62*, 1–11. [CrossRef]
38. Duffy, S.; Turner, P.E.; Burch, C.L. Pleiotropic costs of niche expansion in the RNA bacteriophage Φ6. *Genetics* **2006**, *172*, 751–757. [CrossRef] [PubMed]
39. Avrani, S.; Schwartz, D.A.; Lindell, D. Virus-host swinging party in the oceans: Incorporating biological complexity into paradigms of antagonistic coexistence. *Mob. Gent. Elem.* **2012**, *2*, 88–95. [CrossRef] [PubMed]
40. Bertozzi Silva, J.; Storms, Z.; Sauvageau, D. Host receptors for bacteriophage adsorption. *FEMS Microbiol. Lett.* **2016**, *363*. [CrossRef]
41. Phage Receptor Database. Available online: https://phred.herokuapp.com (accessed on 18 July 2019).
42. Buckling, A.; Brockhurst, M. Bacteria-virus coevolution. *Adv. Exp. Med. Biol.* **2012**, *751*, 347–370. [CrossRef]
43. Tsai, R.; Corrêa, I.R.; Xu, M.Y.; Xu, S.Y. Restriction and modification of deoxyarchaeosine (dG+)-containing phage 9 g DNA. *Sci. Rep.* **2017**, *7*, 8348. [CrossRef]
44. Šimoliunas, E.; Šimoliuniene, M.; Kaliniene, L.; Zajanckauskaite, A.; Skapas, M.; Mešky, S.R.; Kaupinis, A.; Valius, M.; Truncaite, L. *Pantoea* bacteriophage vB_PagS_Vid5: A low-temperature siphovirus that harbors a cluster of genes involved in the biosynthesis of archaeosine. *Viruses* **2018**, *10*, 583. [CrossRef]
45. Ngazoa-Kakou, S.; Shao, Y.; Rousseau, G.M.; Addablah, A.A.; Tremblay, D.M.; Hutinet, G.; Lemire, N.; Plante, P.L.; Corbeil, J.; Koudou, A.; et al. Complete genome sequence of *Escherichia coli* siphophage BRET. *Microbiol. Resour. Announc.* **2019**, *8*. [CrossRef]
46. Hobbs, Z.; Abedon, S.T. Diversity of phage infection types and associated terminology: The problem with 'lytic or lysogenic'. *FEMS Microbiol. Lett.* **2016**, *363*. [CrossRef] [PubMed]
47. Gutiérrez, D.; Fernández, L.; Rodríguez, A.; García, P. Practical method for isolation of phage deletion mutants. *Methods Protoc.* **2018**, *1*, 6. [CrossRef] [PubMed]
48. Dedrick, R.M.; Guerrero-Bustamante, C.A.; Garlena, R.A.; Russell, D.A.; Ford, K.; Harris, K.; Gilmour, K.C.; Soothill, J.; Jacobs-Sera, D.; Schooley, R.T.; et al. Engineered bacteriophages for treatment of a patient with a disseminated drug-resistant *Mycobacterium abscessus*. *Nat. Med.* **2019**, *25*, 730–733. [CrossRef] [PubMed]
49. Keen, E.C.; Bliskovsky, V.V.; Malagon, F.; Baker, J.D.; Prince, J.S.; Klaus, J.S.; Adhya, S.L. Novel "superspreader" bacteriophages promote horizontal gene transfer by transformation. *mBio* **2017**, *8*. [CrossRef] [PubMed]
50. Baig, A.; Colom, J.; Barrow, P.; Schouler, C.; Moodley, A.; Lavigne, R.; Atterbury, R. Biology and genomics of an historic therapeutic *Escherichia coli* bacteriophage collection. *Front. Microbiol.* **2017**, *8*, 1652. [CrossRef] [PubMed]
51. Gill, J.J.; Hyman, P. Phage choice, isolation, and preparation for phage therapy. *Curr. Pharm. Biotechnol.* **2010**, *11*, 2–14. [CrossRef] [PubMed]
52. Speck, P.; Smithyman, A. Safety and efficacy of phage therapy via the intravenous route. *FEMS Microbiol. Lett.* **2016**, *363*. [CrossRef] [PubMed]
53. Salmon, G.G., Jr.; Symonds, M. Staphage lysate therapy in chronic staphylococcal infections. *J. Med. Soc. N. J.* **1963**, *60*, 188–193. [PubMed]
54. Meaden, S.; Koskella, B. Exploring the risks of phage application in the environment. *Front. Microbiol.* **2013**, *4*, 358. [CrossRef]
55. Regulski, K.; Champion-Arnaud, P.; Gabard, J. Bacteriophage manufacturing: From early twentieth-century processes to current GMP. In *Bacteriophages*; Harper, D., Ed.; Springer: Cham, Switzerland, 2018.
56. Jurač, K.; Nabergoj, D.; Podgornik, A. Bacteriophage production processes. *Appl. Microbiol. Biotechnol.* **2019**, *103*, 685–694. [CrossRef]
57. Pirnay, J.P.; Merabishvili, M.; Van Raemdonck, H.; De Vos, D.; Verbeken, G. Bacteriophage production in compliance with regulatory requirements. *Methods Mol. Biol.* **2018**, *1693*, 233–252. [CrossRef] [PubMed]
58. Jończyk, E.; Kłak, M.; Międzybrodzki, R.; Górski, A. The influence of external factors on bacteriophages—Review. *Folia Microbiol.* **2011**, *56*, 191–200. [CrossRef] [PubMed]
59. Ackermann, H.W.; Tremblay, D.; Moineau, S. Long-term bacteriophage preservation. *WFCC Newslett.* **2004**, *38*, 35–40.
60. González-Menéndez, E.; Fernández, L.; Gutiérrez, D.; Rodríguez, A.; Martínez, B.; García, P. Comparative analysis of different preservation techniques for the storage of *Staphylococcus* phages aimed for the industrial development of phage-based antimicrobial products. *PLoS ONE* **2018**, *13*, e0205728. [CrossRef] [PubMed]

61. Hubalek, Z. Protectants used in the cryopreservation of microorganisms. *Cryobiology* **2003**, *46*, 205–229. [CrossRef]
62. Golec, P.; Dabrowski, K.; Hejnowicz, M.S.; Gozdek, A.; Loś, J.M.; Wegrzyn, G.; Lobocka, M.B.; Loś, M. A reliable method for storage of tailed phages. *J. Microbiol. Methods* **2011**, *84*, 486–489. [CrossRef] [PubMed]
63. González-Menéndez, E.; Fernández, L.; Gutiérrez, D.; Pando, D.; Martínez, B.; Rodríguez, A.; García, P. Strategies to encapsulate the *Staphylococcus aureus* bacteriophage phiIPLA-RODI. *Viruses* **2018**, *10*, 495. [CrossRef] [PubMed]
64. Bodier-Montagutelli, E.; Morello, E.; L'Hostis, G.; Guillon, A.; Dalloneau, E.; Respaud, R.; Pallaoro, N.; Blois, H.; Vecellio, L.; Gabard, J.; et al. Inhaled phage therapy: A promising and challenging approach to treat bacterial respiratory infections. *Expert Opin. Drug Deliv.* **2017**, *14*, 959–972. [CrossRef]
65. Leung, S.S.Y.; Parumasivam, T.; Gao, F.G.; Carter, E.A.; Carrigy, N.B.; Vehring, R.; Finlay, W.H.; Morales, S.; Britton, W.J.; Kutter, E.; et al. Effects of storage conditions on the stability of spray dried, inhalable bacteriophage powders. *Int. J. Pharm.* **2017**, *521*, 141–149. [CrossRef]
66. Leung, S.S.; Parumasivam, T.; Gao, F.G.; Carrigy, N.B.; Vehring, R.; Finlay, W.H.; Morales, S.; Britton, W.J.; Kutter, E.; Chan, H.K. Production of inhalation phage powders using spray freeze drying and spray drying techniques for treatment of respiratory infections. *Pharm. Res.* **2016**, *33*, 1486–1496. [CrossRef]
67. Ma, Y.; Pacan, J.C.; Wang, Q.; Xu, Y.; Huang, X.; Korenevsky, A.; Sabour, P.M. Microencapsulation of bacteriophage Felix O1 into chitosan-alginate microspheres for oral delivery. *Appl. Environ. Microbiol.* **2008**, *74*, 4799–4805. [CrossRef] [PubMed]
68. Singla, S.; Harjai, K.; Katare, O.P.; Chhibber, S. Bacteriophage-loaded nanostructured lipid carrier: Improved pharmacokinetics mediates effective resolution of *Klebsiella pneumoniae*—Induced lobar pneumonia. *J. Infect. Dis.* **2015**, *212*, 325–334. [CrossRef] [PubMed]
69. Nieth, A.; Verseux, C.; Barnert, S.; Süss, R.; Römer, W. A first step toward liposome-mediated intracellular bacteriophage therapy. *Expert Opin. Drug Deliv.* **2015**, *12*, 1411–1424. [CrossRef] [PubMed]
70. Nobrega, F.L.; Costa, A.R.; Santos, J.F.; Siliakus, M.F.; van Lent, J.W.; Kengen, S.W.; Azeredo, J.; Kluskens, L.D. Genetically manipulated phages with improved pH resistance for oral administration in veterinary medicine. *Sci. Rep.* **2016**, *6*, 39235. [CrossRef]
71. Esteban, P.P.; Alves, D.R.; Enright, M.C.; Bean, J.E.; Gaudion, A.; Jenkins, A.T.; Young, A.E.; Arnot, T.C. Enhancement of the antimicrobial properties of bacteriophage-K via stabilization using oil-in-water nano-emulsions. *Biotechnol. Prog.* **2014**, *30*, 932–944. [CrossRef]
72. Esteban, P.P.; Jenkins, A.T.; Arnot, T.C. Elucidation of the mechanisms of action of bacteriophage K/nano-emulsion formulations against *Staphylococcus aureus* via measurement of particle size and zeta potential. *Colloids Surf. B Biointerfaces* **2016**, *139*, 87–94. [CrossRef]
73. Merabishvili, M.; Monserez, R.; van Belleghem, J.; Rose, T.; Jennes, S.; de Vos, D.; Verbeken, G.; Vaneechoutte, M.; Pirnay, J.P. Stability of bacteriophages in burn wound care products. *PLoS ONE* **2017**, *12*, e0182121. [CrossRef]
74. Majewska, J.; Beta, W.; Lecion, D.; Hodyra-Stefaniak, K.; Kłopot, A.; Kaźmierczak, Z.; Miernikiewicz, P.; Piotrowicz, A.; Ciekot, J.; Owczarek, B.; et al. Oral application of T4 phage induces weak antibody production in the gut and in the blood. *Viruses* **2015**, *7*, 2845. [CrossRef]
75. Abedon, S.T.; Kuhl, S.J.; Blasdel, B.G.; Kutter, E.M. Phage treatment of human infections. *Bacteriophage* **2011**, *1*, 66–85. [CrossRef]
76. Kucharewicz-Krukowska, A.; Slopek, S. Immunogenic effect of bacteriophage in patients subjected to phage therapy. *Arch. Immunol. Ther. Exp.* **1987**, *35*, 553–561.
77. Kim, K.P.; Cha, J.D.; Jang, E.H.; Klumpp, J.; Hagens, S.; Hardt, W.D.; Lee, K.Y.; Loessner, M.J. PEGylation of bacteriophages increases blood circulation time and reduces T-helper type 1 immune response. *Microb. Biotechnol.* **2008**, *1*, 247–257. [CrossRef] [PubMed]
78. Costerton, J.W.; Stewart, P.S.; Greenberg, E.P. Bacterial biofilms: A common cause of persistent infections. *Science* **1999**, *284*, 1318–1322. [CrossRef] [PubMed]
79. de la Fuente-Núñez, C.; Reffuveille, F.; Fernández, L.; Hancock, R.E.W. Bacterial biofilm development as a multicellular adaptation: Antibiotic resistance and new therapeutic strategies. *Curr. Opin. Microbiol.* **2013**, *16*, 580–589. [CrossRef] [PubMed]
80. Chan, B.K.; Abedon, S.T. Bacteriophages and their enzymes in biofilm control. *Curr. Pharm. Des.* **2015**, *21*, 85–99. [CrossRef] [PubMed]

81. Geredew Kifelew, L.; Mitchell, J.G.; Speck, P. Mini-review: Efficacy of lytic bacteriophages on multispecies biofilms. *Biofouling* **2019**, *35*, 472–481. [CrossRef] [PubMed]
82. González, S.; Fernández, L.; Campelo, A.B.; Gutiérrez, D.; Martínez, B.; Rodríguez, A.; García, P. The behavior of *Staphylococcus aureus* dual-species biofilms treated with bacteriophage phiIPLA-RODI depends on the accompanying microorganism. *Appl. Environ. Microbiol.* **2017**, *83*. [CrossRef] [PubMed]
83. Khalifa, L.; Brosh, Y.; Gelman, D.; Coppenhagen-Glazer, S.; Beyth, S.; Poradosu-Cohen, R.; Que, Y.A.; Beyth, N.; Hazan, R. Targeting *Enterococcus faecalis* biofilms with phage therapy. *Appl. Environ. Microbiol.* **2015**, *81*, 2696–2705. [CrossRef] [PubMed]
84. Yuan, Y.; Qu, K.; Tan, D.; Li, X.; Wang, L.; Cong, C.; Xiu, Z.; Xu, Y. Isolation and characterization of a bacteriophage and its potential to disrupt multi-drug resistant *Pseudomonas aeruginosa* biofilms. *Microb. Pathog.* **2019**, *128*, 329–336. [CrossRef] [PubMed]
85. Wintachai, P.; Naknaen, A.; Pomwised, R.; Voravuthikunchai, S.P.; Smith, D.R. Isolation and characterization of *Siphoviridae* phage infecting extensively drug-resistant *Acinetobacter baumannii* and evaluation of therapeutic efficacy In Vitro and In Vivo. *J. Med. Microbiol.* **2019**, *68*, 1096–1108. [CrossRef]
86. Gu, Y.; Xu, Y.; Xu, J.; Yu, X.; Huang, X.; Liu, G.; Liu, X. Identification of novel bacteriophage vB_EcoP-EG1 with lytic activity against planktonic and biofilm forms of uropathogenic *Escherichia coli*. *Appl. Microbiol. Biotechnol.* **2019**, *103*, 315–326. [CrossRef]
87. Briandet, R.; Lacroix-Gueu, P.; Renault, M.; Lecart, S.; Meylheuc, T.; Bidnenko, E.; Steenkeste, K.; Bellon-Fontaine, M.N.; Fontaine-Aupart, M.P. Fluorescence correlation spectroscopy to study diffusion and reaction of bacteriophages inside biofilms. *Appl. Environ. Microbiol.* **2008**, *74*, 2135–2143. [CrossRef] [PubMed]
88. González, S.; Fernández, L.; Gutiérrez, D.; Campelo, A.B.; Rodríguez, A.; García, P. Analysis of different parameters affecting diffusion, propagation and survival of staphylophages in bacterial biofilms. *Front. Microbiol.* **2018**, *9*, 2348. [CrossRef] [PubMed]
89. Tkhilaishvili, T.; Lombardi, L.; Klatt, A.B.; Trampuz, A.; Di Luca, M. Bacteriophage Sb-1 enhances antibiotic activity against biofilm, degrades exopolysaccharide matrix and targets persisters of *Staphylococcus aureus*. *Int. J. Antimicrob. Agents* **2018**, *52*, 842–853. [CrossRef] [PubMed]
90. Pires, D.P.; Oliveira, H.; Melo, L.D.; Sillankorva, S.; Azeredo, J. Bacteriophage-encoded depolymerases: Their diversity and biotechnological applications. *Appl. Microbiol. Biotechnol.* **2016**, *100*, 2141–2151. [CrossRef] [PubMed]
91. Latka, A.; Maciejewska, B.; Majkowska-Skrobek, G.; Briers, Y.; Drulis-Kawa, Z. Bacteriophage-encoded virion-associated enzymes to overcome the carbohydrate barriers during the infection process. *Appl. Microbiol. Biotechnol.* **2017**, *101*, 3103–3119. [CrossRef] [PubMed]
92. Schmerer, M.; Molineux, I.J.; Bull, J.J. Synergy as a rationale for phage therapy using phage cocktails. *PeerJ* **2014**, *2*, e590. [CrossRef] [PubMed]
93. Lu, T.K.; Collins, J.J. Dispersing biofilms with engineered enzymatic bacteriophage. *Proc. Natl. Acad. Sci. USA* **2007**, *104*, 11197–11202. [CrossRef]
94. Pei, R.; Lamas-Samanamud, G.R. Inhibition of biofilm formation by T7 bacteriophages producing quorum-quenching enzymes. *Appl. Environ. Microbiol.* **2014**, *80*, 5340–5348. [CrossRef]
95. Fernández, L.; Rodríguez, A.; García, P. Phage or foe: An insight into the impact of viral predation on microbial communities. *ISME J.* **2018**, *12*, 1171–1179. [CrossRef]
96. Fernández, L.; González, S.; Campelo, A.B.; Martínez, B.; Rodríguez, A.; García, P. Low-level predation by lytic phage phiIPLA-RODI promotes biofilm formation and triggers the stringent response in *Staphylococcus aureus*. *Sci. Rep.* **2017**, *7*, 40965. [CrossRef]
97. Hosseinidoust, Z.; Tufenkji, N.; van de Ven, T.G. Formation of biofilms under phage predation: Considerations concerning a biofilm increase. *Biofouling* **2013**, *29*, 457–468. [CrossRef] [PubMed]
98. Tan, D.; Dahl, A.; Middelboe, M. Vibriophages differentially influence biofilm formation by *Vibrio anguillarum* strains. *Appl. Environ. Microbiol.* **2015**, *81*, 4489–4497. [CrossRef] [PubMed]

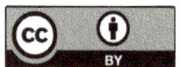

© 2019 by the authors. Licensee MDPI, Basel, Switzerland. This article is an open access article distributed under the terms and conditions of the Creative Commons Attribution (CC BY) license (http://creativecommons.org/licenses/by/4.0/).

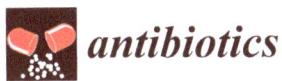

Review

Present and Future of Carbapenem-Resistant *Enterobacteriaceae* (CRE) Infections

Beatriz Suay-García and María Teresa Pérez-Gracia *

Área de Microbiología, Departamento de Farmacia, Instituto de Ciencias Biomédicas, Facultad de Ciencias de la Salud, Universidad Cardenal Herrera-CEU, C/Santiago Ramón y Cajal, 46115 Alfara del Patriarca, Valencia, Spain
* Correspondence: teresa@uchceu.es; Tel.: +34-96-1369000

Received: 29 July 2019; Accepted: 16 August 2019; Published: 19 August 2019

Abstract: Carbapenem-resistant *Enterobacteriaceae* (CRE) have become a public health threat worldwide. There are three major mechanisms by which *Enterobacteriaceae* become resistant to carbapenems: enzyme production, efflux pumps and porin mutations. Of these, enzyme production is the main resistance mechanism. There are three main groups of enzymes responsible for most of the carbapenem resistance: KPC (*Klebsiella pneumoniae* carbapenemase) (Ambler class A), MBLs (Metallo-ß-Lactamases) (Ambler class B) and OXA-48-like (Ambler class D). KPC-producing *Enterobacteriaceae* are endemic in the United States, Colombia, Argentina, Greece and Italy. On the other hand, the MBL NDM-1 is the main carbapenemase-producing resistance in India, Pakistan and Sri Lanka, while OXA-48-like enzyme-producers are endemic in Turkey, Malta, the Middle-East and North Africa. All three groups of enzymes are plasmid-mediated, which implies an easier horizontal transfer and, thus, faster spread of carbapenem resistance worldwide. As a result, there is an urgent need to develop new therapeutic guidelines to treat CRE infections. Bearing in mind the different mechanisms by which *Enterobacteriaceae* can become resistant to carbapenems, there are different approaches to treat infections caused by these bacteria, which include the repurposing of already existing antibiotics, dual therapies with these antibiotics, and the development of new ß-lactamase inhibitors and antibiotics.

Keywords: *Enterobacteriaceae*; carbapenem-resistant; CRE; antibiotic resistance; antimicrobials

1. Introduction

Antibiotic resistance occurs when bacteria causing an infection survive after being exposed to a drug that, under normal conditions, would kill it or inhibit its growth [1]. As a result, these surviving strains multiply and spread due to the lack of competition from other strains sensitive to the same drug. Due to the inappropriate prescription and administration of antibiotics, resistant bacteria have become a public health threat worldwide [2]. In fact, the issue of antibiotic resistant bacteria is such that, according to the World Health Organization (WHO) predictions, if antibiotic resistance continues to increase at this rate, infections caused by resistant bacteria will become the top cause of death worldwide, ahead of cancer, diabetes and cardiovascular diseases [3].

In 2017, WHO published a list of antibiotic resistant bacteria against which there is an urgent need to develop new antibiotics [4]. This list is divided into three categories depending on the urgency with which new antibiotics are needed: critical, high and medium priority. Within the critical priority group are carbapenem and 3rd generation cephalosporin resistant *Enterobacteriaceae*. These bacteria are common pathogens causing severe infections such as bloodstream infections, pneumonia, complicated urinary tract infections and complicated intra-abdominal infections. As a result, antibiotic resistance in *Enterobacteriaceae* has significant clinical and socioeconomic consequences [5,6].

Initially, *Enterobacteriaceae* posed a threat to the public health due to their ability to become resistant to antibiotics by producing extended-spectrum ß-lactamases (ESBLs) [7]. To fight this threat, the medical community turned to drugs such as carbapenems as first-line empirical treatments [8]. This new treatment for resistant bacteria had an unexpected result, as it led to a more serious problem, the emergence of carbapenem-resistant *Enterobacteriaceae* (CRE) [9]. In particular, CRE refer to bacteria belonging to the *Enterobacteriaceae* family that have the ability to survive and grow in the presence of clinically relevant concentrations of carbapenems [10]. Specifically, the Centers for Disease Control and Prevention (CDC) defines CRE as enterobacteria non-susceptible to any carbapenem or documented to produce carbapenemases [11].

This review analyzes the epidemiology of CRE as well as current and future treatment options against these increasingly resistant bacteria. Furthermore, it provides an extensive review of the different mechanisms by which *Enterobacteriaceae* develop resistance against carbapenems. The presence of these three aspects in one article could be used as a key tool for a better understanding of this emerging problem and as guidance to elaborate plans to manage the CRE crisis and develop new active drugs more efficiently.

2. Mechanisms of Drug Resistance

There are three major mechanisms by which *Enterobacteriaceae* become resistant to carbapenems: enzyme production, efflux pumps and porin mutations [12]. Of these, enzyme production is the main resistance mechanism. Gram-negative bacteria generally develop resistances through the production of ß-lactam-hydrolyzing enzymes [13]. Initially, these enzymes inactivated penicillin, however, as different types of antibiotics were introduced in the treatment of infectious diseases, their spectra extended. Thus, cephalosporinases, ESBLs, metallo-ß-lactamases (MBLs) and other carbapenemases appeared [14]. Generally, CRE are divided into two main subgroups: carbapenemase-producing CRE (CP-CRE) and non-carbapenemase-producing CRE (non-CP-CRE) (Figure 1) [15].

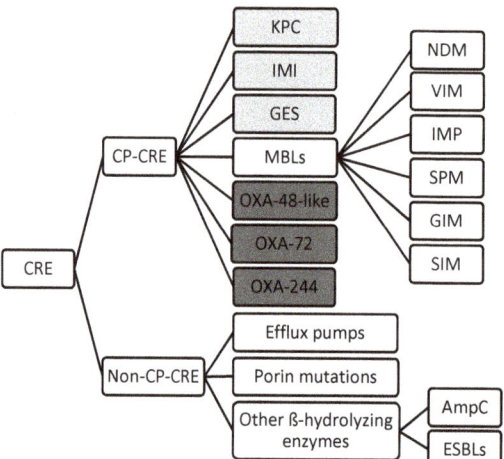

Figure 1. Classification of the different mechanisms of drug resistance in CRE. (Light grey: Ambler class A, White: Ambler class B, Dark grey: Ambler class D) (CRE: Carbapenem-resistant Enterobacteriaceae; CP: carbapenemase producing; KPC: *Klebsiella pneumoniae* carbapenemase; IMI: Imipenem-hydrolyzing ß-lactamase; GES: Guiana extended-spectrum ß-lactamase; MBLs: Metallo-ß-lactamase; OXA: oxacillinase; NDM: New Delhi metallo-ß-lactamase; VIM: Verona integron-borne metallo-ß-lactamase; IMP: Imipenem-resistant *Pseudomonas* carbapenemase; SMP: Sao Paulo metallo-ß-lactamase; GIM: German imipenemase; SIM: Seoul imipenemase; AmpC: Type C ampicillinase; ESBLs: Extended-spectrum ß-lactamase).

2.1. Carbapenemase-producing CRE

CP-CRE can produce a large variety of carbapenemases which can be divided in three groups according to the Ambler classification: class A, class B and class D ß-lactamases [16]. There is a fourth class, Ambler class C, however, its clinical relevance remains unknown [17].

Within class A carbapenemases is the clinically relevant *Klebsiella pneumoniae* carbapenemase (KPC) [18]. This is a plasmid encoded enzyme which actively hydrolyzes carbapenems and is partially inhibited by clavulanic acid [19]. Its clinical relevance is due to the fact that it is the most prevalent and most widely spread worldwide [20] *Enterobacteriaceae* producing KPCs have acquired multidrug resistance to ß-lactams, which limits the therapeutic options to treat infections caused by these bacteria [21]. KPC were originally found in *K. pneumoniae* isolates, however, clinical isolates of KPC-producing *Escherichia coli, Klebsiella oxytoca, Salmonella enterica, Citrobacter freundii, Enterobacter aerogenes, Enterobacter cloacae, Proteus mirabillis* and *Serratia marcescens* have been identified [22–26] (Table 1). According to a study by Perez et al. [27], a total of 12 bla_{KPC} gene variants exist globally.

Table 1. Carbapenemases detected in different species belonging to the *Enterobacteriaceae* family.

Species	Class A	Class B (MBLs)	Class D	Ref.
Klebsiella pneumoniae	KPC-3	NDM-1, VIM-1	OXA-48	Okoche et al. Boutal et al.
Klebsiella oxytoca			OXA-48, OXA-181	Okoche et al. Boutal et al.
Escherichia coli	KPC	NDM-1, NDM-5, NDM-9, VIM	OXA-48, OXA-181, OXA-244	Okoche et al. Boutal et al.
Proteus mirabilis	KPC		OXA-48	Okoche et al. Boutal et al.
Serratia marcescens	KPC	VIM		Okoche et al. Boutal et al.
Enterobacter cloacae	KPC, IMI-1	VIM-4	OXA-48	Okoche et al. Boutal et al.
Enterobacter aerogenes	KPC		OXA-48	Okoche et al. Boutal et al.
Citrobacter freundii		VIM	OXA-48	Okoche et al. Boutal et al.
Citrobacter koseri			OXA-48	Okoche et al. Boutal et al.
Salmonella enterica	KPC-2	NMD-1, NMD-5, VIM-1, VIM-2, IMP-4	OXA-48	Fernández et al.
Morganella morganii		NDM-1	OXA-48	Boutal et al.
Providencia stuartii	KPC-2	VIM-1		Abdallah et al.
Providencia rettgeri		IMP-1	OXA-72	Abdallah et al.

Another major carbapenemase family belonging to class A are MBLs. These enzymes depend on the interaction with zinc ions in the active site of the enzyme [28]. These enzymes are particularly problematic as they have a high potential for horizontal transfer, they lack clinically useful inhibitors, and they have broad hydrolytic properties that affect most ß-lactam antibiotics except for monobactams [29]. However, MBL resistance is usually associated with multidrug-resistance, with MBL-producing isolates often co-expressing ESBLs, which inactivate monobactams [13]. The most common families of MBLs found in *Enterobacteriaceae* were acquired [17]. These families are the New Delhi metallo-ß-lactamase 1 (NDM-1), Imipenem-resistant *Pseudomonas* (IMP)-type carbapenemases and the Verona integron-encoded metallo-ß-lactamases (VIM) [14]. IMP-type carbapenemases were first detected in Japan during the 1990s and have up to 18 varieties [30]. Similarly, VIM was first isolated in Verona, Italy, in 1997 and consists of 14 members [31]. Both MBLs originated in *P. aeruginosa* and were transferred to *Enterobacteriaceae*. In fact, these MBLs share similarities regarding the plasmids they are carried on and their mechanism of action, as both hydrolyze all ß-lactams except for monobactams and are susceptible to all ß-lactam inhibitors [32]. Regarding NDM-1, it is the most recently discovered MBL. It was isolated in India, which is considered the main reservoir of NDM-producing bacteria [33]. Since then, it has spread worldwide, reaching Europe and the United States through tourists [34]. Currently, NDM is predominant in *K. pneumoniae* and *E. coli* [34]. Studies suggest that most plasmids containing bla_{NDM} also harbor other resistance determinants encoding different ß-lactamases, quinolone resistance and 16S rRNA methylases which confer resistance to aminoglycosides [35].

The third clinically relevant group of carbapenemases are OXA-48-like, which belong to Ambler class D. Six OXA-48-like variants have been identified, OXA-48 being the most widespread [36]. The remaining variants are: OXA-162, OXA-163, OXA-181, OXA-204 and OXA-232. They are all grouped within the OXA-48-like category because they only differ on one to five amino acid substitutions or deletions [36]. These plasmid-mediated enzymes are primarily found in *K. pneumoniae*, *E. coli*, *C. freundii* and *E. cloacae* [37]. A major concern with these carbapenemases is that no existing inhibitors work against them and they have an extraordinary ability to mutate and expand their activity spectrum [38]. These enzymes are highly active against penicillins, have low activity against carbapenems and intermediate activity against broad-spectrum cephalosporins [17].

2.2. Non-Carbapenemase-producing CRE

Besides carbapenemase production, *Enterobacteriaceae* have alternative mechanisms by which they can present carbapenem resistance. These are unspecific mechanisms which can result in multi-drug resistance, such as the production of other ß-lactamases, porin loss and efflux pump overexpression [14]. These mechanisms generally appear paired among themselves or with carbapenemase-production [39]. In fact, while carbapenemases specifically target carbapenems and other ß-lactam antibiotics, efflux pump expression or porin changes are associate with multi-drug resistance [40]. All three alternative mechanisms aim to block the penetration of the antibiotic within the bacterial cell.

Firstly, *Enterobacteriaceae* can produce different types of ß-lactamases, such as AmpC-type ß-lactamases. These enzymes do not degrade carbapenems [41] but they form a bond with the carbapenem molecule, preventing it from accessing its target [42]. Specifically, the plasmid-encoded AmpC CMY-2 is frequently found in *E. coli* and other *Enterobacteriaceae* worldwide, causing resistance to carbapenems [43].

Secondly, resistance-nodulation-division (RND) efflux pumps are a major mechanism of multi-drug resistance in *Enterobacteriaceae* [44]. Among the different efflux systems, the AcrAB-TolC RND system is the most common [44]. This RND efflux pump, along with the CusABC efflux complex, belongs to *E. coli* [45]. Similarly, *Campylobacter jejuni* presents multi-drug resistance through the expression of the CmeABC complex [45]. These resistant genes can be easily transmitted from one microorganism to another through plasmids [46].

Lastly, alterations of porin synthesis also contribute to blocking penetration of carbapenems into the bacterial cell [47]. These alterations have been described in AmpC- and carbapenemase-producing *K. pneumoniae*, which suggests that changes in porin expression play a key role in the ß-lactam resistance displayed by multi-drug resistant bacteria [48]. Studies suggest that strains that have their porins mutated or their expression modulated typically do not have potential for mobilization into community settings but may proliferate locally within hospitals [49].

3. Current Resistance Status

Since the detection of the first strain of CRE in the 1980s [50], CRE has rapidly spread worldwide. Epidemiology studies suggest that different carbapenemases predominate in different areas of the world. For that matter, NDM-1 is the main carbapenemase producing resistance in India, Pakistan and Sri Lanka. On the other hand, KPC-producing *Enterobacteriaceae* are endemic in the United States, Colombia, Argentina, Greece and Italy, while OXA-48-like enzyme-producers are endemic in Turkey, Malta, the Middle-East and North Africa [51] (Figure 2).

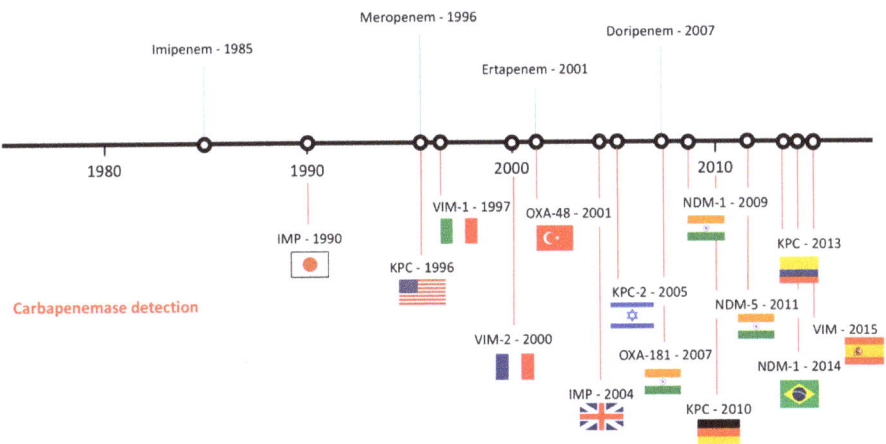

Figure 2. Timeline representing the introduction of carbapenems and the appearance of carbapenemases worldwide.

As mentioned earlier, the first case of CP-CRE was isolated in Japan and corresponded to an IMP-producing *Serratia marcescens* [50]. This strain caused a plasmid-mediated outbreak in seven Japanese hospitals, followed by a widespread dissemination of bla_{IMP-1}-harboring *Enterobacteriaceae* throughout Japan. Since then, 52 variants of IMP genes have been identified and have their endemicity limited to Japan and Taiwan [52]. VIM-type MBLs were described shortly after in *P. aeruginosa* strains [53]. By the early 2000s, cases of VIM-producing *Enterobacteriaceae* were already being reported [17]. *K. pneumoniae* and *E. coli* strains producing VIM-type carbapenemases have their endemicity peak in Greece [28]. However, the major threat of MBL-producing *Enterobacteriaceae* appeared with the discovery of an ST14 *K. pneumoniae* strain producing the NDM enzyme from a Swedish patient who received healthcare in New Delhi, India [54]. Bacteria producing this enzyme is endemic in the Indian subcontinent and generally appears as sporadic cases in the rest of the world [55]. NDM-1 producing *Enterobacteriaceae* have been reported both in hospital and community-acquired infections, including urinary tract infections, septicemia, pulmonary infections, peritonitis, device-associated infections and soft tissue infections [56]. An additional issue with NDM-producing bacteria is their ability to spread via environmental sources in community settings of lower-income countries. In fact, studies carried out in India found that 4% of the drinking water and 30% of seepage samples contained NDM-1-producing bacteria [33].

KPC-producing *Enterobacteriaceae* are categorized as one of the most successful pandemics in the history of Gram-negative bacteria, particularly due to *K. pneumoniae* ST258 [57]. This strain has been reported as endemic in Greece, Israel, Latin America and the United States [39]. The endemic state of KPC-producing *Enterobacteriaceae* is not surprising, seeing as the first case of *K. pneumoniae* producing this enzyme was reported in a patient in a North Carolina hospital in 1996 [18]. Only five years later, an outbreak of KPC-producing bacteria took place throughout northeastern United States within hospitalized patients [58]. On the other hand, Greece has one of the highest CRE rates worldwide. Initially, this resistance was due to VIM enzymes, however, in 2007, a rapid dissemination of KPC-producing bacteria made KPC the main mechanism of resistance against carbapenems in the country [39]. Current studies suggest that around 40% of the carbapenemase-resistant *K. pneumoniae* harbor bla_{KPC} in Greece [59]. Colombia was the first country within Latin America to report an outbreak of KPC-producing *K. pneumoniae*, which originated from a patient who had travelled to Israel [60]. Since then, Argentina, Chile, Mexico and Brazil have also reported the detection of KPC-producing CRE [39].

Finally, regarding OXA-48-like-producing CRE, outbreaks caused by these bacteria have been reported in several countries, however, only Turkey, Japan and Taiwan have reported endemicity [61].

4. Treatment Options

Carbapenems continue to be used for the treatment of infections caused by *Enterobacteriaceae* as suggested by both, EUCAST (European Committee on Antimicrobial Susceptibility Testing) and CLSI (Clinical and Laboratory Standards Institute) guidelines [62,63]. The clinical breakpoints of the carbapenems currently used are presented in Table 2. It must be noted that doripenem has been removed from 2019 EUCAST guidelines due to the lack of availability of this drug in most countries. In those countries where doripenem is still available, 2018 EUCAST guidelines must be used as a reference [64]. However, CRE are an increasingly common issue in the clinical practice, rendering carbapenems useless.

Table 2. Breakpoints for carbapenems against *Enterobacteriaceae* family.

Antibiotic	Guidelines	Disk Content (µg)	Disk Diffusion (mm)			Dilution (µg/mL)		
			S	I	R	S	I	R
Ertapenem	EUCAST [1]	10	≥25	-	≤25	≤0.5	-	0.5
	CLSI [2]		≥23	19–21	≤18	≤0.5	1	≥2
Imipenem	EUCAST [1]	10	22	21–18	≤17	≤2	3	4
	CLSI [2]		≥23	20–22	≤19	≤1	2	≥4
Meropenem	EUCAST [1]	10	22	21–17	16	≤2	3–7	8
	CLSI [2]		≥23	20–22	≤19	≤1	2	≥4
Doripenem	EUCAST [3]	10	22	21–17	≤16	≤1	2–3	4
	CLSI [2]	10	≥23	20–22	≤19	≤1	2	≥4

[1] The European Committee on Antimicrobial Susceptibility Testing. Breakpoint tables for interpretation of minimum inhibitory concentrations (MICs) and zone diameters. Version 9.0, 2019. Available on: http//www.eucast.org [62]. [2] CLSI. Performance Standards for Antimicrobial Susceptibility Testing. 29th ed. CLSI supplement M100. Wayne, PA: Clinical and Laboratory Standards Institute; 2019 [63]. [3] The European Committee on Antimicrobial Susceptibility Testing. Breakpoint tables for interpretation of MICs and zone diameters. Version 8.1, 2018. Available on: http//www.eucast.org [64].

Bearing in mind the different mechanisms by which *Enterobacteriaceae* can become resistant to carbapenems, there are different approaches to treat infections caused by these bacteria. These treatment options include the repurposing of already existing antibiotics, dual therapies with these antibiotics and the development of new ß-lactamase inhibitors and antibiotics [65] (Table 3).

Table 3. Current and future treatment options for infections caused by CRE.

	Drug (Pharmaceutical Company)	Action Mechanism	Structure	Limitations	Ref.
"Old Antibiotics"	Fosfomycin (Merck)	Cell wall synthesis inhibitor		Appearance of resistance	Vardakas et al.
	Aminoglycosides	Protein synthesis inhibitor		Appearance of resistance	Rodriguez-Bano et al. Satlin et al.
	Colistin (Kobayashi Bacteriological Laboratory)	Cell membrane disruptor		Nephrotoxicity and other severe adverse effects	Karaiskos et al. Daikos et al.
	Tigecycline (Pfizer)	Protein synthesis inhibitor		Low concentration in tissue	Ni et al.
Dual Therapies	Ertapenem + Meropenem/ Doripenem	Cell wall synthesis inhibitor		-	Bulik et al.
	Ceftazidime/ Avibactam (Allergan)	Cell wall synthesis inhibitor/ ß-lactamase inhibitor		Appearance of resistance	De Jonge et al.
	Meropenem/ Vaborbactam (Melinta)	Cell wall synthesis inhibitor/ ß-lactamase inhibitor		Insufficient clinical data	Karaiskos et al.

Table 3. Cont.

	Drug (Pharmaceutical Company)	Action Mechanism	Structure	Limitations	Ref.
Novel Drugs	Plazomicin (Achaogen)	Protein synthesis inhibitor		Ineffective against MBL-producers	Landman et al.
	Eravacycline (Tetraphase)	Protein synthesis inhibitor		Currently in clinical trials	Zhanel et al.
	Imipenem/ Relebactam (Merck)	Cell wall synthesis inhibitor/ ß-lactamase inhibitor		Currently in clinical trials	Blizzard et al.
	Cefiderocol (Shionogi)	Cell wall synthesis inhibitor		Currently in clinical trials	Saisho et al.
	Zidebactam (Wockhardt)	ß-lactamase inhibitor		Currently in clinical trials	Karaiskos et al.
	Nacubactam (Roche)	ß-lactamase inhibitor		Currently in clinical trials	Papp-Wallace et al.

Firstly, certain "old antibiotics" which have been included in the therapeutic arsenal for years are still effective against CRE. For example, fosfomycin, frequently used to treat urinary tract infections (UTIs), continues to be effective against approximately 80% of CRE [66]. Similarly, aminoglycosides are still considered first-line therapy for the treatment of carbapenem-resistant *K. pneumoniae* infections [6]. While gentamicin is the most frequently used aminoglycoside, studies report cases where amikacin was the only active molecule [67]. Colistin also remains as a key drug in the treatment of CRE infections [65]. However, CRE, and more particularly *K. pneumoniae*, have started to develop resistance against this drug, decreasing its efficiency as a monotherapy treatment [68]. As a result, colistin has been included as part of a dual therapy with meropenem, which results in a significant reduction of mortality, especially in patients with septic shock, high mortality score or rapidly fatal underlying diseases [69]. Moreover, polymyxins continue to be considered last resort drugs due to their adverse effects, which include nephrotoxicity, neurotoxicity and skin pigmentation [65].

Tigecycline also remains as an option for CRE treatment in certain cases [70]. The particularity with this drug is that it displays low serum concentrations in the approved dosing regimen for the treatment of community-acquired and nosocomial-acquired pneumonia, which hampers clinical outcomes [71]. As a result, a high-dose tigecycline regimen has been investigated and is being used to treat CRE infections. This therapy consists of a 200 mg initial dose and a maintenance dose of 100 mg every

12 h [65]. This high-dose is particularly effective for the treatment of ventilator-associated pneumonia caused by CRE [72]. Furthermore, a systematic review comprising 25 studies reporting the efficacy and safety of tigecycline-based regimens for treating CRE infections concluded that a much lower mortality rate resulted from high-dose tigecycline than standard-dose tigecycline [70].

Lastly, carbapenems continue to be used for the treatment of CRE infections. This is done through the combination of two different carbapenems, which is known as "double carbapenems". Generally, the combination consists of an initial dose of ertapenem followed by a prolonged infusion of meropenem or doripenem over 3 or 4 h with additional 2 g doses of meropenem every 8 h [73]. This therapy is effective against CRE because the greater affinity of ertapenem to KPC makes it play a "sacrificial role", meaning that it is preferentially hydrolyzed by the carbapenemase, allowing the concomitant administration of the second carbapenem to sustain a high concentration [74]. Comparator studies such as those by Oliva et al. [75] and Venugopalan et al. [76] confirm the efficacy of dual carbapenem therapy, reporting clinical success rates of more than 70% in both cases.

Regarding novel antibacterial drugs, they can be differentiated in two groups: newly approved antibiotics and molecules in development stages. The latest antibiotics approved and already being used to treat CRE infections are ceftazidime/avibactam, meropenem/vaborbactam, plazomicin and eravacycline.

Ceftazidime/avibactam (Allergan) is a novel ß-lactam/ß-lactamase inhibitor combination. The novelty of this combination relies on avibactam, which is a synthetic non-ß-lactam ß-lactamase inhibitor active against ß-lactamases from Ambler classes A, C and D [77]. Clinical studies using this combination are still scarce, however, initial results show an improved mortality rate of 9% compared to the 32% obtained when using colistin [78]. Regardless of the promising initial results, ceftazidime/avibactam resistant strains have already been reported during treatment [79,80]. The resistance is due to mutations in the bla_{KPC-2} and bla_{KPC-3} genes affecting omega loop D179Y, down-regulation of ompk35/36 and increase in efflux, which could decrease meropenem activity [81]. This should be taken into account by clinicians when prescribing this treatment.

Similarly, meropenem/vaborbactam (Melinta) is also a new ß-lactam/ß-lactamase inhibitor consisting of a carbapenem and a novel boron-containing serine-ß-lactamase inhibitor that potentiates the activity of meropenem [65]. This combination inhibits Ambler classes A and C serine carbapenemases [82]. There are few clinical data with this combination, however, in vivo results showed that, out of 991 clinical isolates of KPC-producing *Enterobacteriaceae*, 99% were susceptible to meropenem-vaborbactam [83]. Furthermore, results from the Tango II trial, which compared the efficacy and safety of this combination with the best available therapy in CRE infections, showed a higher clinical cure (65.6% vs 33.3%) and 28-day mortality (15.6% vs 33.3%) for meropenem/vaborbactam [84].

Plazomicin (Achaogen) is a next-generation semisynthetic aminoglycoside with activity against bacteria producing aminoglycoside-modifying enzymes [85]. Studies report higher potency of plazomicin compared to other aminoglycosides against KPC-producing *Enterobacteriaceae* [86]. Along these lines, Endimiani et al. [86] analyzed collections of clinically relevant KPC-producers with resistance to aminoglycosides and observed inhibition using plazomicin, with a minimum inhibitory concentration (MIC_{90}) of ≤2 mg/L [87]. Plazomicin has shown broad-spectrum activity against Gram-positive cocci and Gram-negative bacilli [87], however, MBL-producers are resistant to this antibiotic due to the methyltransferase enzymes which are commonly found, especially in NDM-producers [87]. Aminoglycosides are not generally used as monotherapy, however, the broad spectrum of activity along with the low renal toxicity of plazomicin make it an option for a targeted monotherapy against extensively-drug resistant *Enterobacteriaceae* causing urinary tract infections [88].

Lastly, eravacycline (Tetraphase) is a synthetic fluorocycline with broad-spectrum antimicrobial activity against Gram-positive, Gram-negative and anaerobic bacteria, regardless of resistance to other antibiotic classes [89]. This antibiotic has several potential advantages over tigecycline, which include a more potent in vitro antibacterial activity, excellent oral bioavailability, lower potential for drug interactions and superior activity in biofilm [90]. This drug was also studied in cUTI (complicated urinary tract infection) in two Phase 3 trials (IGNITE 2/3), failing to meet endpoints in both studies, which could be explained by an erratic pharmacokinetic in urine [91]. However, eravacycline did meet endpoints in the IGNITE 4 Phase 3 study, in which it demonstrated similar activity to ertapenem (100% cure rate for eravacycline vs 92.3% for ertapenem) in the treatment of complicated intra-abdominal infections [92].

In addition to these already approved drugs, there are six molecules in early developmental stages: imipenem/cilastatin and relebactam (Merck), cediferocol (Shionogi), SPR741 (SperoTherapeutics), zidebactam (Wockhardt), nacubactam (Roche) and VNRX 5133 (VenatoRx Pharmaceuticals). Firstly, imipenem/cilastatin and relebactam shares similarities with previously discussed combinations in that it combines an approved carbapenem with a novel ß-lactamase inhibitor. In fact, the inhibitory mechanism of relebactam is similar to that of avibactam, as it covalently and reversibly binds to classes A and C ß-lactamases [93]. By including relebactam, the activity of imipenem increases considerably against carbapenemase-producing bacteria, up to >16 fold [94]. In fact, the RESTORE-IMI 1 study proved this combination to be as effective and better tolerated than colistin/imipenem for the treatment of infections caused by KPC-producing *Enterobacteriaceae* [95]. Regarding cefiderocol, it is the first siderophore-conjugated cephalosporin antibiotic to advance into late-stage development. This drug has a novel mechanism of action in which the cathecol substituent forms a chelating complex with iron, acting as a trojan horse by using iron active transport systems in gram negative bacteria to bypass the other membrane permeability barrier [96]. This molecule demonstrates potent in vitro and in vivo activity against a variety of Gram-negative bacteria, including CRE [96]. A study analyzed the activity of cefiderocol and comparative agents against 1,022 isolates of carbapenem-nonsusceptible *Enterobacteriaceae*, obtaining MIC_{50} and MIC_{90} for cefiderocol of 1 and 4 µg/mL, respectively [97]. SPR741 is in very early stages of the development process. This molecule is a polymyxin B potentiator that increases ceftazidime and piperazine/tazobactam activity against CRE and ESBLs including OXA-48 [98].

The remaining molecules under development are ß-lactamase inhibitors. Firstly, zidebactam and nacubactam have high affinity to Ambler classes A and C ß-lactamases [99]. Moreover, they also have affinity to PBPs as well as ß-lactam enhancer activity [100]. The cefepime/zidebactam combination is currently in phase 2 clinical trials for the treatment of Gram-negative bacteria. This combination showed potent in vitro activity against carbapenemase-producing *Enterobacteriaceae*, with MIC_{50} of 0.25 mg/L for KPC-producers and 0.5 mg/L for MBL-producers [101]. On the other hand, nacubactam in combination with meropenem is currently in phase 1 trials against Gram-negative bacteria causing UTI infections [102]. Results from this study show improved MIC values for the meropenem/nacubactam combination in comparison with meropenem alone. Furthermore, this combination was active against ceftazidime/avibactam-resistant isolates. Lastly, VNRX 5133 is a cyclic boronate broad spectrum ß-lactamase inhibitor in clinical development with cefepime for the treatment of multidrug-resistant bacteria [103].

5. Conclusions

As highlighted by the Global Priority List published by WHO, carbapenem-resistant *Enterobacteriaceae* pose an exponentially increasing threat for the public health worldwide. These bacteria possess diverse and versatile mechanisms of drug resistance, which makes control and early detection of infections caused by CRE difficult. As a result, a joint effort must be made between the scientific and medical community to slow down the appearance of resistances. Along these lines, there is an urgent need to develop new therapeutic guidelines to treat CRE infections. This includes the repurposing of already existing antibiotics such as fosfomycin, aminoglycosides and colistin and the development of novel drugs such as plazomicin, eravacycline or cefiderocol among others.

Author Contributions: B.S.-G. conceived and wrote the paper and M.T.P.-G. conceived and wrote the paper.

Funding: This research received no external funding.

Conflicts of Interest: The authors declare no conflict of interest.

References

1. Centers for Disease Control and Prevention. About Antimicrobial Resistance. 2018. Available online: https://www.cdc.gov/drugresistance/about.html (accessed on 20 July 2019).
2. Niu, G.; Li, W. Next-Generation Drug Discovery to Combat Antimicrobial Resistance. *Trends Biochem. Sci.* **2019**, in press. [CrossRef] [PubMed]
3. O'Neill, J. Antimicrobial Resistance: Tackling a Crisis for the Health and Wealth of Nations (HM Government and Wellcome Trust). 2014. Available online: https://amr-review.org/sites/default/files/AMR%20Review%20Paper%20-%20Tackling%20a%20crisis%20for%20the%20health%20and%20wealth%20of%20nations_1.pdf (accessed on 20 July 2019).
4. World Health Organization. WHO Priority Pathogens List for R&D of New Antibiotics. 2017. Available online: http://www.who.int/bulletin/volumes/94/9/16-020916.pdf (accessed on 20 July 2019).
5. Lee, C.; Lai, C.C.; Chiang, H.T.; Lu, M.C.; Wang, L.F.; Tsai, T.L.; Kang, M.Y.; Jan, Y.N.; Lo, Y.T.; Ko, W.C.; et al. Presence of multidrug-resistant organisms in the residents and environments of long-term care facilities in Taiwan. *J. Microbiol. Immunol. Infect.* **2017**, *50*, 133–144. [CrossRef] [PubMed]
6. Rodriguez-Bano, J.; Gutierrez-Gutierrez, B.; Machuca, I.; Pascual, A. Treatment of infections caused by extended-spectrum-beta-lactamase-, AmpC-, and carbapenemase-producing *Enterobacteriaceae*. *Clin. Microbiol. Rev.* **2018**, *31*, e00079-17. [CrossRef]
7. Pana, Z.D.; Zaoutis, T. Treatment of extended-spectrum ß-lactamase-producing *Enterobacteriaceae* (ESBLs) infections: What have we learned until now? *F1000Res* **2018**, *7*. [CrossRef]
8. D'Angelo, R.G.; Johnson, J.K.; Bork, J.T.; Heil, E.L. Treatment options for extended-spectrum beta-lactamase (ESBL) and AmpC-producing bacteria. *Expert Opin. Pharmacother.* **2016**, *17*, 953–967. [CrossRef] [PubMed]
9. Sheu, C.C.; Lin, S.Y.; Chang, Y.T.; Lee, C.Y.; Chen, Y.H.; Hsueh, P.R. Management of infections caused by extended-spectrum beta-lactamase-producing *Enterobacteriaceae*: Current evidence and future prospects. *Expert Rev. Anti Infect. Ther.* **2018**, *16*, 205–218. [CrossRef] [PubMed]
10. Durante-Mangoni, E.; Andini, R.; Zampino, R. Management of carbapenem-resistant *Enterobacteriaceae* infections. *Clin. Microbiol. Infect.* **2019**, *25*, 943–950. [CrossRef] [PubMed]
11. Centers for Disease Control and Prevention. Facility Guidance for Control of Carbapenem-Resistant Enterobacteriaceae (CRE)—November 2015 Update CRE Toolkit. Available online: https://www.cdc.gov/hai/organisms/cre/Cre-toolkit/index.html (accessed on 22 July 2019).
12. Haidar, G.; Clancy, C.J.; Chen, L.; Samanta, P.; Shields, R.K.; Kreiswirth, B.N.; Nguyen, M.H. Identifying spectra of activity and therapeutic niches for ceftazidime-avibactam and imipenem-relebactam against carbapenem-resistant *Enterobacteriaceae*. *Antimicrob. Agents Chemother.* **2017**, *61*. [CrossRef]
13. Tooke, C.L.; Hinchliffe, P.; Bragginton, E.C.; Colenso, C.K.; Hirvonen, V.H.A.; Takebayashi, Y.; Spencer, J. ß-Lactamases and ß-Lactamase Inhibitors in the 21st Century. *J. Mol. Biol.* **2019**. [CrossRef]
14. Codjoe, F.S.; Donkor, E.S. Carbapenem Resistance: A review. *Med. Sci.* **2018**, *6*, 1. [CrossRef]
15. Lutgring, J.D.; Limbago, B.M. The Problem of Carbapenemase-Producing-Carbapenem-Resistant-*Enterobacteriaceae* Detection. *J. Clin. Microbiol.* **2016**, *54*, 529–534. [CrossRef]
16. Ambler, R.P. The structure of ß-lactamases. *Philos. Trans. R. Soc. Lond. B* **1980**, *289*, 321–331. [CrossRef]
17. Queenan, A.M.; Bush, K. Carbapenemases: The versatile ß-lactamases. *Clin. Microbiol. Rev.* **2007**, *20*, 440–458. [CrossRef] [PubMed]
18. Yigit, H.; Queenan, A.M.; Anderson, G.J.; Domenech-Sanchez, A.; Biddle, J.W.; Steward, C.D.; Alberti, S.; Bush, K.; Tenover, F.C. Novel carbapenem-hydrolyzing beta-lactamase, KPC-1, from a carbapenem-resistant strain of *Klebsiella pneumoniae*. *Antimicrob. Agents Chemother.* **2001**, *45*, 1151–1161. [CrossRef] [PubMed]
19. Ji, S.; Lv, F.; Du, X.; Wei, Z.; Fu, Y.; Mu, X.; Jiang, Y.; Yu, Y. Cefepime combined with amoxicillin/clavulanic acid: A new choice for the KPC-producing *K. pneumoniae* infection. *Int. J. Infect. Dis.* **2015**, *38*, 108–114. [CrossRef] [PubMed]
20. Porreca, A.M.; Sullivan, K.V.; Gallagher, J.C. The Epidemiology, Evolution, and Treatment of KPC-Producing Organisms. *Curr. Infect. Dis. Rep.* **2018**, *20*, 13. [CrossRef] [PubMed]

21. Nordmann, P.; Cuzon, G.; Naas, T. The real threat of *Klebsiella pneumoniae* carbapenemase-producing bacteria. *Lancet Infect. Dis.* **2009**, *9*, 228–233. [CrossRef]
22. Miriagou, V.; Cornaglia, G.; Edelstein, M.; Galani, I.; Giske, G. Acquired carbapenemases in Gram-negative bacterial pathogens: Detection and surveillance issues. *Clin. Microbiol. Infect.* **2010**, *16*, 112–122. [CrossRef] [PubMed]
23. Okoche, D.; Asiimwe, B.B.; Katabazi, F.A.; Kato, L.; Najjuka, C.F. Prevalence and Characterization of Carbapenem-Resistant *Enterobacteriaceae* Isolated from Mulago National Referral Hospital, Uganda. *PLoS ONE* **2015**, *10*, e0135745. [CrossRef]
24. Boutal, H.; Vogel, A.; Bernabeu, S.; Devilliers, K.; Creton, E.; Cotellon, G.; Plaisance, M.; Oueslati, S.; Dortet, L.; Jousset, A.; et al. A multiplex lateral flow immunoassay for the rapid identification of NDM-, KPC-, IMP- and VIM-type and OXA-48-like carbapenemase-producing *Enterobacteriaceae*. *J. Antimicrob. Chemother.* **2018**, *73*, 909–915. [CrossRef]
25. Fernández, J.; Guerra, B.; Rodicio, M.R. Resistance to Carbapenems in Non-Typhoidal *Salmonella enterica* Serovars from Humans, Animals and Food. *Vet. Sci.* **2018**, *5*, 40. [CrossRef] [PubMed]
26. Abdallah, M.; Balshi, A. First literature review of carbapenem-resistant *Providencia*. *New Microb. New Infect.* **2018**, *25*, 16–23. [CrossRef] [PubMed]
27. Perez, F.; van Duin, D. Carbapenem-resistant *Enterobacteriaceae*: A menace to our most vulnerable patients. *Clevel Clin. J. Med.* **2013**, *80*, 225–233. [CrossRef] [PubMed]
28. Walsh, T.R.; Toleman, M.A.; Piorel, L.; Nordman, P. Metallo-b-lactamases: The quiet before the storm? *Clin. Microbiol. Rev.* **2005**, *18*, 306–325. [CrossRef] [PubMed]
29. Van Duin, D.; Doi, Y. The global epidemiology of carbapenemase-producing *Enterobacteriaceae*. *Virulence* **2017**, *8*, 460–469. [CrossRef] [PubMed]
30. Livermore, D.M.; Woodford, N. Carbapenemases: A problem in waiting? *Curr. Opin. Microbiol.* **2000**, *3*, 489–495. [CrossRef]
31. Gupta, V. Metallo-b-lactamases in *Pseudomonas aeruginosa* and *Acinetobacter* species. *Expert Opin. Investig. Drugs* **2008**, *17*, 131–143. [CrossRef]
32. Bush, K. Past and Present Perspectives on ß-Lactamases. *Antimicrob. Agents Chemother.* **2018**, *62*, e01076-18. [CrossRef]
33. Walsh, T.R.; Weeks, J.; Livermore, D.M.; Toleman, M.A. Dissemination of NDM-1 positive bacteria in the New Delhi environment and its implications for human health: An environmental point prevalence study. *Lancet Infect. Dis.* **2011**, *11*, 355–362. [CrossRef]
34. Poirel, L.; Hombrouck-Alet, C.; Freneaux, C.; Bernabeu, S.; Nordmann, P. Global spread of New Delhi metallo-ß-lactamase 1. *Lancet Infect. Dis.* **2010**, *10*, 832. [CrossRef]
35. Ivanov, I.; Sabtcheva, S.; Dobreva, E.; Todorova, B.; Velinov, T.Z.; Borissova, V.; Kantardijev, T. Prevalence of carbapenemase genes among 16S rRNA methyltransferase-producing *Enterobacteriaceae* isolated for cancer patients. *Probl. Infect. Parasit. Dis.* **2014**, *42*, 10–13.
36. Poirel, L.; Potron, A.; Nordmann, P. OXA-48-like carbapenemases: The phantom menace. *J. Antimicrob. Chemother.* **2012**, *67*, 1597–1606. [CrossRef] [PubMed]
37. Rasmussen, J.W.; Hoiby, N. OXA-type carbapenemases. *J. Antimicrob. Chemother.* **2006**, *57*, 373–383. [CrossRef] [PubMed]
38. Stewart, A.; Harris, P.; Henderson, A.; Paterson, D. Treatment of Infections by OXA-48-Producing *Enterobacteriaceae*. *Antimicrob. Agents Chemother.* **2018**, *62*, e01195-18. [CrossRef] [PubMed]
39. Logan, L.K.; Weinstein, R.A. The Epidemiology of Carbapenem-Resistant *Enterobacteriaceae*: The Impact and Evolution of a Global Menace. *J. Infect. Dis.* **2017**, *215* (Suppl. 1), S28–S36. [CrossRef]
40. Tzouvelekis, L.S.; Marjogiannakis, A.; Psichogiou, M.; Tassios, P.T.; Daikos, G.L. Carbapenemases in *Klebsiella pneumoniae* and other *Enterobacteriaceae*: An evolving crisis of global dimensions. *Clin. Microbiol. Rev.* **2012**, *25*, 682–707. [CrossRef]
41. Queenan, A.M.; Shang, W.; Flamm, R.; Bush, K. Hydrolysis and inhibition profiles of ß-lactamases from molecular classes A to D with doripenem, imipenem, and meropenem. *Antimicrob. Agents Chemother.* **2010**, *54*, 565–569. [CrossRef]
42. Goessens, W.H.F.; van der Bij, A.K.; van Boxtel, R.; Pitout, J.D.D.; van Ulsen, P.; Melles, D.C.; Tommassen, J. Antibiotic trapping by plasmid-encoded CMY-2 ß-lactamase combined with reduced outer membrane

permeability as a mechanism of carbapenem resistance in *Escherichia coli*. *Antimicrob. Agents Chemother.* **2013**, *57*, 3941–3949. [CrossRef]
43. Philippon, A.; Arlet, G.; Jacoby, G.A. Plasmid-determined AmpC-type ß-lactamases. *Antimicrob. Agents Chemother.* **2002**, *46*, 1–11. [CrossRef]
44. Weston, N.; Sharma, P.; Ricci, V.; Piddock, L.J.V. Regulation of the AcrAB-TolC efflux pump in *Enterobacteriaceae*. *Res. Microbiol.* **2018**, *169*, 425–431. [CrossRef]
45. Routh, M.D.; Zalucki, Y.; Su, C.C.; Zhang, Q.; Shager, W.M.; Yu, E.W. Efflux pumps of the resistance-nodulation-division family: A perspective of their structure, function, and regulation in gram-negative bacteria. *Adv. Enzymol. Relat. Areas Mol. Biol.* **2011**, *77*, 109–146. [PubMed]
46. Courvalin, P. Transfer of antibiotic resistance genes between gram-positive and gram-negative bacteria. *Antimicrob. Agents Chemother.* **1994**, *38*, 1447–1451. [CrossRef] [PubMed]
47. Bialek-Davenet, S.; Mayer, N.; Vergalli, J.; Duprilot, M.; Brisse, S.; Pagès, J.M.; Nicolas-Chanoine, M.H. In-vivo loss of carbapenem resistance by extensively drug-resistant *Klebsiella pneumoniae* during treatment via porin expression modification. *Sci. Rep.* **2017**, *7*, 6722. [CrossRef] [PubMed]
48. Masi, M.; Réfrigiers, M.; Pos, K.M.; Pagès, J.M. Mechanisms of envelope permeability and antibiotic influx and efflux in Gram-negative bacteria. *Nat. Microbiol.* **2017**, *2*, 17001. [CrossRef] [PubMed]
49. Walsh, C. Molecular mechanisms that confer antibacterial drug resistance. *Nature* **2000**, *406*, 775–781. [CrossRef] [PubMed]
50. Ito, H.; Arakawa, Y.; Oshuka, S.; Wacharotayankun, R.; Kato, N.; Ohta, M. Plasmid-mediated dissemination of the metallo-beta-lactamase gene blaIMP among clinically isolated strains of *Serratia marcescens*. *J. Antimicrob. Chemother.* **1995**, *50*, 503–511. [CrossRef] [PubMed]
51. Nordmann, P.; Poirel, L. The difficult-to-control spread of carbapenemase producers among *Enterobacteriaceae* worldwide. *Clin. Microbiol. Infect.* **2014**, *20*, 821–830. [CrossRef]
52. Nordmann, P.; Naas, T.; Poirel, L. Global spread of carbapenemase-producing *Enterobacteriaceae*. *Emerg. Infect. Dis.* **2011**, *17*, 1791–1798. [CrossRef]
53. Lauretti, L.; Riccio, M.K.; Mazzariol, A.; Cornaglia, G.; Amicosante, G.; Fontana, R.; Rossolini, G.M. Cloning and characterization of blaVIM, a new integron-borne metallo-beta-lactamase gene from a *Pseudomonas aeruginosa* clinical isolate. *Antimicrob. Agents Chemother.* **1999**, *43*, 1584–1590. [CrossRef]
54. Yong, D.; Toleman, M.A.; Giske, C.G.; Cho, H.S.; Sundman, K.; Lee, K.; Walsh, T.R. Characterization of new metallo-beta-lactamase gene, bla(NDM-1), and a novel erythromycin esterase gene carried on a unique genetic structure in *Klebsiella pneumoniae* sequence type 14 from India. *Antimicrob. Agents Chemother.* **2009**, *53*, 5046–5054. [CrossRef]
55. Dortet, L.; Poirel, L.; Nordmann, P. Worldwide dissemination of the NDM-type carbapenemases in Gram-negative bacteria. *Biomed. Res. Int.* **2014**, *2014*, 249856. [CrossRef] [PubMed]
56. Poirel, L.; Savov, E.; Nazli, A.; Trifonova, A.; Todorova, I.; Gergova, I.; Nordmann, P. Outbreak caused by NDM-1- and RmtB- producing *Escherichia coli* in Bulgaria. *Antimicrob. Agents Chemother.* **2012**, *58*, 2472–2474. [CrossRef] [PubMed]
57. Patel, G.; Bonomo, R.A. Stormy waters ahead: Global emergence of carbapenemases. *Front. Microbiol.* **2013**, *4*, 1–17. [CrossRef] [PubMed]
58. Bradford, P.A.; Bratu, S.; Urban, C.; Visalli, M.; Mariano, N.; Landman, D.; Rahal, J.J.; Brooks, S.; Cebular, S.; Quale, J. Emergence of carbapenem-resistant *Klebsiella* species possessing the class a carbapenem-hydrolyzing KPC-2 and inhibitor-resistant TEM-30 ß-lactamases in New York City. *Clin. Infect. Dis.* **2004**, *39*, 55–60. [CrossRef] [PubMed]
59. Munoz-Price, L.S.; Poirel, L.; Bonomo, R.A.; Schwaber, M.J.; Daikos, G.L.; Cormican, M.; Cornaglia, G.; Garau, J.; Gniadkowski, M.; Hayden, M.K. Clinical epidemiology of the global expansion of *Klebsiella pneumoniae* carbapenemases. *Lancet Infect. Dis.* **2013**, *13*, 785–796. [CrossRef]
60. Maya, J.J.; Ruiz, S.J.; Blanco, V.M.; Gotuzzo, E.; Guzman-Blanco, M.; Labarca, J.; Salles, M.; Quinn, J.P.; Villegas, M.V. Current status of carbapenemases in Latin America. *Expert Rev. Anti Infect. Ther.* **2013**, *11*, 657–667. [CrossRef]
61. Poirel, L.; Bonnin, R.A.; Nordmann, P. Genetic features of the widespread plasmid coding for the carbapenemase OXA-48. *Antimicrob. Agents Chemother.* **2012**, *56*, 559–562. [CrossRef]
62. The European Committee on Antimicrobial Susceptibility Testing. *Breakpoint Tables for Interpretation of MICs and Zone Diameters*, Version 9.0; 2019. Available online: http//www.eucast.org (accessed on 25 July 2019).

63. CLSI. *Performance Standards for Antimicrobial Susceptibility Testing*, 29th ed.; CLSI supplement M100; Clinical and Laboratory Standards Institute: Wayne, PA, USA, 2019.
64. The European Committee on Antimicrobial Susceptibility Testing. *Breakpoint Tables for Interpretation of MICs and Zone Diameters*, Version 8.1; 2018. Available online: http//www.eucast.org (accessed on 25 July 2019).
65. Karaiskos, I.; Lagou, S.; Pontikis, K.; Rapti, V.; Poulakou, G. The "Old" and the "New" antibiotics for MDR gram-negative pathogens: For whom, when and how. *Front. Public Health* **2019**, *7*, 151. [CrossRef]
66. Vardakas, K.Z.; Legakis, N.J.; Triarides, N.; Falagas, M.E. Susceptibility of contemporary isolates to Fosfomycin: A systematic review of the literature. *Int. J. Antimicrob. Agents* **2016**, *47*, 269–285. [CrossRef]
67. Satlin, M.J.; Kubin, C.J.; Blumental, J.S.; Cohen, A.B.; Furuya, E.Y.; Wilson, S.J.; Jenkins, S.G.; Calfee, D.P. Comparative effectiveness of aminoglycosides, polymyxin B and tigecycline for clearance of carbapenem resistant *Klebsiella pneumoniae* from urine. *Antimicrob. Agents Chemother.* **2011**, *55*, 2528–2531. [CrossRef]
68. Sader, H.S.; Castanheira, M.; Duncan, L.R.; Flamm, R.K. Antimicrobial susceptibility of *Enterobacteriaceae* and *Pseudomonas aeruginosa* isolates from United States medical centers stratified by infection type: Results from the international network for optimal resistance monitoring (INFORM) surveillance program, 2015–2016. *Diagn. Microbiol. Infect. Dis.* **2018**, *92*, 69–74. [CrossRef] [PubMed]
69. Daikos, G.L.; Tsaousi, S.; Tzouvelekis, L.S.; Anyfantis, I.; Psichogiou, M.; Argyropoulou, A.; Stefanou, I.; Sypsa, V.; Miriagou, V.; Nepka, M. Carbapenemase-producing *Klebsiella pneumoniae* bloodstream infections: Lowering mortality by antibiotic combination schemes and the role of carbapenems. *Antimicrob. Agents Chemother.* **2014**, *58*, 2322–2328. [CrossRef] [PubMed]
70. Ni, W.; Han, Y.; Liu, J.; Wei, C.; Zhao, J.; Cui, J.; Wang, R.; Liu, Y. Tigecycline treatment for carbapenem-resistant *Enterobacteriaceae* infections: A systematic review and meta-analysis. *Medicine* **2016**, *95*, e3126. [CrossRef] [PubMed]
71. Giamarellou, H.; Poulakou, G. Pharmakokinetic and pharmacodynamic evaluation of tigecycline. *Expert Opin. Drug Metab. Toxicol.* **2011**, *7*, 1459–1470. [CrossRef] [PubMed]
72. De Pascale, G.; Montini, L.; Pennisi, M.; Bernini, V.; Maviglia, R.; Bello, G.; Spanu, T.; Tumbarello, M.; Antonelli, M. High dose tigecycline in critically ill patients with severe infections due to multidrug-resistant bacteria. *Crit. Care* **2014**, *18*, R90. [CrossRef] [PubMed]
73. Bulik, C.C.; Nicolau, D.P. Double-carbapenem therapy for carbapenemase-producing *Klebsiella pneumoniae*. *Antimicrob. Agents Chemother.* **2011**, *55*, 3002–3004. [CrossRef] [PubMed]
74. Anderson, K.F.; Lonsway, D.R.; Rasheed, J.K.; Biddle, J.; Jensen, B.; McDougal, L.K.; Carey, R.B.; Thompson, A.; Stocker, S.; Limbago, B.; et al. Evaluation of methods to identify the *Klebsiella pneumoniae* carbapenemase in *Enterobacteriaceae*. *J. Clin. Microbiol.* **2007**, *45*, 2723–2725. [CrossRef] [PubMed]
75. Oliva, A.; Scorzolini, L.; Castaldi, D.; Gizzi, F.; De Angelis, M.; Sotrto, M.; D'Abramo, A.; Aloj, F.; Mascellino, M.T.; Mastroianni, C.M.; et al. Double-carbapenem regimen, alone or in combination with colistin, in the treatment of infections caused by carbapenem-resistant *Klebsiella pneumoniae* (CR-Kp). *J. Infect.* **2017**, *74*, 103–106. [CrossRef]
76. Venugopalan, V.; Nogid, B.; Le, T.N.; Rahman, S.M.; Bias, T.E. Double carbapenem therapy (DCT) for bacteremia due to carbapenem-resistant *Klebsiella pneumoniae* (CRKP): From the test tube to clinical practice. *Infect. Dis.* **2017**, *49*, 867–870. [CrossRef]
77. De Jonge, B.L.; Karlowsky, J.A.; Kazmierczak, K.M.; Biedenbach, D.J.; Sahm, D.F.; Nichols, W.W. In vitro susceptibility to ceftazidime-avibactam of carbapenem-nonsusceptible *Enterobacteriaceae* isolates collected during the INFORM Global Surveillance Study (2012 to 2014). *Antimicrob. Agents Chemother.* **2016**, *60*, 3163–3169. [CrossRef]
78. Van Duin, D.; Lok, J.J.; Earley, M.; Cober, E.; Richter, S.S.; Perez, F.; Salata, R.A.; Kalayjian, R.C.; Watkins, R.R.; Doi, Y.; et al. Colistin Versus Ceftazidime-Avibactam in the Treatment of Infections Due to Carbapenem-Resistant *Enterobacteriaceae*. *Clin. Infect. Dis.* **2018**, *66*, 163–171. [CrossRef] [PubMed]
79. Nelson, K.; Hemarajata, P.; Sun, D.; Rubio-Aparicio, D.; Tsivokovski, R.; Yang, S.; Sebra, R.; Kasarskis, A.M.; Nguyen, H.; Hanson, B.M.; et al. Resistance to Ceftazidime-Avibactam Is Due to Transposition of KPC in a Porin-Deficient Strain of *Klebsiella pneumoniae* with Increased Efflux Activity. *Antimicrob. Agents Chemother.* **2017**, *61*, e00989-17. [CrossRef] [PubMed]
80. Venditti, C.; Nisii, C.; D'Arezzo, S.; Vulcano, A.; Capone, A.; Antonini, M.; Ippolito, G.; Di Caro, A. Molecular and phenotypical characterization of two cases of antibiotic-driven ceftazidime-avibactam resistance in bla_{KPC-3}-harboring *Klebsiella pneumoniae*. *Infect. Drug Resist.* **2019**, *12*, 1935–1940. [CrossRef] [PubMed]

81. Humphries, R.M. *Mechanisms of Resistance to Ceftazidime-Avibactam*, 28th ed.; European Congress of Clinical Microbiology & Infectious Diseases (ECCMID): Madrid, Spain, 2018.
82. Petty, L.A.; Henig, O.; Patel, T.S.; Pogue, J.M.; Kaye, K.S. Overview of meropenem-vaborbactam and newer antimicrobial agents for the treatment of carbapenem-resistant *Enterobacteriaceae*. *Infect. Drug Resist.* **2018**, *11*, 1461–1472. [CrossRef] [PubMed]
83. Lomovskaya, O.; Sun, D.; Rubio-Aparicio, D.; Nelson, K.; Tsivkovski, R.; Griffith, D.C.; Dudley, M.N. Vaborbactam: Spectrum of beta-lactamase inhibition and impact of resistance mechanisms on activity in *Enterobacteriaceae*. *Antimicrob. Agents Chemother.* **2017**, *61*, 1–15. [CrossRef] [PubMed]
84. Wunderink, R.G.; Giamarellos-Bourboulis, E.J.; Rahav, G.; Mathers, A.J.; Bassetti, M.; Vazquez, J.; Cornely, O.A.; Solomkin, J.; Bhowmick, T.; Bishara, J.; et al. Effect and safety of meropenem-vaborbactam versus best-available therapy in patients with carbapenem-resistant *Enterobacteriaceae* infections: The TANGO II randomized clinical trial. *Infect. Dis. Ther.* **2018**, *7*, 439–455. [CrossRef]
85. Landman, D.; Babu, E.; Shah, N.; Kelly, P.; Backer, M.; Bratu, S.; Quale, J. Activity of a novel aminoglycoside, ACHN-490, against clinical isolates of *Escherichia coli* and *Klebsiella pneumoniae* from New York City. *J. Antimicrob. Chemother.* **2010**, *65*, 2123–2127. [CrossRef]
86. Endimiani, A.; Hujer, K.M.; Hujer, A.M.; Armstrong, E.S.; Choudhary, Y.; Aggen, J.B.; Bonomo, R.A. ACHN-490, a neoglycoside with potent in vitro activity against multidrug-resistant *Klebsiella pneumoniae* isolates. *Antimicrob. Agents Chemother.* **2009**, *53*, 4504–4507. [CrossRef]
87. Walkty, A.; Adam, H.; Baxter, M.; Denisuik, A.; Lagace-Wiens, P.; Karlowsky, J.A.; Hoban, D.J.; Zhanel, G.G. In vitro activity of plazomicin against 5,015 Gram-negative and Gram-positive clinical isolates obtained from patients in Canadian hospitals as part of the CANWARD study, 2011–2012. *Antimicrob. Agents Chemother.* **2014**, *58*, 2554–2563. [CrossRef]
88. Castanheira, M.; Deshpande, L.M.; Woosley, L.N.; Serio, A.W.; Krause, K.M.; Flamm, R.K. Activity of plazomicin compared with other aminoglycosides against isolates from European and adjacent countries, including *Enterobacteriaceae* molecularly characterized for aminoglycoside-modifying enzymes and other resistance mechanisms. *J. Antimicrob. Chemother.* **2018**, *73*, 3346–3354. [CrossRef]
89. Zhanel, G.G.; Cheung, D.; Adam, H.; Zelenitsky, S.; Golden, A.; Schweizer, F.; Gorityala, B.; Lagacé-Wiens, P.R.; Walkty, A.; Gin, A.S.; et al. Review of eravacycline, a novel fluorocycline antibacterial agent. *Drugs* **2016**, *76*, 567–588. [CrossRef] [PubMed]
90. Bassetti, M.; Righi, E. Eravacycline for the treatment of intra-abdominal infections. *Expert Opin. Investig. Drugs* **2014**, *23*, 1575–1584. [CrossRef] [PubMed]
91. XERAVA (Eravacycline) for Injection. XERAVA (Eravacycline) IGNITE1 and IGNITE4 Trial Results. 2019. Available online: https://www.xerava.com/efficacy (accessed on 25 July 2019).
92. Solomkin, J.S.; Ramesh, M.K.; Cesnauskas, G.; Novikovs, N.; Stefanova, P.; Sutcliffe, J.A.; Walpole, S.M.; Horn, P.T. Phase 2, randomized, double-blind study of the efficacy and safety of two dose regimens of eravacycline versus ertapenem for adult community-acquired complicated intra-abdominal infections. *Antimicrob. Agents Chemother.* **2014**, *58*, 1847–1854. [CrossRef]
93. Blizzard, T.A.; Chen, H.; Kim, S.; Wu, J.; Bodner, R.; Gude, C.; Imbriglio, J.; Young, K.; Park, Y.W.; Ogawa, A.; et al. Discovery of MK-7655, a beta-lactamase inhibitor for combination with Primaxin®. *Bioorg. Med. Chem. Lett.* **2014**, *24*, 780–785. [CrossRef] [PubMed]
94. Zhanel, G.G.; Lawrence, C.K.; Adam, H.; Schweizer, F.; Zelenitsky, S.; Zhanel, M.; Lagacé-Wiens, P.R.S.; Walkty, A.; Denisuik, A.; Golden, A.; et al. Imipenem-Relebactam and Meropenem-Vaborbactam: Two Novel Carbapenem-ß-Lactamase Inhibitor Combinations. *Drugs* **2018**, *78*, 65–98. [CrossRef] [PubMed]
95. Motsch, J.; Oliveira, C.; Stus, V.; Koksal, I.; Lyulko, O.; Boucher, H.W.; Kaye, K.S.; File, T.M.; Brown, M.L.; Khan, I.; et al. *RESTORE-IMI 1: A Multicenter, Randomized, Double-Blind, Comparator-Controlled Trial Comparing the Efficacy and Safety of Imipenem/Relebactam Versus Colistin Plus Imipenem in Patients with Imipenem-Non-Susceptible Bacterial Infections*, 28th ed.; ECCMID: Madrid, Spain, 2018.
96. Saisho, Y.; Katsube, T.; White, S.; Fukase, H.; Shimada, J. Pharmacokinetics, safety, and tolerability of cefiderocol, a novel siderophore cephalosporin for Gram-negative bacteria, in healthy subjects. *Antimicrob. Agents Chemother.* **2018**, *62*, e-02163-17. [CrossRef] [PubMed]
97. Hackel, M.A.; Tsuji, M.; Yamano, Y.; Echols, R.; Karlowsky, J.A.; Sahm, D.F. In Vitro Activity of the Siderophore Cephalosporin, Cediferocol, against Carbapenem-Nonsusceptible and Multidrug-Resistant

Isolates of Gram-Negative Bacilli Collected Worldwide in 2014 to 2016. *Antimicrob. Agents Chemother.* **2018**, *62*, e01968-17. [CrossRef]
98. Corbett, D.; Wise, A.; Langley, T.; Skinner, K.; Trimby, E.; Birchall, S.; Dorali, A.; Sandiford, S.; Williams, J.; Warn, P.; et al. Potentiation of Antibiotic Activity by a Novel Cationic Peptide: Potency and Spectrum of Activity of SPR741. *Antimicrob. Agents Chemother.* **2017**, *61*. [CrossRef]
99. Karaiskos, I.; Galani, I.; Souli, M.; Giamarellou, H. Novel ß-lactam-ß-lactamase inhibitor combinations: Expectations for the treatment of carbapenem-resistant Gram-negative pathogens. *Expert Opin. Drug Metab. Toxicol.* **2019**, *15*, 133–149. [CrossRef]
100. Papp-Wallace, K.M.; Nguyen, N.Q.; Jacobs, M.R.; Bethel, C.R.; Barnes, M.D.; Kumar, V.; Bajaksouzian, S.; Rudin, S.D.; Bhavsar, S.; et al. Strategic Approaches to Overcome Resistance against Gram-Negative Pathogens Using ß-lactamase Inhibitors and ß-Lactam Enhancers: Activity of Three Novel Diazabicyclooctanes WCK 5153, Zidebactam (WCK 5107), and WCK 4234. *J. Med. Chem.* **2018**, *61*, 4067–4086. [CrossRef]
101. Sader, H.S.; Rhomberg, P.R.; Flamm, R.K.; Jones, R.N.; Castanheira, M. WCK 5222 (cefepime/zidebactam) antimicrobial activity tested against Gram-negative organisms producing clinically relevant ß-lactamases. *J. Antimicrob. Chemother.* **2017**, *72*, 1696–1703. [CrossRef] [PubMed]
102. Monogue, M.L.; Giovagnoli, S.; Bissantz, C.; Zampaloni, C.; Nicolau, D.P. In Vivo Efficacy of Meropenem with a Novel Non-ß-Lactam-ß-Lactamase Inhibitor, Nacubactam, against Gram-Negative Organisms Exhibiting Various Resistance Mechanisms in a Murine Complicated Urinary Tract Infection Model. *Antimicrob. Agents Chemother.* **2018**, *62*, e02596-17. [CrossRef] [PubMed]
103. Daigle, D.; Hamrick, J.; Chatwin, C.; Kurepina, N.; Kreiswirth, B.N.; Shields, R.K.; Oliver, A.; Clancy, C.J.; Nguyen, M.H.; Pevear, D.; et al. Cefepime/VNRX-5133 Borad-Spectrum Activity Is Mantained Against Emerging KPC- and PDC-Variants in Multidrug-Resistant *K. pneumoniae* and *P. aeruginosa*. *Open Forum Infect. Dis.* **2018**, *5* (Suppl. 1), S419–S420. [CrossRef]

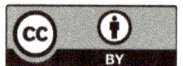

© 2019 by the authors. Licensee MDPI, Basel, Switzerland. This article is an open access article distributed under the terms and conditions of the Creative Commons Attribution (CC BY) license (http://creativecommons.org/licenses/by/4.0/).

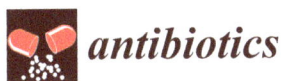

Commentary

Challenges for Economic Evaluation of Health Care Strategies to Contain Antimicrobial Resistance

Emily A. F. Holmes * and Dyfrig A. Hughes

Centre for Health Economics and Medicines Evaluation (CHEME), Bangor University, Normal Site, Bangor, Gwynedd LL57 2PZ, UK; d.a.hughes@bangor.ac.uk
* Correspondence: e.holmes@bangor.ac.uk; Tel.: +44-1248-382-709

Received: 20 August 2019; Accepted: 24 September 2019; Published: 27 September 2019

Abstract: The threat of antimicrobial resistance has global health and economic consequences. Medical strategies to reduce unnecessary antibiotic prescribing, to conserve the effectiveness of current antimicrobials in the long term, inevitably result in short-term costs to health care providers. Economic evaluations of health care interventions therefore need to consider the short-term costs of interventions, to gain future benefits. This represents a challenge for health economists, not only in terms of the most appropriate methods for evaluation, but also in attributing the potential budget impact over time and considering health impacts on future populations. This commentary discusses the challenge of accurately capturing the cost-effectiveness of health care interventions aimed at tackling antimicrobial resistance. We reflect on methods to capture and incorporate the costs and health outcomes associated with antimicrobial resistance, the appropriateness of the quality-adjusted-life year (QALY), individual time preferences, and perspectives in economic evaluation.

Keywords: antimicrobial resistance; economic evaluation; cost-utility analysis; cost-effectiveness analysis; antibiotics

1. Introduction

Antimicrobial resistance encapsulates the loss of effectiveness of any anti-infective medicine, including antiviral, antifungal, antibacterial, and antiparasitic medicines [1,2]. The threat of antimicrobial resistance has global health and economic consequences; resistant infections are responsible for an estimated 700,000 deaths annually worldwide which, if no action is taken, could result in a cumulative cost of $100 trillion by 2050 [3]. Urgent threats include *Clostridioides difficile*, carbapenem-resistant *Enterobacteriaceae* (CRE), and drug-resistant *Neisseria gonorrhoeae* [4]. The current rate of *Clostridioides difficile* infection in the United States (US) alone is 500,000 cases and 15,000 deaths per year. The urgency of addressing antimicrobial resistance is recognised widely [4,5], and a range of containing strategies have been implemented, including antimicrobial stewardship, which has become a central aspect of delivering safe and effective health care [6]. Antimicrobial stewardship involves a coordinated approach to promote and monitor the judicious use of antimicrobials to preserve their future effectiveness [6]. The UK's five-year action plan outlines three key targets for tackling antimicrobial resistance: (i) reducing need and unintentional exposure, (ii) optimizing use, and (iii) investing in innovation, supply, and access [3]. A key strategy to achieve these aims includes more appropriate prescribing, which includes reducing unnecessary antibiotic prescribing [7–10]. Not only is unnecessary antibiotic prescribing costly for little or no therapeutic benefit, it places patients at risk of adverse effects [8,11] and contributes to the development of antibiotic resistance [7–10]. The potential for improved health outcomes and lower costs are easily recognised; however, health care strategies may also include trade-offs between short-term outcomes and long-term gains, for example, not using the most effective anti-infective medicine, in order to preserve future effectiveness. This represents a shift of focus of evaluation, from clinical decision making for an individual patient in the present, to a longer-term (intergenerational) public health agenda. Similarly, there has been a shift of focus in the pharmaceutical industry, with strategies incentivizing the pharmaceutical industry to develop new drugs, using funding mechanisms not linked to volume [3].

Economic evidence is central to understanding the value of competing health care strategies to lessen the probability of resistance development [12,13]. Interventions or services are typically evaluated using standard methods of health technology assessment, including cost-effectiveness or cost-utility analyses. Economic evaluations inform judgements on whether the value of additional health benefits exceed the opportunity cost; where opportunity cost is the next best alterative foregone. As conventionally applied, health benefits relate to the effectiveness of interventions in relation to managing infections less any adverse effects, which are typically confined to adverse drug reactions. However, the application of such methods in the context of antimicrobial resistance poses several unique methodological challenges, not least in quantifying the costs and externality effects (impacts on other patients) of future reductions in antimicrobial effectiveness (Table 1).

Table 1. Examples of challenges for the economic evaluation of health care strategies to contain antimicrobial resistance.

Item	Example of Challenges	Recommendations
Population	Population extends beyond those receiving the intervention. This is also likely to extend across health technology agency (HTA) boundaries.	Where appropriate, extend the population beyond the cohort receiving the intervention and consider other/future patients who become infected by a resistant pathogen, or who have not experienced resistant infection but receive alternative agents due to increased resistance of common pathogens.
Clinical	Adequate measurement of the expected rate of growth of antimicrobial resistance and associated outcomes over time. Clinical parameters in the present are more easily captured than those associated with future global consequences.	Use both empirical data and secondary data to forecast long-term clinical consequences. Ensure appropriate assessment of uncertainty.
Costs	Resource implications most likely to be short-term. Difficult to capture long-term resource use and the cost of negative externalities. Cost of health care intervention impacts different budgets to the return, e.g., primary care cost in short-term, for long-term secondary care gains.	Application of robust resource use data collection methods [14]. Include costs of treating patients not receiving the intervention (see population). Use threshold analysis as an alternative to specifying attaching an actual cost to antimicrobial resistance.
Health outcomes	Health states associated with acute infection may be perceived as transient, which limits the validity of trade-off exercises typically used for utility valuation. Utility measures, such as the EQ-5D, measure health "today" and fail to capture the value (utility) associated with future health gains.	Cautious interpretation of quality-adjusted-life year (QALY) gains. Consider alternative or multiple frameworks for analysis, e.g., disability-adjusted-life year (DALYs) to assess global burden, cost-benefit analysis, using contingent valuation. Where appropriate include the disutility for patients with resistant infection and the disutility of alternative agents.
Perspective	Economic evaluations of health care intervention are often restricted to direct health effects and costs with the health technology program considering the evidence. Antimicrobial resistance is a societal issue and extends beyond individual HTA jurisdictions.	Consider a societal perspective to reflect the true range of costs and outcomes. Acknowledge the limitations of HTA by individual agencies.
Time horizon	Evaluations often adopt inadequate time horizons. Time preference may be paradoxical for antimicrobial consumption. Costs and outcomes extend to future generations.	Adopt a lifetime horizon of analysis, use appropriate discounting rates, and conduct empirical research on time preferences for antimicrobial preferences.

2. Challenges

2.1. Capturing the Benefits of Strategies to Contain Antimicrobial Resistance

How best to assess the value of any intervention to reduce antimicrobial resistance is a methodological challenge, which requires adequate measurement of the expected rate of growth of antimicrobial resistance and associated outcomes over time [15]. Economic evaluation of health care strategies to reduce antibiotic prescribing, for instance, ought to value their impact on antimicrobial resistance. Most economic evaluations in this area, however, fail to consider the costs and outcomes relating to antimicrobial resistance—or where they have, consideration has been restricted to projected financial costs and was not reflective of population health [16,17]. In order to achieve this, data are required on the long-term health outcomes of both current patients and future cohorts of patients who may be prescribed antimicrobial therapy in the future. This includes the health outcome of patients who become infected by a resistant pathogen, or who have not experienced resistant infection but receive alternative agents due to increased resistance of common pathogens. The disutility of potentially less effective treatment represents an important economic parameter that is required in addition to the capturing the more obvious morbidity and mortality associated with short-term health outcomes of the patient presenting with an infection.

Measure of Health Outcome

Economic evaluations of health care interventions to tackle antimicrobial resistance may consider different measures of health outcomes, ranging from the number of prescriptions avoided, to years of life gained and quality-adjusted-life years (QALYs). Cost-utility analyses, which yield incremental costs per QALY gained, measure value in terms of health utility and survival. Utility represents the value or desirability of a given health state, most typically based on indirect, multi-attribute, preference-based measures, such as the EQ-5D [18,19]. The appropriateness of QALYs for use in evaluation of acute conditions, such as respiratory tract infections, a common focus of intervention aimed at tacking antimicrobial resistance, has both measurement and evaluation problems. Health state utilities used to calculate the QALY are typically elicited using trade-off exercises, and the issue with acute infection is that when trading quality and quantity of life, the ill-health state may be perceived as transient, thus questioning the reliability of this method [20]. Furthermore, health care strategies to contain antimicrobial resistance—by design—are only unlikely to concern the outcomes of today. The valuation of future health outcomes is also important and represents a challenge for health economists. An alternative evaluative framework may be required to capture the complexity of health outcomes over time.

The disability-adjusted-life year (DALY) represents an alternative health index used in cost-effectiveness analyses. The DALY captures the number of healthy years lost, by incorporating reduction in life expectancy with years lost to disability; as such health care interventions seek to avert the DALY (as opposed to increasing the QALY). The DALY provides an estimate of the burden of disease, such as infectious diseases, that is useful in global health prioritization. Cassini and colleagues reported the DALYs caused by five infections with antibiotic-resistant bacteria across populations in Europe and found this to be substantive compare to other infectious diseases [21]. From a global health perspective, the DALY is an oft-used measure that can be utilised in economic evaluations.

Cost-benefit analysis (CBA) is an approach to economic evaluation that places a monetary valuation on the consequences as well as the costs of interventions. This may be achieved using methods such as willingness to pay, which has been suggested as an alternative to the QALY when evaluating acute disease [20]. The willingness to pay method is based on contingent valuation to elicit monetary value for items not typically traded, such as health, and therefore accounts for both health and non-health effects. Whilst this is considered more comprehensive, in many jurisdictions patients may be unfamiliar with purchasing health care directly, and this may have an impact on the reliability of the methods. A further challenge is the potential association with ability to pay, based on income and wealth. In the context of health care strategies to tackle antimicrobial resistance, however, cost-benefit analysis offers a feasible method for capturing the cost of the negative externalities, on a global scale, to represent the true value future benefits. Where applied with robust formative work, there is potential for this method to be used to elicit individuals' willingness to pay to avoid an illness (resistant infection) or obtain the benefits of a future treatment.

2.2. Perspective

Prior to conducting any economic valuation, the perspective needs to be defined [22]. The perspective of the valuation, e.g., whether it is conducted from the point of view of the patient, health care payer, or society, will determine the costs and outcomes that need to be included in the analysis. In the UK, the National Institute for Health and Care Excellence (NICE) recommends the perspective on outcomes should be all direct health effects, whether for patients or other people; and the perspective adopted on costs within its Technology Appraisal programme should be that of the National Health Service (NHS) and personal and social services (PSS) [23]. Benefits are the assigned general population's valuation of health outcome (obtained from surveys), and costs include the cost of treatment and associated health service resource use (e.g., GP visits, hospitalisation, etc.). Whilst this provides a reference case for comparison of different health technologies, such Technology Appraisals consider individual patients or cohorts of patients, whereas antimicrobial resistance should consider populations. Evaluation of containment strategies may necessitate a broader perspective, and evidence in other areas suggests that assessment of the same strategy from different perspectives can arrive at different conclusions [24].

The broadest perspective adopted in economic evaluation is the societal perspective. This should reflect the full range of social opportunity costs associated with different interventions [22], for example, productivity losses due to patients' inability to work. However, there is a paucity of evidence on the long-term indirect impact of antimicrobial resistance on costs and outcomes [25], and this represents a significant challenge for health economists evaluating containment strategies. Economic evaluations with restrictive perspectives have potential to overestimate the value of interventions or services. Where the perspective for costs is limited to hospital or health service, indirect costs to current and future patients, such as working days lost due to resistant infection, or treatment toxicity, fail to be captured.

To fully assess the cost-effectiveness of strategies to contain antimicrobial resistance and to avoid the inefficient allocation of scarce health service resources, decision makers require economic evaluations that incorporate costs and outcomes beyond the patient and hospital and consider the full ramification of antimicrobial resistance. Defining the "society" then becomes a challenge within itself, as antimicrobial resistance impacts populations that extends across jurisdictions. Adoption of a global multiagency perspective represents new territory and a limitation of conventional health technology assessment (HTA) and health-economic approaches. In the absence of long-term data, economists have taken a pragmatic approach; for example, our evaluation of C-reactive protein testing to guide antibiotic prescribing for lower respiratory tract infection in Wales, included a sensitivity analysis of the cost of the long term global cost of antibiotic resistance [17]. A challenge for future economic evaluation is to incorporate more robust measurement and modelling of longer-term indirect costs and outcomes—that go beyond today's cohorts of patients to consider the population of tomorrow.

2.3. Capturing the Long-Term Costs of Antimicrobial Resistance

The resource implications of antimicrobial resistance are most likely to accumulate in the long-term. Short-term, direct health effects may only include the effect of the intervention on the affected patient; however, longer-term effects on both the patient and others are more likely. It is therefore important that all costs are captured and incorporated into economic evaluations across adequate time-horizons. Whilst interventions to reduce unnecessary prescribing in a clinical setting may represent a short time horizon, e.g., prescribing outcomes and re-consultation over 28-days, the longer-term effects of unnecessary antibiotic prescribing extend to current and future patients' lifetimes [10,26]. Initially, resource use and costs associated with interventions that aim to contain resistance would typically be captured using health records and/or patient reports in the short-term. Estimating long-term direct and indirect cost and the cost consequences to others, however, may present more of a challenge. The cost impact has potential to go beyond the lifetime horizon of the patient and impact the population of tomorrow, and in some situations the product life-cycle [27] may be more relevant than the life time of the patients being treated.

Where long-term costs have been considered in existing economic evaluations, these have relied on estimates of per-prescription costs of antimicrobial resistance based on rudimentary calculations of the global costs of resistance divided by the annual number of prescriptions in each geographic region [16]. Oppong et al. 2013 [16], reported three estimates for the cost of antibiotic resistance, based on the annual cost of resistance in the US ($55 billion) [28], the cost of multidrug resistance in the European Union (EU) (€1.5 billion) [29], and the cost of global resistance over a 35-year period (US$2.8 trillion annually) [5]. This method assumes that antibiotic prescribing is the main cause of resistance, but whilst more robust estimates are required, it is widely acknowledged that this would require complex modelling methods [15]. Robust estimates of other long-term health conditions, such as increased risk of *Clostridioides difficile* infection, also require consideration. Indirect costs are also often difficult to estimate, as they may bias against people who are not in employment and may fluctuate over time.

A further challenge is that both direct and indirect costs may be attributable to different systems and payers at different time points. For example, even when restricting analysis to direct health service costs, the initial outlay for point of care C-reactive protein testing to avoid unnecessary antibiotic prescribing may be borne by a local health service provider; however, the longer-term cost savings are likely to be at a secondary level. Data collection should not be restricted to a single source, such as primary care databases, but should utilise appropriate methods (e.g., self-report, hospital episode data) to collect comprehensive data reflective of all costs incurred [14].

2.4. Time Preference

An individual's time preference represents the extent to which they are willing to trade between short-term costs and/or benefits and long-term costs and/or benefits, attributable with a health-related behaviour, such as the consumption of antimicrobials. The time preference rate (discount rate) quantifies the difference between the perceived value of future outcomes relative to more immediate ones. Individuals with lower time preference rates have a higher value for future utility and therefore discount the future less; and conversely, individuals with higher time preference rates have a lower value for future utility and so require greater future reward for their behaviour. Time preference rates for health are typically between 3–6% per annum [30]. In the UK a consistent societal discount rate of 3.5% per annum is applied as recommended in guidance issued by HM Treasury on how to appraise policies, programs, and projects [31]. Variation in the choice of discount rate has a marked effect on studies with long time horizons and is therefore an important consideration for evaluations of strategies aimed to contain resistance—an issue defined by long-term impacts. Given the future value of antibiotics, a lower (zero or perhaps even negative in some circumstances) discount rate may be more relevant for health outcomes [32]. This issue also applies to vaccination, where differential discounting in model-based cost-effectiveness evaluations is being explored [33]. Empirical evidence on time preference rates can be estimated using stated preference techniques that rely on hypothetical scenarios [34]. Participants are typically required to imagine a health state and choose between future outcomes related to that hypothetical health state; this method would generate empirical evidence on individuals time preferences to inform future economic evaluations. A further challenge that will need to be addressed is that in the context of antimicrobial resistance, the future health state to be valued is not that of the respondent but is more likely to be the future health of others. Sensitive analysis using a range of discount rates is recommended.

3. Conclusions

Ascertaining the most clinically and cost-effective interventions and services to reduce antimicrobial resistance will require a multifaceted approach, from incentivizing pharmaceutical companies to co-production of patient-centred acceptable interventions that maximise the utility of both patients and society. Economic evidence is central to understanding the value of competing strategies to lessen the probability of resistance development, although the application of such methods poses several methodological challenges. When assessment and interpreting the results of existing economic evaluations of health care interventions in the context of antimicrobial resistance, careful consideration is required, of the perspective, costs, and externality effects (impacts on other patients) of future reductions in antimicrobial effectiveness. We have presented just some of the challenges of accurately estimating the cost-effectiveness of interventions to tackle antimicrobial resistance. Further research is required to capture the effects of antimicrobial resistance in economic evaluations to reflect the value of preserving effective medicines for future use. This requires appropriate consideration of the wider externalities and methodological approaches which differ from standard "reference" case of NICE and other HTA organizations.

Author Contributions: Conceptualization, E.A.F.H. and D.A.H.; Writing—Original draft preparation, E.A.F.H.; Writing—Review and editing, D.A.H.

Funding: This research received no external funding.

Acknowledgments: The authors acknowledge discussion of these issues at the Welsh Health Economics Group (WHEG) Meeting October 2018.

Conflicts of Interest: The authors declare no conflict of interest.

References

1. Coates, A.; Hu, Y.; Bax, R.; Page, C. The future challenges facing the development of new antimicrobial drugs. *Nat. Rev. Drug Discov.* **2002**, *1*, 895. [CrossRef] [PubMed]
2. World Health Organization. *Antimicrobial Resistance: Global Report on Surveillance*; World Health Organization: Geneva, Switzerland, 2014.
3. HM Government. Tackling Antimicrobial Resistance 2019–2024. The UK's Five-Year National Action Plan. Published 24 January 2019. Available online: https://assets.publishing.service.gov.uk/government/uploads/system/uploads/attachment_data/file/784894/UK_AMR_5_year_national_action_plan.pdf (accessed on 15 August 2019).
4. CDC. Antibiotic Resistance Threats in the United States 2013. Available online: https://www.cdc.gov/drugresistance/biggest_threats.html (accessed on 14 September 2019).
5. O'Neill, J. Tackling Drug-Resistant Infections Globally: Final Report and Recommendations. 2016. Available online: https://amr-review.org/sites/default/files/160525_Final%20paper_with%20cover.pdf (accessed on 26 June 2018).
6. National Institute of Health and Care Excellence (NICE) Guidelines on Antimicrobial Stewardship. Quality Standard [QS121]. Available online: https://www.nice.org.uk/guidance/qs121 (accessed on 13 March 2018).
7. Currie, C.J.; Berni, E.; Jenkins-Jones, S.; Poole, C.D.; Ouwens, M.; Driessen, S.; de Voogd, H.; Butler, C.C.; Morgan, C.L. Antibiotic treatment failure in four common infections in UK primary care 1991–2012: Longitudinal analysis. *BMJ* **2014**, *349*, g5493. [CrossRef] [PubMed]
8. Llor, C.; Bjerrum, L. Antimicrobial resistance: Risk associated with antibiotic overuse and initiatives to reduce the problem. *Ther. Adv. Drug Saf.* **2014**, *5*, 229–241. [CrossRef] [PubMed]
9. Costelloe, C.; Metcalfe, C.; Lovering, A.; Mant, D.; Hay, A.D. Effect of antibiotic prescribing in primary care on antimicrobial resistance in individual patients: Systematic review and meta-analysis. *BMJ* **2010**, *340*, c2096. [CrossRef] [PubMed]
10. Bell, B.G.; Schellevis, F.; Stobberingh, E.; Goossens, H.; Pringle, M. A systematic review and meta-analysis of the effects of antibiotic consumption on antibiotic resistance. *BMC Infect. Dis.* **2014**, *14*, 13. [CrossRef] [PubMed]

11. Owens, R.C., Jr.; Donskey, C.J.; Gaynes, R.P.; Loo, V.G.; Muto, C.A. Antimicrobial-associated risk factors for Clostridium difficile infection. *Clin. Infect. Dis.* **2008**, *46*, S19–S31. [CrossRef] [PubMed]
12. Megiddo, I.; Drabik, D.; Bedford, T.; Morton, A.; Wesseler, J.; Laxminarayan, R. Investing in antibiotics to alleviate future catastrophic outcomes: What is the value of having an effective antibiotic to mitigate pandemic influenza? *Health Econ.* **2019**, *28*, 556–571. [CrossRef] [PubMed]
13. Attema, A.E.; Lugnér, A.K.; Feenstra, T.L. Investment in antiviral drugs: A real options approach. *Health Econ.* **2010**, *19*, 1240–1254. [CrossRef] [PubMed]
14. Franklin, M.; Thorn, J. Self-reported and routinely collected electronic healthcare resource-use data for trial-based economic evaluations: The current state of play in England and considerations for the future. *BMC Med. Res. Methodol.* **2019**, *19*, 8. [CrossRef]
15. Rothery, C.; Woods, B.; Schmitt, L.; Claxton, K.; Palmer, S.; Sculpher, M. *Framework for Value Assessment of New Antimicrobials*; Policy Research Unit in Economic Evaluations of Health & Care Interventions: New York, NY, USA, 2018; Available online: http://www.eepru.org.uk/wp-content/uploads/2017/11/eepru-report-amr-oct-2018-059.pdf (accessed on 19 November 2018).
16. Oppong, R.; Smith, R.D.; Little, P.; Verheij, T.; Butler, C.C.; Goossens, H.; Coenen, S.; Moore, M.; Coast, J. Cost effectiveness of amoxicillin for lower respiratory tract infections in primary care: An economic evaluation accounting for the cost of antimicrobial resistance. *Br. J. Gen. Pract.* **2016**, *66*, e633–e639. [CrossRef]
17. Holmes, E.A.F.; Harris, S.D.; Hughes, A.; Craine, N.; Hughes, D.A. Cost-effectiveness analysis of the use of point of care C-reactive protein testing to reduce antibiotic prescribing in primary care. *Antibiotics* **2018**, *7*, 106. [CrossRef] [PubMed]
18. Euroqol Group. EQ-5D. Available online: https://euroqol.org/ (accessed on 14 September 2019).
19. Wisloff, T.; Hagen, G.; Hamidi, V.; Movik, E.; Klemp, M.; Olsen, J.A. Estimating QALY gains in applied studies: A review of cost-utility analyses published in 2010. *Pharmacoeconomics* **2014**, *32*, 367–375. [CrossRef] [PubMed]
20. Bala, M.V.; Zarkin, G.A. Are QALYs an appropriate measure for valuing morbidity in acute diseases? *Health Econ.* **2000**, *9*, 177–180. [CrossRef]
21. Cassini, A.; Högberg, L.D.; Plachouras, D.; Quattrocchi, A.; Hoxha, A.; Simonsen, G.S.; Colomb-Cotinat, M.; Kretzschmar, M.E.; Devleesschauwer, B.; Cecchini, M.; et al. Attributable deaths and disability-adjusted life-years caused by infections with antibiotic-resistant bacteria in the EU and the European Economic Area in 2015: A population-level modelling analysis. *Lancet Infect. Dis.* **2019**, *19*, 56–66. [CrossRef]
22. Byford, S.; Raftery, J. Perspectives in economic evaluation. *BMJ* **1998**, *316*, 1529–1530. [CrossRef] [PubMed]
23. National Institute for Health and Care Excellence. *Guide to the Methods of Technology Appraisal 2013. Process and Methods [PMG9]*; National Institute for Health and Care Excellence: London, UK, 2013.
24. Drummond, M.; Weatherly, H.; Ferguson, B. Economic evaluation of health interventions. *BMJ* **2008**, *337*, 1204. [CrossRef] [PubMed]
25. Eliopoulos, G.M.; Cosgrove, S.E.; Carmeli, Y. The impact of antimicrobial resistance on health and economic outcomes. *Clin. Infect. Dis.* **2003**, *36*, 1433–1437. [CrossRef]
26. Wilcox, M.H.; Ahir, H.; Coia, J.E.; Dodgson, A.; Hopkins, S.; Llewelyn, M.J.; Settle, C.; Mclain-Smith, S.; Marcella, S.W. Impact of recurrent Clostridium difficile infection: Hospitalization and patient quality of life. *J. Antimicrob. Chemother.* **2017**, *72*, 2647–2656. [CrossRef]
27. Hoyle, M. Accounting for the drug life cycle and future drug prices in cost-effectiveness analysis. *Pharmacoeconomics* **2011**, *29*, 1–15. [CrossRef]
28. Centers for Disease Control and Prevention. Antimicrobial Resistance: No Action Today, No Cure Tomorrow. Available online: http://www.cdc.gov/media/releases/2011/f0407_antimicrobialresistance.pdf (accessed on 19 November 2018).
29. European Centre for Disease Prevention and Control, European Medicines Agency. The Bacterial Challenge: Time to React. Joint Technical Report. 2009. Available online: https://ecdc.europa.eu/sites/portal/files/media/en/publications/Publications/0909_TER_The_Bacterial_Challenge_Time_to_React.pdf (accessed on 19 November 2018).
30. Cairns, J.A.; van der Pol, M.M. The estimation of marginal time preference in a UK-wide sample (TEMPUS) project. *Health Technol. Assess.* **2000**, *4*, i–iv. [CrossRef]
31. HM Treasury. *The Green Book Appraisal and Evaluation in Central Government: Treasury Guidance*; TSO: Norwich, UK, 2003.

32. Roope, L.S.; Tonkin-Crine, S.; Butler, C.C.; Crook, D.; Peto, T.; Peters, M.; Walker, A.S.; Wordsworth, S. Reducing demand for antibiotic prescriptions: Evidence from an online survey of the general public on the interaction between preferences, beliefs and information, United Kingdom, 2015. *Eurosurveillance* **2018**, *23*, 1700424. [CrossRef] [PubMed]
33. Jit, M.; Mibei, W. Discounting in the evaluation of the cost-effectiveness of a vaccination programme: A critical review. *Vaccine* **2015**, *33*, 3788–3794. [CrossRef] [PubMed]
34. Van der Pol, M.; Cairns, J. Estimating time preferences for health using discrete choice experiments. *Soc. Sci. Med.* **2001**, *52*, 1459–1470. [CrossRef]

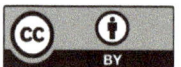

© 2019 by the authors. Licensee MDPI, Basel, Switzerland. This article is an open access article distributed under the terms and conditions of the Creative Commons Attribution (CC BY) license (http://creativecommons.org/licenses/by/4.0/).

MDPI
St. Alban-Anlage 66
4052 Basel
Switzerland
Tel. +41 61 683 77 34
Fax +41 61 302 89 18
www.mdpi.com

Antibiotics Editorial Office
E-mail: antibiotics@mdpi.com
www.mdpi.com/journal/antibiotics

www.ingramcontent.com/pod-product-compliance
Lightning Source LLC
LaVergne TN
LVHW070140100526
838202LV00015B/1855